Respiratory Medicine

Series editors
Sharon I.S. Rounds
Department of Medicine, Pathology, and Laboratory Medicine
Albert Medical School of Brown University
Providence, Rhode Island
USA

Anne Dixon
Department of Medicine
University of Vermont College of Medicine
Burlington, Vermont
USA

Lynn M. Schnapp
Pulmonary, Critical Care, Allergy
Medical University of South Carolina
Charleston, South Carolina
USA

Respiratory Medicine offers clinical and research-oriented resources for pulmonologists and other practitioners and researchers interested in respiratory care. Spanning a broad range of clinical and research issues in respiratory medicine, the series covers such topics as COPD, asthma and allergy, pulmonary problems in pregnancy, molecular basis of lung disease, sleep disordered breathing, and others.

More information about this series at http://www.springer.com/series/7665

Anna Maria Hibbs • Marianne S. Muhlebach

Editors

Respiratory Outcomes in Preterm Infants

From Infancy through Adulthood

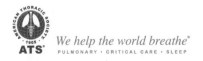

We help the world breathe®
PULMONARY · CRITICAL CARE · SLEEP

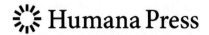

Editors
Anna Maria Hibbs
Department of Pediatrics
Case Western Reserve University
Cleveland
Ohio
USA

Marianne S. Muhlebach
Department of Pediatrics
University of North Carolina Chapel Hill
Chapel Hill
North Carolina
USA

ISSN 2197-7372   ISSN 2197-7380   (electronic)
Respiratory Medicine
ISBN 978-3-319-84026-0   ISBN 978-3-319-48835-6   (eBook)
DOI 10.1007/978-3-319-48835-6

Printed on acid-free paper

This Humana Press imprint is published by Springer Nature
The registered company is Springer International Publishing AG
The registered company address is: Gewerbestrasse 11, 6330 Cham, Switzerland

Preface

Premature birth has lifelong consequences for respiratory health. These consequences have long been recognized for the extreme premature infants, especially the early life morbidities associated with bronchopulmonary dysplasia (BPD) in very low birthweight (VLBW) infants. Additionally, a growing body of data indicates lifelong sequelae of prematurity in moderately preterm and late-preterm infants (32–37 weeks gestation). Lung parenchyma, vasculature, and airways are affected. With at least one in ten people in the United States born preterm, the long-lasting sequelae of prematurity may impact persons of all ages. This book is intended for physicians and nurses caring for these patients. We take an evidence-based approach, highlighting both what is known and where further research is needed.

The chapters are written by neonatologists, pediatric and adult pulmonologists, and otolaryngologists with expertise in the care of patients born preterm. This range of authors highlights the variety of known or latent effects of prematurity on the respiratory system throughout the life span. The chapters present complementary perspectives, from bench research to population-based studies. We address the anatomy, physiology, epidemiology, and public health consequences of the respiratory sequelae of prematurity. We summarize proven strategies for prevention and treatment, as well as highlight key knowledge gaps.

In Chap. 1, Drs. Mcgrath-Morrow and Collaco provide an overview of the clinical problems facing the preterm respiratory system. The next two chapters tackle the problem of wheezing in persons born prematurely, highlighting epidemiologic data and risk factors (Dr. Vrijilandt) and pathophysiology based on airway and neuronal development pre- and postnatally (Drs. Martin and Raffay). Chapters 4 and 5 address the problem of BPD. Dr. Keller reviews the utility and limitations of different clinical and research definitions of BPD. Drs. Bancalari and Wu then go on to describe normal lung development and the structural and functional derangements seen with prematurity, with a focus on BPD. In Chap. 6, Drs. Davis, Ren, and Cristea address the different testing modalities available to assess airway and lung disease from infancy to adolescence. Chapter 7 provides a key resource for caregivers of adolescent of adolescent and adult patients; Drs. Bush and Bolton review the long-term sequelae of prematurity that may impact the lung and respiratory system, even into the geriatric years and highlight potential relationship to COPD. Public health aspects of prematurity are addressed in Chaps. 8 and 9. Dr. Lorch reviews the public health impact of prematurity and Dr. McEvoy addresses primary prevention strategies for prematurity-associated respiratory diseases. Chapter 10, written by Drs. Redline and Ross, reviews the myriad changes in sleep associated with prematurity, as experienced throughout different life stages. In Chap. 11, Drake, Fleischman, and McClain address aspects of large airway abnormalities from the ENT perspective with emphasis on the sequelae of prematurity. Dr. Abman reviews the pathophysiology and therapies for BPD-associated pulmonary hypertension in Chap. 12. Finally, Drs. Sanchez, Wozniak, and Moallem review the role of infection in augmenting pulmonary pathology in preterm infants, as well as the subsequent vulnerability of preterm infants to infection.

The care of patients born preterm requires an awareness of how prematurity may impact respiratory health throughout the lifetime. Whether the patient is an infant with BPD dependent on home oxygen, a young child with wheezing, or an adult with early symptoms of COPD, their care will be enhanced by understanding the pathophysiology and prognosis of prematurity-related diseases. This book serves as a valuable compendium for those caring for patients or engaging in research, as well as a call for future research to better understand how prematurity can impact pulmonary health and how these processes can best be treated and prevented.

Cleveland, OH, USA   Anna Maria Hibbs
Chapel Hill, NC, USA   Marianne S. Muhlebach

Contents

Contributors

Steven H. Abman, MD Department of Pediatrics, University of Colorado School of Medicine and Children's Hospital Colorado, Aurora, CO, USA

Eduardo Bancalari, MD Department of Pediatrics/Division of Neonatology, University of Miami School of Medicine, Miami, FL, USA

Charlotte Bolton, BM, BS, MD, FRCP University of Nottingham, Nottingham, UK Nottingham University Hospitals Trust, Nottingham, UK

Andrew Bush, MD, FRCP, FRCPCH, FERS Department of Paediatric Respiratory Medicine, Royal Brompton Hospital, London, UK

Shawna Calhoun, MPH Center for Outcomes Research, The Children's Hospital of Philadelphia, Philadelphia, PA, USA

Joseph M. Collaco, MD, MPH Johns Hopkins Medical Institutions, Eudowood Division of Pediatric Respiratory Sciences, Baltimore, MD, USA

Ioana Cristea Department of Pediatrics, Section of Pediatric Pulmonology, Allergy and Sleep Medicine, Riley Hospital for Children at Indiana University Health, Indianapolis, IN, USA

Stephanie D. Davis Department of Pediatrics, Section of Pediatric Pulmonology, Allergy and Sleep Medicine, Riley Hospital for Children at Indiana University Health, Indianapolis, IN, USA

Amelia F. Drake, MD Department of Otolaryngology/Head and Neck Surgery, University of North Carolina School of Medicine, Chapel Hill, NC, USA

Gita M. Fleischman, MD Department of Otolaryngology/Head and Neck Surgery, University of North Carolina School of Medicine, Chapel Hill, NC, USA

Roberta L. Keller, MD Department of Pediatrics/Neonatology, UCSF Benioff Children's Hospital, San Francisco, CA94143, USA

Scott A. Lorch, MD, MSCE Center for Outcomes Research, The Children's Hospital of Philadelphia, Philadelphia, PA, USA

Richard J. Martin, MD Case Western Reserve University School of Medicine, Cleveland, OH, USA

Rainbow Babies & Children's Hospital, Cleveland, OH, USA

Wade G. McClain, DO Department of Otolaryngology/Head and Neck Surgery, University of North Carolina School of Medicine, Chapel Hill, NC, USA

Cindy T. McEvoy, MD, MCR Department of Pediatrics, Oregon Health & Science University, Portland, OR, USA

Sharon A. McGrath-Morrow, MD, MBA Johns Hopkins Medical Institutions, Eudowood Division of Pediatric Respiratory Sciences, Baltimore, MD, USA

Mohannad Moallem, MD Department of Pediatrics, Nationwide Children's Hospital – The Ohio State University, Columbus, OH, USA

Thomas M. Raffay, MD Case Western Reserve University school of Medicine, Cleveland, OH, USA

Rainbow Babies and Children's Hospital, Cleveland, OH, USA

Susan Redline, MD, MPH Harvard Medical School, Brigham and Women's Hospital and Beth Israel Deaconess Medical Center, Boston, MA, USA

Clement L. Ren Department of Pediatrics, Section of Pediatric Pulmonology, Allergy and Sleep Medicine, Riley Hospital for Children at Indiana University Health, Indianapolis, IN, USA

Kristie R. Ross, MD, MS Case Western Reserve University School of Medicine, Cleveland, OH, USA

Rainbow Babies and Children's Hospital, Cleveland, OH, USA

Pablo J. Sánchez, MD Department of Pediatrics, Division of Neonatology and Pediatric Infectious Diseases, Nationwide Children's Hospital – The Ohio State University, Columbus, OH, USA

Elianne Vrijlandt, MD, PhD Department of Pediatric Pulmonology and Pediatric Allergology, Beatrix Children's Hospital, Groningen, The Netherlands

University of Groningen, GRIAC Research Institute, University Medical Center Groningen, Groningen, the Netherlands

Phillip S. Wozniak, BA Division of Neonatology, Nationwide Children's Hospital – The Ohio State University, Columbus, OH, USA

Shu Wu, MD Department of Pediatrics/Division of Neonatology, University of Miami School of Medicine, Batchelor Children's Research Institute, Miami, FL, USA

The Problem of the Preterm Lung: Definitions, History, and Epidemiology

Joseph M. Collaco and Sharon A. McGrath-Morrow

Lung Parenchymal Disease

The archetypal lung disease in preterm infants and one of the more common complications of preterm birth is bronchopulmonary dysplasia (BPD), which may include both parenchymal and small airway components. Common clinical manifestations of BPD include hypoxia, hypercarbia, tachypnea, and asthma-like symptoms [7]. "Classic" or "old" BPD was first described in 1967 by Northway et al. [8], and was characterized by inflammation with airway injury and alveolar fibrosis. Over time, BPD has evolved ("new" BPD), particularly with use of newer ventilation strategies and exogenous surfactant, to a phenotype characterized by fewer and larger simplified alveoli with dysnaptic growth of the pulmonary vascular bed [9, 10]. Although several definitions of BPD or chronic lung disease of prematurity have been used since 1967 [11], currently the most widely agreed upon definition of BPD was developed at a NICHD workshop published in 2001 [12]. At this workshop, the diagnosis and severity of BPD in premature infants were based on gestational age (<32 weeks or ≥32 weeks) and need for oxygen and/or respiratory support at specified time points. This definition was subsequently validated in 2005 [11]. It should be recognized that this oxygen-based definition could overestimate or underestimate the incidence of BPD as goal oxygen saturations remain controversial [13, 14] and can vary among clinical centers [15]. Additionally, this oxygen-based definition may overestimate the incidence of BPD in clinical sites at higher altitudes where the partial pressure of oxygen is decreased [16, 17]. Furthermore, many preterm infants are placed on supplemental oxygen for apnea of prematurity who may or may not have moderate or severe

J.M. Collaco, MD, MPH (✉) • S.A. McGrath-Morrow, MD, MBA
Eudowood Division of Pediatric Respiratory Sciences, Johns Hopkins Medical Institutions,
David M. Rubenstein Building, 200 North Wolfe Street, Baltimore, MD 21287, USA
e-mail: mcollac1@jhmi.edu; smcgrath@jhmi.edu

© Springer International Publishing AG 2017
A.M. Hibbs, M. S. Muhlebach (eds.), *Respiratory Outcomes in Preterm Infants*,
Respiratory Medicine, DOI 10.1007/978-3-319-48835-6_1

BPD. In addition, these criteria do not define the BPD severity with reference to emerging respiratory support technologies, such as high-flow nasal cannulas.

In comparison to many of the other pulmonary manifestations of prematurity, more data exist on the epidemiology of BPD. Approximately 25 % of infants born with a birth weight of less than 1500 g are diagnosed with BPD [18], although the frequency of BPD reported may vary by center [5, 18]. Assuming that 1.4 % births in the United States annually are born with a birth weight less than 1500 g [4], this extrapolates to 14,000 infants who develop BPD in the United States annually. Although rates for preterm births have declined slightly in recent years [4], rates of BPD may not be mirroring this decline [19].

Infants with BPD frequently experience hypoxemia and many require supplemental oxygen at home, usually delivered via nasal cannula. A validation study of the NICHD BPD criteria in 4866 infants born at less than 32 weeks gestation and weighing less than 1000 g at birth observed that 2.8 % of infants with no or mild BPD were discharged on oxygen, while 64.4 % of those with moderate or severe BPD were discharged to home on supplemental oxygen [11]. These data would suggest that 31.6 % of these extremely low birth weight preterm infants are discharged to home on oxygen. Also, in this validation study, infants with no BPD or mild/moderate BPD were discontinued from home-supplemental oxygen between 7–8 months of age on average, whereas infants with severe BPD were discontinued from oxygen at 9.7 months of age [11].

Infants and children with the most severe BPD resulting in chronic respiratory failure may require tracheostomy placement for long-term ventilation with varying published estimates on the incidence. A 2010 study from Riley Children's Hospital estimated the incidence to be 4.77 per 100,000 live births with a median duration of home ventilator support of 24 months of age [20], which extrapolates to 400 patients with BPD on home ventilation in the United States at any given time. However, a 2011 study from the Ventilator Assisted Children's Home Program in Pennsylvania estimated that 8000 children in the United States are receiving home-invasive ventilation, and in this program, 36 % of ventilator-dependent children have chronic lung disease, with 77 % of these diagnosed with BPD [21], which extrapolates approximately 2200 patients with BPD on home ventilation in the United States at any given time. One single site study of 102 infants with BPD requiring home ventilation found an 81.4 % survival rate with 83.1 % of survivors being weaned from ventilation at a median age of 24 months, and 87.0 % of those weaned from ventilation being decannulated at a median age of 37.5 months [20].

Contributing to the difficulty of formulating algorithms for the management of BPD is its multifactorial development. Identified risk factors certainly include gestational age at birth, with infants born at earlier gestational ages experiencing a higher incidence of BPD [19]. Fetal growth also plays a role as infants with lower birth weights corrected for gestational age (fetal growth restriction) have higher rates of BPD [22, 23], and a large Swedish cohort found a 2.7 times higher risk of developing BPD with being born small for gestational age (2 standard deviations below the mean) [24]. Some prenatal risk factors for the development of BPD could include preeclampsia [25, 26], chorioamnionitis [26, 27], and the premature rupture of membranes [24, 28]. However, there remains controversy regarding the role of preeclampsia, as other studies have found preeclampsia to be protective [29] or not a risk factor at all [23, 30]. Likewise, studies of chorioamnionitis as a risk factor have also produced conflicting results [31, 32]. Postnatal risk factors may include patent ductus arteriosus [24, 33, 34] (and again, this is not definitively clear) [35], late-onset infections [24, 34, 36], pneumothorax [24], and mechanical ventilation [24, 34, 37]. In terms of postnatal therapies that may alter the incidence of BPD, retrospective data suggest that prophylactic use of caffeine within the first few days of life may reduce the likelihood of developing BPD [38–40]. However, while ante-natal corticosteroids administered to women at risk of preterm birth can accelerate fetal lung maturation [41], neither the use of postnatal systemic or inhaled cortico-steroids has been shown to reduce the incidence of BPD [42–45].

In addition, genetic factors may predispose individual infants to develop BPD based on heritability studies of twins [46, 47], but genomewide association studies have not confirmed positive findings from candidate gene studies [48]. Three genomewide association studies have been performed among infants with BPD, and one performed in European and African populations identified *SPOCK2*, which may have a potential role in alveolar development, to be associated with BPD [49], but two North American studies did not identify any SNPs meeting genomewide significance, including *SPOCK2* [50, 51]. Pathway analyses in one of the GWAS studies found an association with BPD and known pathways of lung development and repair (CD44, phosphorus oxygen lyase activity) as well as novel pathways (adenosine deaminase, targets of miR-219) [51]. In addition to genetic factors, an emerging risk factor for the development of BPD may be epigenetic changes (non-nucleotide changes to the genome) that alter gene expression [52]. One study of umbilical cord blood demonstrated that preterm infants that developed BPD had distinct patterns of chromatin remodeling and histone acetylation pathways com-pared to those who did not ($n = 54$) [53].

Small Airways Disease

Another frequently seen pulmonary sequelae of preterm infants is small airways disease, which is often secondary to BPD, and can manifest as wheezing and cough-ing among patients of all ages, and obstructive findings on pulmonary function test-ing in older children. Computed tomography of the chest in preterm children with a prior history of BPD may reveal emphysema, hyperexpansion, and fibrous/intersti-tial changes [54].

Objective data regarding the incidence of small airways disease in infants are difficult to capture, as infant pulmonary function testing is only available in a small number of centers and carries the risks attendant to sedating an infant with known respiratory disease. In older children, spirometry can routinely be carried out as a marker of obstructive lung function secondary to small airways disease. A meta-analysis of lung function in former preterm and full-term infants published in 2013 demonstrated that the percent predicted forced expiratory volume in 1 s (FEV$_1$), a commonly used marker of obstructive lung disease, in former preterm infants has been steadily improving in later birth cohorts, although still is approximately 90 % that of former full-term infants [55].

Although the small airways disease associated with prematurity is not necessarily equivalent to asthma, the prototypical obstructive lung disorder in children, the diagnosis of asthma can serve as a marker of small airways disease among preterm infants. Although the risk of asthma is highest in preterm infants born at ≤32 weeks gestation (adjusted OR: 3.9) compared to full-term infants born at 39–40 weeks gestation, even late preterm infants born at 33–36 weeks gestation and early term infants born at 37–38 weeks gestation may be at higher risk as well (adjusted ORs: 1.7 and 1.2, respectively) [56]. It should be noted that the association between asthma and late preterm births has not been consistently observed [57], and that the strength of this association may decrease with age [58]. Nevertheless, given that the prevalence of asthma is 9.5 % among children aged 0–17 years within the general population in the United States [59] and there is an increased odds ratio of asthma of ~3.9 among early preterm infants [56, 58], the prevalence of asthma among these infants may approach 40 %.

Large Airways Disease

Large airways disease in preterm infants is most likely to manifest as tracheomalacia and/or bronchomalacia. Typically, infants with large airway malacia present with respiratory distress (often with abrupt cyanosis), or persistent atelectasis or hyperinflation on imaging [60, 61]. A common clinical scenario of infants with severe large airway malacia may be the onset of sudden respiratory distress and profound desaturations in the setting of agitation or vagal stimulation, and may require use of a bag valve mask for resuscitation.

In terms of the epidemiology of large airway disease in preterm infants, the prevalence is less well characterized and may be underdiagnosed, perhaps due to the difficulties in diagnosis. Classically, direct visualization with bronchoscopy is utilized for diagnosis, which may not be readily available at all NICUs, and may include the attendant risks of sedation and intubation. Newer modalities of imaging, such as CT scanning, may be helpful in the diagnosis of evaluating tracheomalacia [62], but may be only available at select tertiary care institutions and may not be reliable in all patients [61].

One prospective study of 117 preterm infants with a history of intubation for >7 days found that 16.2 % had tracheomalacia, which was associated with severe BPD, hypercarbia, and apnea [63]. Of these patients with moderate to severe tracheomalacia, 21 % required tracheostomies for management.

Vascular Disease

Over the past decade, there has been emerging recognition of pulmonary vascular disease in preterm infants in the form of pulmonary hypertension, which is defined as a resting mean pulmonary artery pressure >25 mm Hg after 2–3 months of age [64]. Pulmonary hypertension in preterm infants is almost always associated with severe lung disease and secondary to a reactive or diminished pulmonary vascular bed, a fact reflected in recent international classifications of pulmonary hypertension [65–67]. However, pulmonary hypertension can also be secondary to cardiovascular lesions; for example, pulmonary vein stenosis has also been reported in preterm infants with pulmonary hypertension and can be associated with poorer outcomes [68, 69]. Although the gold standard for diagnosis of pulmonary hypertension is cardiac catheterization [64], many cases are screened or diagnosed via echocardiograms. Among young children with chronic lung disease, including BPD, echocardiography has been shown to diagnose pulmonary hypertension, but may not be reliable in determining severity [70].

Pulmonary hypertension in preterm infants can manifest as persistent BPD symptoms poorly responsive to therapies or evidence of right heart insufficiency or failure [71]. Also, patients with baseline pulmonary hypertension can experience acute hypertensive crises, which present with an acute increase in work of breathing, hypoxemia, and/or, in the most severe instances, cardiorespiratory failure or arrest [71]. These sometimes life-threatening episodes can be triggered by anesthesia induction [72] or respiratory tract infections [73], possibly through changes in gas exchange leading to hypoxemia or hypercarbia [74–76].

Prospective and retrospective studies have demonstrated a range in prevalence of pulmonary hypertension ranging from 14 to 43 % of preterm infants with BPD [77–82]. Unfortunately, the mortality with patients with pulmonary hypertension remains high, ranging from 14 to 38 % [77–82]. In addition, these patients also experience additional morbidity in the form of longer initial hospital stays, with infants with pulmonary hypertension having a 2.2 month longer initial NICU admission compared to infants with BPD without pulmonary hypertension, which may result in at least an additional $198,000 in health care expenditures [83].

Pulmonary hypertension likely arises from a series of complex interactions between multiple factors, including genetic and prenatal/postnatal environmental factors [84]. These factors may include alterations in angiogenic pathways [85–88], possible genetic modifiers [46, 89], intrauterine growth [78, 81, 90–92], oligohydramnios [79, 92], patent ductus arteriosus [77], and placental vascularity [93, 94]. Although most cases of pulmonary hypertension arise as a function of reactive or diminished pulmonary vascular bed, pulmonary hypertension can occur as a function of pulmonary vein stenosis [68, 69], for which umbilical catheters may be a risk factor [95].

Control of Breathing

Infants born prematurely frequently demonstrate issues with immature control of breathing manifesting as central apneas. These apneas, if prolonged, can be accompanied by bradycardia and oxygen desaturations. The oxygen desaturations may be more prominent in infants with poor pulmonary reserve (i.e., parenchymal disease) and can occur with brief central apneas that last only a few seconds [96]. In addition, preterm infants with BPD may have blunted chemoreflex responses to both hypoxia [97] and/or hyperoxia [98]. Limited data suggest that infants with a history of posthemorrhagic hydrocephalus are more likely to have apneic events [99, 100], and certainly untreated or inadequately treated elevated intracranial pressures from hydrocephalus may cause bradypnea or apnea.

Although central apneas may be isolated events, they also may occur in rapid successive sequence with periodic breathing. Periodic breathing is commonly observed in infants, including preterm infants, but may frequently lead to oxygen desaturations in preterm infants [101]. The incidence of disordered control of breathing is likely underestimated, as the use of supplemental oxygen or augmented airflow may also mask control of breathing abnormalities [102]. Nevertheless, the frequency of such events and time to resolution are associated with gestational age at birth with infants born earlier at a higher risk of demonstrating apnea and a later age of resolution [103, 104].

Data from apnea monitor downloads suggest that preterm infants may be at a risk of more extreme events until 43 weeks postconceptional age [105]. Overnight polysomnography data obtained on infants and toddlers born prematurely also demonstrate a decrease in central apneas after 12 months of age [96]. Although there are no published data regarding sleep-disordered breathing in adults born prematurely, alterations in ventilatory control, including both hypoventilation and hyperventilation, in exercising children and adults born prematurely have been observed compared to term controls [106] as well as in adults born prematurely exposed to hypoxic and hyperoxic conditions [107].

Upper Airway Obstruction

Upper airway obstruction leading to obstructive apneas or hypopneas can occur in several anatomic locations in preterm infants. During infancy, obstruction in the palatal or retroglossal regions may be more common, in addition to laryngeal lesions such as vocal cord paresis and subglottic stenosis, whereas in toddlers, anatomic obstruction is more likely to be secondary to adenotonsillar hypertrophy [108]. In addition, a relatively larger tongue size for preterm infants has been postulated to contribute to narrowing of the upper airway based on respiration-timed radiographs [109]. Although the gold standard for diagnosis of upper airway obstruction is overnight polysomnography with specialist evaluation [110], specific diagnoses are often made by direct visualization by an otolaryngologist.

The risk factors and prevalence for upper airway obstruction in preterm infants are dependent on the site of the obstruction. Acquired subglottic stenosis is often associated with intubation, and pertinent risk factors may include duration of intubation, endotracheal tube size, and the occurrence of traumatic intubation [111]. Acquired subglottic cysts may also be more likely to occur with traumatic or prolonged intubation [112, 113]. In at least one prospective study, subglottic cysts were identified in 7.2 % of preterm infants after prolonged intubation ($n = 153$) [113]. Although it can be postulated that gastroesophageal reflux (which is not uncommon in preterm infants) could be associated with obstructive apnea through upper airway inflammation or laryngeal chemoreflexes [114], the association between reflux and apnea is not well established in infants, regardless of prematurity [115, 116]. Vocal cord paresis may occur as a complication of cardiac surgeries, including PDA ligation. In one meta-analysis, the weighted pooled proportion of unilateral vocal fold paralysis in studies that assessed the vocal folds postoperatively was 29.8 % for any congenital cardiac surgery (11 studies; $n = 584$) and 39 % for patent ductus arteriosus ligation (6 studies; $n = 274$) [117].

Although there are limited data regarding the prevalence of sleep-disordered breathing among former preterm infants, a US-based population cohort study of 850 children aged 8–11 years, of whom 46 % were born preterm, found that sleep-disordered breathing was 3–5 times more common among those born prematurely compared to those born at term [118]. Other retrospective chart reviews have also found an association between prematurity and obstructive sleep apnea [119].

Conclusions

Preterm infants can manifest a variety of respiratory complications, which providers who care for preterm infants should be aware of. The diverse elements of the respiratory tract that may be involved and the varying severity of presentations make it difficult to apply common algorithms for prevention and management. Further research is necessary to more clearly delineate the scope of disease as well as best practices for diagnosis and treatment.

References

1. Stoll BJ, Hansen NI, Bell EF, Walsh MC, Carlo WA, Shankaran S, et al. Trends in care practices, morbidity, and mortality of extremely preterm neonates, 1993-2012. JAMA. 2015;314(10):1039–51. PubMed PMID: 26348753.
2. Liu L, Oza S, Hogan D, Perin J, Rudan I, Lawn JE, et al. Global, regional, and national causes of child mortality in 2000-13, with projections to inform post-2015 priorities: an updated systematic analysis. Lancet. 2015;385(9966):430–40. PubMed PMID: 25280870.
3. Martin JA, Hamilton BE, Osterman MJ. Births in the United States, 2014. NCHS Data Brief. 2015;216:1–8. PubMed PMID: 26460599.

4. Hamilton BE, Martin JA, Osterman MJ, Curtin SC, Matthews TJ. Births: final data for 2014. National vital statistics reports: from the Centers for Disease Control and Prevention, National Center for Health Statistics. Natl Vital Stat Syst. 2015;64(12):1–64. PubMed PMID: 26727629.

5. Guaman MC, Gien J, Baker CD, Zhang H, Austin ED, Collaco JM. Point prevalence, clinical characteristics, and treatment variation for infants with severe bronchopulmonary dysplasia. Am J Perinatol. 2015;32(10):960–7. PubMed PMID: 25738785. Pubmed Central PMCID: 4617756.

6. Lapcharoensap W, Gage SC, Kan P, Profit J, Shaw GM, Gould JB, et al. Hospital variation and risk factors for bronchopulmonary dysplasia in a population-based cohort. JAMA Pediatr. 2015;169(2):e143676. PubMed PMID: 25642906.

7. Baraldi E, Filippone M. Chronic lung disease after premature birth. N Engl J Med. 2007;357(19):1946–55. PubMed PMID: 17989387.

8. Northway Jr WH, Rosan RC, Porter DY. Pulmonary disease following respirator therapy of hyaline-membrane disease. Bronchopulmonary dysplasia. N Engl J Med. 1967;276(7):357–68. PubMed PMID: 5334613.

9. Jobe AJ. The new BPD: an arrest of lung development. Pediatr Res. 1999;46(6):641–3. PubMed PMID: 10590017.

10. Thebaud B, Abman SH. Bronchopulmonary dysplasia: where have all the vessels gone? Roles of angiogenic growth factors in chronic lung disease. Am J Respir Crit Care Med. 2007;175(10):978–85. PubMed PMID: 17272782. Pubmed Central PMCID: 2176086.

11. Ehrenkranz RA, Walsh MC, Vohr BR, Jobe AH, Wright LL, Fanaroff AA, et al. Validation of the National Institutes of Health consensus definition of bronchopulmonary dysplasia. Pediatrics. 2005;116(6):1353–60. PubMed PMID: 16322158.

12. Jobe AH, Bancalari E. Bronchopulmonary dysplasia. Am J Respir Crit Care Med. 2001;163(7):1723–9. PubMed PMID: 11401896.

13. Group BIUKC, Group BIAC, Group BINZC, Stenson BJ, Tarnow-Mordi WO, Darlow BA, et al. Oxygen saturation and outcomes in preterm infants. N Engl J Med. 2013;368(22):2094–104. PubMed PMID: 23642047.

14. Network SSGotEKSNNR, Carlo WA, Finer NN, Walsh MC, Rich W, Gantz MG, et al. Target ranges of oxygen saturation in extremely preterm infants. N Engl J Med. 2010;362(21):1959–69. PubMed PMID: 20472937. Pubmed Central PMCID: 2891970.

15. Ellsbury DL, Acarregui MJ, McGuinness GA, Klein JM. Variability in the use of supplemental oxygen for bronchopulmonary dysplasia. J Pediatr. 2002;140(2):247–9. PubMed PMID: 11865280.

16. Britton JR. Altitude, oxygen and the definition of bronchopulmonary dysplasia. J Perinatol Off J California Perinat Assoc. 2012;32(11):880–5. PubMed PMID: 22343395.

17. Fernandez CL, Fajardo CA, Favareto MV, Hoyos A, Jijon-Letort FX, Carrera MS, et al. Oxygen dependency as equivalent to bronchopulmonary dysplasia at different altitudes in newborns 1500 g at birth from the SIBEN network. J Perinatol Off J California Perinat Assoc. 2014;34(7):538–42. PubMed PMID: 24699220.

18. Jensen EA, Schmidt B. Epidemiology of bronchopulmonary dysplasia. Birth Defects Res Part A Clin Mol Teratol. 2014;100(3):145–57. PubMed PMID: 24639412.

19. Stoll BJ, Hansen NI, Bell EF, Shankaran S, Laptook AR, Walsh MC, et al. Neonatal outcomes of extremely preterm infants from the NICHD Neonatal Research Network. Pediatrics. 2010;126(3):443–56. PubMed PMID: 20732945. Pubmed Central PMCID: 2982806.

20. Cristea AI, Carroll AE, Davis SD, Swigonski NL, Ackerman VL. Outcomes of children with severe bronchopulmonary dysplasia who were ventilator dependent at home. Pediatrics. 2013;132(3):e727–34. PubMed PMID: 23918888. Pubmed Central PMCID: 3876749.

21. Boroughs D, Dougherty JA. Decreasing accidental mortality of ventilator-dependent children at home: a call to action. Home Healthc Nurse. 2012;30(2):103–11. quiz 12-3. PubMed PMID: 22306756.

22. Bose C, Van Marter LJ, Laughon M, O'Shea TM, Allred EN, Karna P, et al. Fetal growth restriction and chronic lung disease among infants born before the 28th week of gestation. Pediatrics. 2009;124(3):e450–8. PubMed PMID: 19706590. Pubmed Central PMCID: 2891899.

23. Torchin H, Ancel PY, Goffinet F, Hascoet JM, Truffert P, Tran D, et al. Placental complications and bronchopulmonary dysplasia: EPIPAGE-2 cohort study. Pediatrics. 2016;137(3):e20152163. PubMed PMID: 26908662.

24. Eriksson L, Haglund B, Odlind V, Altman M, Ewald U, Kieler H. Perinatal conditions related to growth restriction and inflammation are associated with an increased risk of bronchopulmonary dysplasia. Acta Paediatr. 2015;104(3):259–63. PubMed PMID: 25469645.

25. Hansen AR, Barnes CM, Folkman J, McElrath TF. Maternal preeclampsia predicts the development of bronchopulmonary dysplasia. J Pediatr. 2010;156(4):532–6. PubMed PMID: 20004912.

26. Eriksson L, Haglund B, Odlind V, Altman M, Kieler H. Prenatal inflammatory risk factors for development of bronchopulmonary dysplasia. Pediatr Pulmonol. 2014;49(7):665–72. PubMed PMID: 24039136.

27. Hartling L, Liang Y, Lacaze-Masmonteil T. Chorioamnionitis as a risk factor for bronchopulmonary dysplasia: a systematic review and meta-analysis. Arch Dis Child Fetal Neonatal Ed. 2012;97(1):F8–F17. PubMed PMID: 21697236.

28. Hanke K, Hartz A, Manz M, Bendiks M, Heitmann F, Orlikowsky T, et al. Preterm prelabor rupture of membranes and outcome of very-low-birth-weight infants in the German Neonatal Network. PLoS One. 2015;10(4):e0122564. PubMed PMID: 25856083. Pubmed Central PMCID: 4391753.

29. Yen TA, Yang HI, Hsieh WS, Chou HC, Chen CY, Tsou KI, et al. Preeclampsia and the risk of bronchopulmonary dysplasia in VLBW infants: a population based study. PLoS One. 2013;8(9):e75168. PubMed PMID: 24073247. Pubmed Central PMCID: 3779258.

30. O'Shea JE, Davis PG, Doyle LW, Victorian Infant Collaborative Study G. Maternal preeclampsia and risk of bronchopulmonary dysplasia in preterm infants. Pediatr Res. 2012;71(2):210–4. PubMed PMID: 22258134.

31. Plakkal N, Soraisham AS, Trevenen C, Freiheit EA, Sauve R. Histological chorioamnionitis and bronchopulmonary dysplasia: a retrospective cohort study. J Perinatol Off J California Perinat Assoc. 2013;33(6):441–5. PubMed PMID: 23238570.

32. Lacaze-Masmonteil T. That chorioamnionitis is a risk factor for bronchopulmonary dysplasia – the case against. Paediatr Respir Rev. 2014;15(1):53–5. PubMed PMID: 24120077.

33. Schena F, Francescato G, Cappelleri A, Picciolli I, Mayer A, Mosca F, et al. Association between hemodynamically significant patent ductus arteriosus and bronchopulmonary dysplasia. J Pediatr. 2015;166(6):1488–92. PubMed PMID: 25882876.

34. Tapia JL, Agost D, Alegria A, Standen J, Escobar M, Grandi C, et al. Bronchopulmonary dysplasia: incidence, risk factors and resource utilization in a population of South American very low birth weight infants. J Pediatr. 2006;82(1):15–20. PubMed PMID: 16532142.

35. Clyman RI. The role of patent ductus arteriosus and its treatments in the development of bronchopulmonary dysplasia. Semin Perinatol. 2013;37(2):102–7. PubMed PMID: 23582964. Pubmed Central PMCID: 3627220.

36. Shah J, Jefferies AL, Yoon EW, Lee SK, Shah PS, Canadian Neonatal N. Risk factors and outcomes of late-onset bacterial sepsis in preterm neonates born at <32 weeks' gestation. Am J Perinatol. 2015;32(7):675–82. PubMed PMID: 25486288.

37. Keszler M, Sant'Anna G. Mechanical ventilation and bronchopulmonary dysplasia. Clin Perinatol. 2015;42(4):781–96. PubMed PMID: 26593078.

38. Patel RM, Leong T, Carlton DP, Vyas-Read S. Early caffeine therapy and clinical outcomes in extremely preterm infants. J Perinatol Off J California Perinat Assoc. 2013;33(2):134–40. PubMed PMID: 22538326.

39. Dobson NR, Patel RM, Smith PB, Kuehn DR, Clark J, Vyas-Read S, et al. Trends in caffeine use and association between clinical outcomes and timing of therapy in very low birth weight

infants. J Pediatr. 2014;164(5):992–8. e3.PubMed PMID: 24461786. Pubmed Central PMCID: 3992195.

40. Lodha A, Seshia M, McMillan DD, Barrington K, Yang J, Lee SK, et al. Association of early caffeine administration and neonatal outcomes in very preterm neonates. JAMA Pediatr. 2015;169(1):33–8. PubMed PMID: 25402629.

41. Roberts D, Dalziel S. Antenatal corticosteroids for accelerating fetal lung maturation for women at risk of preterm birth. Cochrane Database Syst Rev. 2006;3:CD004454. PubMed PMID: 16856047.

42. Onland W, Offringa M, van Kaam A. Late (>/= 7 days) inhalation corticosteroids to reduce bronchopulmonary dysplasia in preterm infants. Cochrane Database Syst Rev. 2012;4:CD002311. PubMed PMID: 22513906.

43. Shah VS, Ohlsson A, Halliday HL, Dunn M. Early administration of inhaled corticosteroids for preventing chronic lung disease in ventilated very low birth weight preterm neonates. Cochrane Database Syst Rev. 2012;5:CD001969. PubMed PMID: 22592680.

44. Shah SS, Ohlsson A, Halliday HL, Shah VS. Inhaled versus systemic corticosteroids for preventing chronic lung disease in ventilated very low birth weight preterm neonates. Cochrane Database Syst Rev. 2012;5:CD002058. PubMed PMID: 22592683.

45. Shah SS, Ohlsson A, Halliday HL, Shah VS. Inhaled versus systemic corticosteroids for the treatment of chronic lung disease in ventilated very low birth weight preterm infants. Cochrane Database Syst Rev. 2012;5:CD002057. PubMed PMID: 22592682.

46. Bhandari V, Bizzarro MJ, Shetty A, Zhong X, Page GP, Zhang H, et al. Familial and genetic susceptibility to major neonatal morbidities in preterm twins. Pediatrics. 2006;117(6):1901–6. PubMed PMID: 16740829.

47. Lavoie PM, Pham C, Jang KL. Heritability of bronchopulmonary dysplasia, defined according to the consensus statement of the national institutes of health. Pediatrics. 2008;122(3):479–85. PubMed PMID: 18762515. Pubmed Central PMCID: 4631604.

48. Lal CV, Ambalavanan N. Genetic predisposition to bronchopulmonary dysplasia. Semin Perinatol. 2015;39(8):584–91. PubMed PMID: 26471063. Pubmed Central PMCID: 4644695.

49. Hadchouel A, Durrmeyer X, Bouzigon E, Incitti R, Huusko J, Jarreau PH, et al. Identification of SPOCK2 as a susceptibility gene for bronchopulmonary dysplasia. Am J Respir Crit Care Med. 2011;184(10):1164–70. PubMed PMID: 21836138.

50. Wang H, St Julien KR, Stevenson DK, Hoffmann TJ, Witte JS, Lazzeroni LC, et al. A genome-wide association study (GWAS) for bronchopulmonary dysplasia. Pediatrics. 2013;132(2):290–7. PubMed PMID: 23897914. Pubmed Central PMCID: 3727675.

51. Ambalavanan N, Cotten CM, Page GP, Carlo WA, Murray JC, Bhattacharya S, et al. Integrated genomic analyses in bronchopulmonary dysplasia. J Pediatr. 2015;166(3):531–7. e13. PubMed PMID: 25449221. Pubmed Central PMCID: 4344889.

52. Piersigilli F, Bhandari V. Biomarkers in neonatology: the new "omics" of bronchopulmonary dysplasia. J Matern Fetal Neonatal Med Off J Eur Assoc Perinat Med Feder Asia Oceania Perinat Soc Int Soc Perinat Obstet. 2015;2015:1–7. PubMed PMID: 26135768.

53. Cohen J, Van Marter LJ, Sun Y, Allred E, Leviton A, Kohane IS. Perturbation of gene expression of the chromatin remodeling pathway in premature newborns at risk for bronchopulmonary dysplasia. Genome Biol. 2007;8(10):R210. PubMed PMID: 17916252. Pubmed Central PMCID: 2246284.

54. Ochiai M, Hikino S, Yabuuchi H, Nakayama H, Sato K, Ohga S, et al. A new scoring system for computed tomography of the chest for assessing the clinical status of bronchopulmonary dysplasia. J Pediatr. 2008;152(1):90–5. 5 e1-3. PubMed PMID: 18154907.

55. Kotecha SJ, Edwards MO, Watkins WJ, Henderson AJ, Paranjothy S, Dunstan FD, et al. Effect of preterm birth on later FEV1: a systematic review and meta-analysis. Thorax. 2013;68(8):760–6. PubMed PMID: 23604458.

56. Harju M, Keski-Nisula L, Georgiadis L, Raisanen S, Gissler M, Heinonen S. The burden of childhood asthma and late preterm and early term births. J Pediatr. 2014;164(2):295–9. e1. PubMed PMID: 24210922.

57. Crump C, Winkleby MA, Sundquist J, Sundquist K. Risk of asthma in young adults who were born preterm: a Swedish national cohort study. Pediatrics. 2011;127(4):e913–20. PubMed PMID: 21422091. Pubmed Central PMCID: 3387891.

58. Damgaard AL, Hansen BM, Mathiasen R, Buchvald F, Lange T, Greisen G. Prematurity and prescription asthma medication from childhood to young adulthood: a Danish national cohort study. PLoS One. 2015;10(2):e0117253. PubMed PMID: 25651521. Pubmed Central PMCID: 4317188.

59. Moorman JE, Akinbami LJ, Bailey CM, Zahran HS, King ME, Johnson CA, et al. National surveillance of asthma: United States, 2001-2010. Series 3, Analytical and epidemiological studies / [US Dept of Health and Human Services, Public Health Service, National Center for Health Statistics]. Vital Health Stat. 2012;2012(35):1–58. PubMed PMID: 24252609.

60. Miller RW, Woo P, Kellman RK, Slagle TS. Tracheobronchial abnormalities in infants with bronchopulmonary dysplasia. J Pediatr. 1987;111(5):779–82. PubMed PMID: 3668747.

61. Mok Q, Negus S, McLaren CA, Rajka T, Elliott MJ, Roebuck DJ, et al. Computed tomography versus bronchography in the diagnosis and management of tracheobronchomalacia in ventilator dependent infants. Arch Dis Child Fetal Neonatal Ed. 2005;90(4):F290–3. PubMed PMID: 15857878. Pubmed Central PMCID: 1721907.

62. Long FR, Castile RG. Technique and clinical applications of full-inflation and end-exhalation controlled-ventilation chest CT in infants and young children. Pediatr Radiol. 2001;31(6):413–22. PubMed PMID: 11436888.

63. Downing GJ, Kilbride HW. Evaluation of airway complications in high-risk preterm infants: application of flexible fiberoptic airway endoscopy. Pediatrics. 1995;95(4):567–72. PubMed PMID: 7700760.

64. Abman SH, Hansmann G, Archer SL, Ivy DD, Adatia I, Chung WK, et al. Pediatric pulmonary hypertension: guidelines from the American Heart Association and American Thoracic Society. Circulation. 2015;132(21):2037–99. PubMed PMID: 26534956.

65. Simonneau G, Gatzoulis MA, Adatia I, Celermajer D, Denton C, Ghofrani A, et al. Updated clinical classification of pulmonary hypertension. J Am Coll Cardiol. 2013;62(25 Suppl):D34–41. PubMed PMID: 24355639.

66. Lammers AE, Adatia I, Cerro MJ, Diaz G, Freudenthal AH, Freudenthal F, et al. Functional classification of pulmonary hypertension in children: report from the PVRI pediatric taskforce, Panama 2011. Pulm Circ. 2011;1(2):280–5. PubMed PMID: 21874157. Pubmed Central PMCID: 3161406.

67. Cerro MJ, Abman S, Diaz G, Freudenthal AH, Freudenthal F, Harikrishnan S, et al. A consensus approach to the classification of pediatric pulmonary hypertensive vascular disease: report from the PVRI Pediatric Taskforce, Panama 2011. Pulm Circ. 2011;1(2):286–98. PubMed PMID: 21874158. Pubmed Central PMCID: 3161725.

68. Laux D, Rocchisani MA, Boudjemline Y, Gouton M, Bonnet D, Ovaert C. Pulmonary hypertension in the preterm infant with chronic lung disease can be caused by pulmonary vein stenosis: a must-know entity. Pediatr Cardiol. 2016;37(2):313–21. PubMed PMID: 26573816.

69. Smith SC, Rabah R. Pulmonary venous stenosis in a premature infant with bronchopulmonary dysplasia: clinical and autopsy findings of these newly associated entities. Pediatr Dev Pathol Off J Soc Pediatr Pathol Paediatr Pathol Soc. 2012;15(2):160–4. PubMed PMID: 22313395.

70. Mourani PM, Sontag MK, Younoszai A, Ivy DD, Abman SH. Clinical utility of echocardiography for the diagnosis and management of pulmonary vascular disease in young children with chronic lung disease. Pediatrics. 2008;121(2):317–25. PubMed PMID: 18245423. Pubmed Central PMCID: 3121163.

71. Collaco JM, Romer LH, Stuart BD, Coulson JD, Everett AD, Lawson EE, et al. Frontiers in pulmonary hypertension in infants and children with bronchopulmonary dysplasia. Pediatr Pulmonol. 2012;47(11):1042–53. PubMed PMID: 22777709. Pubmed Central PMCID: 3963167.

72. Carmosino MJ, Friesen RH, Doran A, Ivy DD. Perioperative complications in children with pulmonary hypertension undergoing noncardiac surgery or cardiac catheterization. Anesth Analg. 2007;104(3):521–7. PubMed PMID: 17312201. Pubmed Central PMCID: 1934984.
73. Farquhar M, Fitzgerald DA. Pulmonary hypertension in chronic neonatal lung disease. Paediatr Respir Rev. 2010;11(3):149–53. PubMed PMID: 20692628.
74. Shukla AC, Almodovar MC. Anesthesia considerations for children with pulmonary hypertension. Pediatr Crit Care Med J Soc Crit Care Med World Feder Pediatr Inten Crit Care Soc. 2010;11(2 Suppl):S70–3. PubMed PMID: 20216167.
75. van der Griend BF, Lister NA, McKenzie IM, Martin N, Ragg PG, Sheppard SJ, et al. Postoperative mortality in children after 101,885 anesthetics at a tertiary pediatric hospital. Anesth Analg. 2011;112(6):1440–7. PubMed PMID: 21543787.
76. Friesen RH, Williams GD. Anesthetic management of children with pulmonary arterial hypertension. Paediatr Anaesth. 2008;18(3):208–16. PubMed PMID: 18230063.
77. An HS, Bae EJ, Kim GB, Kwon BS, Beak JS, Kim EK, et al. Pulmonary hypertension in preterm infants with bronchopulmonary dysplasia. Korean Circ J. 2010;40(3):131–6. PubMed PMID: 20339498. Pubmed Central PMCID: 2844979.
78. Khemani E, McElhinney DB, Rhein L, Andrade O, Lacro RV, Thomas KC, et al. Pulmonary artery hypertension in formerly premature infants with bronchopulmonary dysplasia: clinical features and outcomes in the surfactant era. Pediatrics. 2007;120(6):1260–9. PubMed PMID: 18055675.
79. Kumar VH, Hutchison AA, Lakshminrusimha S, Morin 3rd FC, Wynn RJ, Ryan RM. Characteristics of pulmonary hypertension in preterm neonates. J Perinatol Off J California Perinat Assoc. 2007;27(4):214–9. PubMed PMID: 17330053.
80. Slaughter JL, Pakrashi T, Jones DE, South AP, Shah TA. Echocardiographic detection of pulmonary hypertension in extremely low birth weight infants with bronchopulmonary dysplasia requiring prolonged positive pressure ventilation. J Perinatol Off J California Perinat Assoc. 2011;31(10):635–40. PubMed PMID: 21311503.
81. Bhat R, Salas AA, Foster C, Carlo WA, Ambalavanan N. Prospective analysis of pulmonary hypertension in extremely low birth weight infants. Pediatrics. 2012;129(3):e682–9. PubMed PMID: 22311993. Pubmed Central PMCID: 3289526.
82. Mourani PM, Sontag MK, Younoszai A, Miller JI, Kinsella JP, Baker CD, et al. Early pulmonary vascular disease in preterm infants at risk for bronchopulmonary dysplasia. Am J Respir Crit Care Med. 2014;191(1):87–95. PubMed PMID: 25389562.
83. Stuart BD, Sekar P, Coulson JD, Choi SE, McGrath-Morrow SA, Collaco JM. Health-care utilization and respiratory morbidities in preterm infants with pulmonary hypertension. J Perinatol Off J California Perinat Assoc. 2013;33(7):543–7. PubMed PMID: 23328926.
84. Mourani PM, Abman SH. Pulmonary hypertension and vascular abnormalities in bronchopulmonary dysplasia. Clin Perinatol. 2015;42(4):839–55. PubMed PMID: 26593082.
85. Lassus P, Turanlahti M, Heikkila P, Andersson LC, Nupponen I, Sarnesto A, et al. Pulmonary vascular endothelial growth factor and Flt-1 in fetuses, in acute and chronic lung disease, and in persistent pulmonary hypertension of the newborn. Am J Respir Crit Care Med. 2001;164(10 Pt 1):1981–7. PubMed PMID: 11734455.
86. Maniscalco WM, Watkins RH, Pryhuber GS, Bhatt A, Shea C, Huyck H. Angiogenic factors and alveolar vasculature: development and alterations by injury in very premature baboons. Am J Physiol Lung Cell Mol Physiol. 2002;282(4):L811–23. PubMed PMID: 11880308.
87. Tang JR, Karumanchi SA, Seedorf G, Markham N, Abman SH. Excess soluble vascular endothelial growth factor receptor-1 in amniotic fluid impairs lung growth in rats: linking preeclampsia with bronchopulmonary dysplasia. Am J Physiol Lung Cell Mol Physiol. 2012;302(1):L36–46. PubMed PMID: 22003089. Pubmed Central PMCID: 3349373.
88. Li F, Hagaman JR, Kim HS, Maeda N, Jennette JC, Faber JE, et al. eNOS deficiency acts through endothelin to aggravate sFlt-1-induced pre-eclampsia-like phenotype. J Am Soc Nephrol. 2012;23(4):652–60. PubMed PMID: 22282588. Pubmed Central PMCID: 3312503.

89. Trittmann JK, Nelin LD, Zmuda EJ, Gastier-Foster JM, Chen B, Backes CH, et al. Arginase I gene single-nucleotide polymorphism is associated with decreased risk of pulmonary hypertension in bronchopulmonary dysplasia. Acta Paediatr. 2014;103(10):e439–43. PubMed PMID: 24919409. Pubmed Central PMCID: 4180790.
90. Bruno CJ, Meerkov M, Capone C, Vega M, Sutton N, Kim M, et al. CRIB scores as a tool for assessing risk for the development of pulmonary hypertension in extremely preterm infants with bronchopulmonary dysplasia. Am J Perinatol. 2015;32(11):1031–7. PubMed PMID: 26368789.
91. Check J, Gotteiner N, Liu X, Su E, Porta N, Steinhorn R, et al. Fetal growth restriction and pulmonary hypertension in premature infants with bronchopulmonary dysplasia. J Perinatol Off J California Perinat Assoc. 2013;33(7):553–7. PubMed PMID: 23328924. Pubmed Central PMCID: 3633609.
92. Kim DH, Kim HS, Choi CW, Kim EK, Kim BI, Choi JH. Risk factors for pulmonary artery hypertension in preterm infants with moderate or severe bronchopulmonary dysplasia. Neonatology. 2012;101(1):40–6. PubMed PMID: 21791938.
93. Yallapragada S, Mestan KK, Palac HL, Porta NF, Gotteiner NL, Hamvas A, et al. Placental villous vascularity is decreased in premature infants with bronchopulmonary dysplasia-associated pulmonary hypertension. Pediatr Dev Pathol Off J Soc Pediatr Pathol Paediatr Pathol Soc. 2015;19(2):101–7. PubMed PMID: 26366786.
94. Mestan KK, Check J, Minturn L, Yallapragada S, Farrow KN, Liu X, et al. Placental pathologic changes of maternal vascular underperfusion in bronchopulmonary dysplasia and pulmonary hypertension. Placenta. 2014;35(8):570–4. PubMed PMID: 24906549. Pubmed Central PMCID: 4119480.
95. Jaillard SM, Godart FR, Rakza T, Chanez A, Lequien P, Wurtz AJ, et al. Acquired pulmonary vein stenosis as a cause of life-threatening pulmonary hypertension. Ann Thorac Surg. 2003;75(1):275–7. PubMed PMID: 12537232.
96. McGrath-Morrow SA, Ryan T, McGinley BM, Okelo SO, Sterni LM, Collaco JM. Polysomnography in preterm infants and children with chronic lung disease. Pediatr Pulmonol. 2012;47(2):172–9. PubMed PMID: 21815283.
97. Calder NA, Williams BA, Smyth J, Boon AW, Kumar P, Hanson MA. Absence of ventilatory responses to alternating breaths of mild hypoxia and air in infants who have had bronchopulmonary dysplasia: implications for the risk of sudden infant death. Pediatr Res. 1994;35(6):677–81. PubMed PMID: 7936817.
98. Katz-Salamon M, Jonsson B, Lagercrantz H. Blunted peripheral chemoreceptor response to hyperoxia in a group of infants with bronchopulmonary dysplasia. Pediatr Pulmonol. 1995;20(2):101–6. PubMed PMID: 8570299.
99. Mancini MC, Barbosa NE, Banwart D, Silveira S, Guerpelli JL, Leone CR. Intraventricular hemorrhage in very low birth weight infants: associated risk factors and outcome in the neonatal period. Rev Hosp Clin. 1999;54(5):151–4. PubMed PMID: 10788836.
100. Robles P, Poblano A, Hernandez G, Ibarra J, Guzman I, Sosa J. Cortical, brainstem and autonomic nervous system dysfunction in infants with post-hemorrhagic hydrocephalus. Rev Invest Clin. 2002;54(2):133–8. PubMed PMID: 12053811.
101. Razi NM, DeLauter M, Pandit PB. Periodic breathing and oxygen saturation in preterm infants at discharge. J Perinatol Off J California Perinat Assoc. 2002;22(6):442–4. PubMed PMID: 12168119.
102. Coste F, Ferkol T, Hamvas A, Cleveland C, Linneman L, Hoffman J, et al. Ventilatory control and supplemental oxygen in premature infants with apparent chronic lung disease. Arch Dis Child Fetal Neonatal Ed. 2015;100(3):F233–7. PubMed PMID: 25716677. Pubmed Central PMCID: 4732273.
103. Henderson-Smart DJ. The effect of gestational age on the incidence and duration of recurrent apnoea in newborn babies. Aust Paediatr J. 1981;17(4):273–6. PubMed PMID: 7347216.
104. Eichenwald EC, Aina A, Stark AR. Apnea frequently persists beyond term gestation in infants delivered at 24 to 28 weeks. Pediatrics. 1997;100(3 Pt 1):354–9. PubMed PMID: 9282705.

105. Ramanathan R, Corwin MJ, Hunt CE, Lister G, Tinsley LR, Baird T, et al. Cardiorespiratory events recorded on home monitors: comparison of healthy infants with those at increased risk for SIDS. JAMA. 2001;285(17):2199–207. PubMed PMID: 11325321.
106. Bates ML, Pillers DA, Palta M, Farrell ET, Eldridge MW. Ventilatory control in infants, children, and adults with bronchopulmonary dysplasia. Respir Physiol Neurobiol. 2013;189(2):329–37. PubMed PMID: 23886637. Pubmed Central PMCID: 3812402.
107. Bates ML, Farrell ET, Eldridge MW. Abnormal ventilatory responses in adults born prematurely. N Engl J Med. 2014;370(6):584–5. PubMed PMID: 24499235. Pubmed Central PMCID: 4769592.
108. Don GW, Kirjavainen T, Broome C, Seton C, Waters KA. Site and mechanics of spontaneous, sleep-associated obstructive apnea in infants. J Appl Physiol. 2000;89(6):2453–62. PubMed PMID: 11090602.
109. Tonkin SL, McIntosh C, Gunn AJ. Does tongue size contribute to risk of airway narrowing in preterm infants sitting in a car safety seat? Am J Perinatol. 2014;31(9):741–4. PubMed PMID: 24338121.
110. Wise MS, Nichols CD, Grigg-Damberger MM, Marcus CL, Witmans MB, Kirk VG, et al. Executive summary of respiratory indications for polysomnography in children: an evidence-based review. Sleep. 2011;34(3):389–98. AW. PubMed PMID: 21359088. Pubmed Central PMCID: 3041716.
111. Amin RS, Rutter MJ. Airway disease and management in bronchopulmonary dysplasia. Clin Perinatol. 2015;42(4):857–70. PubMed PMID: 26593083.
112. Watson GJ, Malik TH, Khan NA, Sheehan PZ, Rothera MP. Acquired paediatric subglottic cysts: a series from Manchester. Int J Pediatr Otorhinolaryngol. 2007;71(4):533–8. PubMed PMID: 17239962.
113. Downing GJ, Hayen LK, Kilbride HW. Acquired subglottic cysts in the low-birth-weight infant. Characteristics, treatment, and outcome. Am J Dis Child. 1993;147(9):971–4. PubMed PMID: 8362815.
114. Qubty WF, Mrelashvili A, Kotagal S, Lloyd RM. Comorbidities in infants with obstructive sleep apnea. J Clin Sleep Med Off Pub Am Acad Sleep Med. 2014;10(11):1213–6. PubMed PMID: 25325583. Pubmed Central PMCID: 4224722.
115. Arad-Cohen N, Cohen A, Tirosh E. The relationship between gastroesophageal reflux and apnea in infants. J Pediatr. 2000;137(3):321–6. PubMed PMID: 10969254.
116. Di Fiore J, Arko M, Herynk B, Martin R, Hibbs AM. Characterization of cardiorespiratory events following gastroesophageal reflux in preterm infants. J Perinatol Off J California Perinat Assoc. 2010;30(10):683–7. PubMed PMID: 20220760. Pubmed Central PMCID: 2891417.
117. Strychowsky JE, Rukholm G, Gupta MK, Reid D. Unilateral vocal fold paralysis after congenital cardiothoracic surgery: a meta-analysis. Pediatrics. 2014;133(6):e1708–23. PubMed PMID: 24843065.
118. Rosen CL, Larkin EK, Kirchner HL, Emancipator JL, Bivins SF, Surovec SA, et al. Prevalence and risk factors for sleep-disordered breathing in 8- to 11-year-old children: association with race and prematurity. J Pediatr. 2003;142(4):383–9. PubMed PMID: 12712055.
119. Cote V, Ruiz AG, Perkins J, Sillau S, Friedman NR. Characteristics of children under 2 years of age undergoing tonsillectomy for upper airway obstruction. Int J Pediatr Otorhinolaryngol. 2015;79(6):903–8. PubMed PMID: 25912628.

Why Do Preterm Infants Wheeze? Clues from Epidemiology

Elianne Vrijlandt

Definitions

In accordance with the World Health Organization (WHO), preterm birth is defined as a live birth before 37 completed weeks of pregnancy. On the basis of gestational age, three subcategories of preterm birth are distinguished:

Extremely preterm (<28 weeks)
Very preterm (28 to <32 weeks)
Moderate to late preterm (32 to <37 weeks)

Bronchopulmonary Dysplasia

The classic diagnosis of BPD may be assigned at 28 days of life, provided the following criteria are met:

1. Supplemental oxygen is required beyond 28 days of age in order to maintain PaO_2 above 50 mmHg
2. Chest radiograph with diffuse abnormal findings characteristic of BPD

E. Vrijlandt, MD, PhD
Department of Pediatric Pulmonology and Pediatric Allergology, Beatrix Children's Hospital, Groningen, the Netherlands

University of Groningen, GRIAC Research Institute, University Medical Center Groningen, Groningen, the Netherlands
e-mail: e.j.l.e.vrijlandt@umcg.nl

© Springer International Publishing AG 2017
A.M. Hibbs, M. S. Muhlebach (eds.), *Respiratory Outcomes in Preterm Infants*,
Respiratory Medicine, DOI 10.1007/978-3-319-48835-6_2

Newer Criteria

The newer criteria for BPD, issued by the National Institute of Health (USA) and applicable to neonates treated with more than 21 % oxygen for at least 28 days, are as follows:

Mild Breathing room air at 36 weeks' postmenstrual age or at discharge (whichever comes first) for infants born before 32 weeks or Breathing room air by 56 days postnatal age or at discharge (whichever comes first) for infants born after 32 weeks' gestation

Moderate The need for <30 % oxygen at 36 weeks' postmenstrual age or at discharge (whichever comes first) for infants born before 32 weeks, or The need for <30 % oxygen until 56 days' postnatal age or at discharge (whichever comes first)

Severe The need for >30 % oxygen, with or without positive pressure ventilation or continuous positive pressure, at 36 weeks' postmenstrual age or at discharge (whichever comes first) for infants born before 32 weeks, or The need for >30 % oxygen, with or without positive pressure ventilation or continuous positive pressure, at 56 days' postnatal age or at discharge (whichever comes first) for infants born after 32 weeks' gestation

Currently, the most commonly used clinical definition of BPD is the need for supplemental oxygen at 36 weeks' corrected gestational age, often referred to as the Shennan definition [1]. Newer definitions, incorporating a physiological test of room air saturation at 36 weeks and a severity grade based on the extent of respiratory support required, have also been proposed and are used both clinically and for research purposes [2].

Wheeze

Wheezing is a high-pitched whistling sound heard during breathing caused by air being forced through airways that are narrower than normal. Wheezing is commonly more prominent when breathing out than when breathing in.

Asthma (WHO Definition; See http://www.who.int/respiratory/asthma/definition/en/)

Asthma is a disease characterized by recurrent attacks of breathlessness and wheezing that vary in severity and frequency from person to person. In one individual such attacks may occur every hour, and in another they are a daily occurrence. This condition is due to inflammation of the air passages in the lungs and affects the sensitivity of the nerve endings in the airways so they become easily irritated. During an attack, the lining of the passages swell, causing the airways to narrow and thus the flow of air in and out of the lungs is reduced.

Introduction

Worldwide, the WHO has estimated that more than 15 million infants are born preterm, that is, 11 % of live births. Rates of preterm births are increasing in most countries with reliable data [3]. Across 184 countries, the rate of preterm births ranges from 5 to 18 % of live births. In 2010, it was estimated that the rate of preterm births in the USA was 12 %, accounting for 42 % of all preterm births in developed regions [4]. Approximately, 90 % of preterm infants survived [5]. In 2014, in the USA, the preterm birth rate declined to 9.57 %, while the low birth weight rate remained essentially unchanged at 8 % [6].

In this chapter, we discuss respiratory outcomes of preterm infants and the impact of the diagnosis BPD later in life. It is important to realize, however, that not only respiratory problems may play a role later on, but cardiovascular diseases and developmental problems also play a role. Many survivors face a lifetime of disability, including learning disabilities, visual, and hearing problems. The significant associations of preterm birth with adult health and health-related problems have become increasingly recognized thanks to epidemiological research and clinical observations [7]. In the light of the increasing numbers of survivors of preterm birth, with or without BPD, and the lack of a clear understanding of the etiology of sequelae in later life, the goal of this chapter is to review the published literature to determine the effects of preterm birth on different stages during the course of life. We address the following questions:

1. Which respiratory symptoms are described in preterm-born infants?
2. Does wheezing occur in former preterm-born children, adolescents, or adults?
3. Does gestational age matter?
4. Which putative mechanisms are to be expected?
5. Which risk factors are described for respiratory problems in former preterm-born children?

Which Respiratory Symptoms Are Described in Preterm-Born Infants?

Preterm birth predisposes individuals to the development of chronic respiratory diseases in infancy, childhood, and adulthood, including asthma and chronic obstructive pulmonary disease (COPD) [8]. Beyond the neonatal period, the major respiratory problems during infancy and early childhood that require hospitalization are respiratory exacerbations caused by infections, viral infections particular. Signs and symptoms of severe respiratory infections may include fever, a barking cough, wheezing, tachypnea, chest wall retractions, nasal flaring, difficulty with drinking, lethargy, and sometimes, cyanosis. These symptoms become milder in school-age children. Nevertheless, a group of children remains – even as they grow older – who have recurrent episodes of wheezing and decreased lung function tests, that is, decreased forced expiratory volume [9].

Other respiratory symptoms associated with preterm birth are noisy breathing and stridor due to laryngomalacia or postintubation, subglottic stenosis, vocal cord paralysis, or tracheomalacia. Although preterm infants do not necessarily have a higher incidence of laryngomalacia, they do tend to develop the more severe form of this condition [10]. Left vocal cord paralysis is not uncommon in patients exposed to persistent ductus arteriosus surgery as preterm infants. The condition may be easily overlooked, and the symptoms may be confused with those of other diseases. Laryngoscopy should be offered on the basis of liberal indications after persistent ductus arteriosus ligation [11].

BPD develops in approximately 10–40 % of infants born with very low birth weight (VLBW) and extremely low birth weight, amounting to 5000 to 10,000 new cases in the USA each year, depending on the definition applied [12]. Although mortality attributable to BPD has declined over the past decade [13], BPD places a significant demand on health services [12] and constitutes a significant health burden long after the neonatal period.

On first presentation in 1967, infants with BPD showed persistent respiratory signs and symptoms; they required supplemental oxygen to treat hypoxemia, displayed persistent abnormal lung fields on chest radiograph; and histopathological changes, such as interstitial thickening, lung fibrosis, airway epithelial metaplasia, and smooth muscle hypertrophy occurred [14]. Following the increased use of antenatal steroids for lung maturation and the development of exogenous surfactant replacement therapy, the severity of infant lung diseases decreased and the survival of preterm newborns improved, particularly at lower gestational ages. These medical advancements resulted in the evolution of the disorder to a new form of the condition, one that predominantly occurs in the group of extremely preterm infants. BPD, in the contemporary era of perinatal care, is characterized by persistent decreases in alveolar counts, with enlarged alveoli, resulting in an overall reduction of the surface area available for gas exchange. It is, therefore, considered a consequence of disrupted or arrested lung development [15, 16].

Several studies have shown that infants who develop BPD experience more problems during infancy, childhood, adolescence, and adult age than preterm-born infants who do not develop BPD and healthy controls [17–19]. These problems emerge in different areas of functioning. Chronic respiratory signs in infants with

BPD include tachypnea with shallow breathing retractions, a paradoxical breathing pattern with rhonchi, crackles, and wheeze. Pulmonary function tests show decreased tidal volume, increased airway resistance, decreased dynamic lung compliance with increasing ventilation/perfusion mismatch, and decreased V'maxFRC (that worsen during the first year of life) [20, 21]. Uneven airway obstruction leads to gas trapping and hyperinflation with abnormal distribution of ventilation [20]. Because of increased vascular resistance in the lungs, children with BPD may develop right ventricular hypertrophy. Left ventricular hypertrophy is also seen, possibly associated with systemic hypertension, a condition commonly found in children with BPD [22–24]. With persisting lung impairment, survivors of BPD may be at risk of developing chronic obstructive physiologic impairments later in life, such as fixed airflow obstruction and hyperinflation.

Does Wheezing Occur in Former Preterm-Born Children, Adolescents, or Adults?

Been et al. performed a systematic review and a meta-analysis on preterm birth and childhood wheezing disorders. The symptoms they studied included wheezing, coughing, chest tightness, and shortness of breath [9].

The researchers identified 30 studies that investigated the association between preterm birth and asthma or wheezing disorders in more than 1.5 million children between 1995 and the present. This time span was chosen to allow for recent changes in the management of preterm birth. Of the 30 major studies on the association published worldwide, nearly a third reported no effect, whereas the others reported significant associations, with odds ratios (ORs) ranging from 1.2 to 4.9. Across the studies, 13.7 % of the preterm-born infants developed asthma or wheezing disorders during childhood, compared to only 8.3 % of infants born at term. Overall, therefore, the risk of preterm infants developing either asthma or a wheezing disorder during childhood was 1.71 times higher than the risk of full-term infants developing these conditions (an unadjusted OR of 1.71) [9]. Inconsistencies in the preterm birth–asthma association in part reflected differences among studies in three key domains: definitions of asthma, degree of prematurity, and the age at which asthma was assessed.

The pulmonary outcome of extremely preterm and very preterm children (born before 32 weeks' gestational age) has been studied extensively [5, 25]. The residual respiratory problems of these children include cough and wheeze and/or other asthma-like symptoms [26, 27]. In contrast to the pulmonary problems of extremely and very preterm infants, the pulmonary outcomes of former moderate to late preterm children are largely unknown, even though this group is much larger [6]. It remains uncertain whether the risk of long-term respiratory morbidity is larger in late preterm- born children than in full-term born children [28]. There are reports of increased hospitalization for respiratory problems in the first year of life, a higher rate of respiratory symptoms, for example, nocturnal coughing or wheezing without having a cold during early childhood, and a higher likelihood of abnormal pulmonary function studies [28, 29].

The Lollipop study showed that moderate to late preterm-born children had more respiratory problems during their first 5 years of life than their full-term born counterparts [29]. At the age of 5 years, rates of respiratory symptoms between former moderate to late preterms and extremely and very preterm children were similar and both were higher than in full-term born children. The symptoms resulted in more medication used and more absenteeism from school (see Table 1).

Other studies, however, found that late preterm birth was not associated with a diagnosis of asthma in early childhood [30, 31].

The EPICure study is a good example of considering respiratory symptoms during preadolescence and adolescence in children born extremely preterm. This study defined extremely preterm as <25 completed weeks of gestation. It showed increased respiratory morbidity at 11 years of age, especially among those children who had been diagnosed with BPD [32]. When compared to classmates, children born extremely preterm were more likely to have a current diagnosis of asthma (25 % versus 13 %; $P < .01$), recent respiratory symptoms, and medication. Among members of the extremely preterm group, significantly more with prior BPD reported wheeze in the past 12 months (see Table 2).

For some former preterm-born adolescents, particularly those who suffered BPD, obstructive lung disease persists into adulthood. Wong et al. reported significantly increased respiratory symptoms in a young adult population born at a time prior to the routine use of surfactant and who had all survived moderate to severe BPD [33]. During adolescence and adulthood, the balance of evidence suggested that preterm infants either with or without subsequent BPD have excess respiratory symptoms, including cough, wheeze, and asthma [34]. Functional pulmonary abnormalities consist of airway obstruction, airway hyperreactivity, and

Table 1 Prevalence of respiratory symptoms at 5 years of age [29]

Symptoms	Early preterms (%)	Moderate to late preterms (%)	Full-term born children (%)
Wheeze	34	28	19
Cough	34	33	24
Treatment for respiratory symptoms	21	18	9
Current asthma	9	10	6
Absent from school due to respiratory symptoms	22	21	11

Table 2 Prevalence of respiratory symptoms at the age of 11 years in extremely preterm children [32]

Symptoms	Extremely preterm, with BPD (%)	Extremely preterm, without BPD (%)	Full-term born children (%)
Wheeze	25	12	14
Nocturnal cough	22	15	11
Current asthma	28	19	13
Asthma medication	27	19	11

hyperinflation as well as exercise restriction [14, 35]. In these patients, a program of lung function monitoring and pulmonary prophylaxis by means of elimination of specific risk factors, such as smoking, in adulthood is advisable.

Does Gestational Age Matter?

Complications of preterm birth (<37 completed weeks of gestation) are most often seen in very preterm infants (28–31 weeks' gestation) and extremely preterm infants (<28 weeks' gestation), although it is increasingly recognized that even moderate to late preterm infants are at increased risk of adverse health and developmental outcomes [36]. This increased risk of respiratory morbidity in late preterm infants is probably related to immature lung structure, since lung development of the terminal respiratory sacs and alveoli continues between gestational weeks 34 and 36.

Infants born most extremely preterm, during the late canalicular or saccular stage of lung development, carry the greatest burden of early respiratory disease, putting them at greatest risk of later pulmonary morbidity. Indeed, despite medical advances in neonatal care that has led to improvements in the survival rate of extremely preterm infants, the prevalence of the neonatal chronic lung disease, BPD, has not diminished [18]. It remains the most common complication of extremely preterm birth. Later in life, the risk of asthma or wheezing disorders increases as the degree of prematurity increases [9]. The risk was considerably higher among children born very preterm, (OR 3.00, 95 % CI 2.61–3.44), when compared to moderately preterm children (OR 1.49, 95 % CI 1.34–1.66) [9].

Which Putative Mechanisms Are to Be Expected?

What is the pathophysiology of respiratory symptoms, such as wheezing disorders, in former preterms? There is the assumption of asthmatics wheeze due to airflow obstruction as a result of the cumulative effects of smooth muscle constriction around airways, airway wall edema, intraluminal mucus accumulation, inflammatory cell infiltration of the submucosa, and basement membrane thickening [37]. Inflammation can cause airway hyperresponsiveness and airflow obstruction.

Is this also the case for preterms? They are often labeled asthmatic, although the underlying mechanisms are likely to be very different. Several mechanisms, such as lung growth, inflammation, and structural changes might play a role in putative mechanisms for wheezing in patients born prematurely.

Lung Growth

The respiratory system undergoes significant growth and development during the third trimester of fetal life and throughout the first year of infancy. Postnatally, the pattern of physiological airway development is best characterized by the global lung initiative (http://www.lungfunction.org/). In healthy children, lung volume and function (FVC and FEV_1) continue to increase throughout childhood and reach a plateau at 20 to 25 years [38]. Subsequently, lung volume and function decline steadily with age. In individuals who experienced early lung injury or maldevelopment during infancy, a reduction in peak lung growth may appear [8]. The outcome of poor lung development depends on the type and severity of the insult as well as the developmental stage of the lung at the time it occurred [39]. Longitudinal studies show temporal tracking of small airway diseases among preterm-born individuals [40, 41].

The "new" BPD is often described with pathologic changes of large, simplified alveolar structures, a dysmorphic capillary configuration, and variable interstitial cellularity and/or fibroproliferation [15]. Airway and vascular lesions, when present, tend to be present in infants who develop more severe diseases over time [42]. The concept that "new" BPD results in an arrest in alveolization should be modified to that of an impairment in alveolarization since evidence shows that short ventilatory times and/or the use of nCPAP allow continued alveolar formation [42]. An area of emerging interest in the field of lung imaging is 3He diffusion MRI. With this technique, alveolar damage was studied in survivors of extreme preterm birth by comparing alveolar dimensions between full-term born and preterm-born school children [43]. Alveolar size at school age was similar in survivors of extreme prematurity and full-term born children. Because extreme preterm birth is associated with deranged alveolar structure in infancy, the most likely explanation for this finding is catch-up alveolarization.

Therefore, prematurity per se may have an impact on lung growth, but neonatal events and treatment, for example, supplemental oxygen or mechanical ventilation, may cause inflammatory responses followed by a repair process. The repair process may be "healing" but may also become chronic in response to continued inflammation, resulting in structural changes in the airways that are referred to as remodeling. These structural changes may result in irreversible narrowing of the airways. Over time, in most children, with or without BPD, pulmonary function improves. Whether this improvement represents repair of damaged lung tissue or growth of new lung tissue, or both, has yet to be determined.

Children and adolescents with severe BPD, however, show evidence of chronic obstructive pulmonary disease. Kotecha et al. systematically reviewed the literature to determine whether the percentage predicted forced expiratory volume during 1 s (%FEV$_1$) is lower in preterm-born subjects, with or without BPD, in comparison to full-term born controls. They found that %FEV$_1$ is decreased in preterm-born survivors, even in individuals who did not develop BPD. For the preterm-born group without BPD, the mean difference %FEV$_1$ in comparison to full-term born controls is −7.2 %, and for the BPD groups, it was −16.2 % to −18.9 %, respectively (according to the definition of BPD) [44].

Inflammation

Former preterm-born children show little evidence of eosinophilic inflammation [45]. Exhaled nitric oxide concentrations are significantly lower in BPD survivors than in asthmatic cases, suggesting that different pathogenetic mechanisms characterize these two chronic obstructive lung diseases [46].

When inflammation plays a role, treatment with inhaled corticosteroids might be effective. A recent systematic review studied whether inhaled bronchodilators and inhaled corticosteroids improve long-term outcomes in neonates with BPD. No meta-analysis was attempted due to the large degree of heterogeneity and quality assessment of the studies included. The conclusion was that although these inhaled therapies seem to have some benefit, very limited data are available suggesting that these treatments at neonatal age improve long-term outcomes of infants with BPD [47].

Kotecha et al. systematically reviewed the evidence for bronchodilator treatment in former preterm-born children and adults. They concluded that the majority of the studies reported short-term effects of a single-dose administration with an improvement in %FEV$_1$ after bronchodilator treatment. There is, however, a paucity of data on the effect of longer term administration of bronchodilators on the lung function of former preterm-born children [48]. The number of studies with inhaled corticosteroids is small in older preterm-born children and these studies show no effect [49]. There is no current evidence to advocate widespread use of bronchodilators or inhaled corticosteroids, even though a component of variable airflow obstruction may be present. Additional evidence for optimal treatment is required [50].

Acute inflammation due to respiratory tract infections, such as respiratory syncytial virus (RSV) infection, could be an important mechanism of recurrent wheeze during the first year of life in preterm-born infants [51]. A connection between viral infections and exaggerated cell death and inflammatory pathways in the developing lung was recently revealed [52].

Structural Changes

In contrast to early lung development, a process exemplified by the branching of the developing airways, the later development of the immature lung remains poorly understood. A key event in late lung development is secondary septation, in which secondary septa arise from primary septa, creating a greater number of alveoli of a smaller size. This phase in lung development dramatically expands the surface area over which gas exchange can take place [52]. Secondary septation, together with architectural changes to the vascular structure of the lung that minimize the distance between inspired air and blood, is the objective of late lung development. When late lung development is disturbed, lung architecture is malformed. Depending on the severity of the architectural malformation, there may be serious consequences in terms of respiratory function, as well as long-term consequences in later life [52]. It is not clear whether early preterm lung injury is associated with structural damage to surrounding lung tissue because it is difficult to obtain histological tissue for study purposes. Nevertheless, a crucial mechanism that secures airway patency and thus adequate maintenance of functional residual capacity (FRC) is airway tethering [53–55]. Tethering is the element that couples lung volume to airway patency. Thus, as lung volumes increase, airway diameter and hence expiratory flows increase. Maturation of the alveolar network improves parenchymal elastance and, as a consequence, airway tethering. Immaturity adds up to the elements constituting the vulnerability of preterm infants [53].

Radiologic studies in older and more severe cases with BPD showed structural changes such as emphysema on high-resolution CT scans [33, 56, 57]. There seems to be an association between the extent of radiological abnormality on high-resolution CT scans and the severity of lung function impairment [33].

Which Risk Factors Are Described for Respiratory Problems in Former Preterm-Born Children?

On the one hand, there are several factors that may cause a preterm birth and that, additionally, are likely to affect fetal lung development and adult outcome. On the other hand, there are several postnatal factors that affect the risk of continuing respiratory problems in a former preterm-born child.

Preterm delivery is the most common cause of abnormal lung development and can itself lead to lifelong sequelae. As described above, compared to full-term born children, children born very preterm (before 32 weeks' gestation) approximately run a three times higher risk of developing asthma and/or wheezing disorders in unadjusted and adjusted analyses [9].

Factors that may result in poor lung development prenatally include inadequate nutrition or specific nutrient deficiencies, maternal alcohol consumption, exposure to tobacco smoke, chorioamnionitis, and intrauterine infection. Postnatal factors include being ventilated with high oxygen concentrations, BPD, respiratory infections, and exposure to environmental pollution [8, 52]. Hypoxia also represents a potent stimulus that has a negative impact on late lung development. The impact of corticosteroids on lung development is complicated, since the positive anti-inflammatory and lung maturation impact of corticosteroids is counterbalanced by growth retardation and other effects on the lung [52].

With regard to the respiratory tract infections, "the chicken or the egg" debate is ongoing. Human RSV is the most common cause of severe lower respiratory tract illnesses in both preterm and full-term newborns and young children, and it is associated with subsequent recurrent wheeze. Observational studies cannot determine whether RSV infection is the cause of recurrent wheeze or the first indication of preexistent pulmonary vulnerability in preterm infants. Several studies showed increased susceptibility of preterm-born children (with and without BPD) to RSV [58]. In the Lollipop study, the rates of hospitalization due to proven RSV infection are higher in both preterm groups than in full terms. No difference in disease severity was observed. Among moderate–late preterms, the rate of RSV hospitalization was higher for lower gestational ages and if the infants had been exposed to passive smoking [59].

Nonrandomized trials in preterm infants (approximately 30 ± 2 weeks' gestational age) suggested that the prevention of lower respiratory tract illness caused by RSV reduces subsequent recurrent wheeze in infants without a family history of atopy, while no effect was found in infants with a family history of atopy [60, 61]. In another study, in otherwise healthy 33–35 weeks' gestational age preterm infants, palivizumab treatment resulted in a significant reduction in wheezing days during the first year of life, even after treatment had stopped. These findings might implicate RSV infection as an important mechanism of recurrent wheeze during the first year of life in such infants [51]. Other risk factors for continuing respiratory problems in moderate to late preterm children were found to be eczema during the first year of life, passive smoking during the first year, higher social class, and a positive family history of asthma [29].

Conclusion

The major respiratory problems for preterm-born infants (with or without BPD) that need hospitalization are respiratory exacerbations caused by infections, particularly viral infections. The most common symptoms in former preterm-born children are cough, wheeze, and/or other asthma-like symptoms. Overall, the risk of former preterm children developing asthma or a wheezing disorder during childhood is almost twice that of full-term infants. As children grow older, the symptoms become milder. Nevertheless, a group of adolescents and adults remains who still present with chronic airway obstruction defined by recurrent episodes of wheezing and decreased lung function tests, that is, decreased forced expiratory volume. The risk of asthma and/or wheezing disorders increases as the degree of prematurity increases. Putative mechanisms for wheeze may include early lung injury or maldevelopment during infancy, respiratory infections during the first year of life, and structural changes of the lung parenchyma. Patients are often labeled asthmatic although the underlying mechanisms are likely to be very different. Characterizing airway diseases in adult survivors of preterm birth in terms of extent and nature of airflow obstruction, pattern of any inflammation, and presence of airway reactivity is very important to prevent over or under treatment.

References

1. Shennan AT, Dunn MS, Ohlsson A, Lennox K, Hoskins EM. Abnormal pulmonary outcomes in premature infants: prediction from oxygen requirement in the neonatal period. Pediatrics. 1988;82(4):527–32.
2. Walsh MC, Yao Q, Gettner P, Hale E, Collins M, Hensman A, et al. Impact of a physiologic definition on bronchopulmonary dysplasia rates. Pediatrics. 2004;114(1098–4275; 5):1305–11.
3. Lawn JE, Blencowe H, Oza S, You D, Lee AC, Waiswa P, et al. Every newborn: progress, priorities, and potential beyond survival. Lancet. 2014;384(9938):189–205.
4. Blencowe H, Cousens S, Oestergaard MZ, Chou D, Moller AB, Narwal R, et al. National, regional, and worldwide estimates of preterm birth rates in the year 2010 with time trends since 1990 for selected countries: a systematic analysis and implications. Lancet. 2012;379(9832):2162–72.
5. Gibson AM, Doyle LW. Respiratory outcomes for the tiniest or most immature infants. Semin Fetal Neonatal Med. 2014;19(2):105–11.
6. Hamilton BE, Martin JA, Osterman MJ, Curtin SC, Matthews TJ. Births: final data for 2014. Natl Vital Stat Rep. 2015;64(12):1–64.
7. Gluckman PD, Hanson MA, Cooper C, Thornburg KL. Effect of in utero and early-life conditions on adult health and disease. N Engl J Med. 2008;359(1):61–73.
8. Stocks J, Hislop A, Sonnappa S. Early lung development: lifelong effect on respiratory health and disease. Lancet Respir Med. 2013;1(9):728–42.
9. Been JV, Lugtenberg MJ, Smets E, van Schayck CP, Kramer BW, Mommers M, et al. Preterm birth and childhood wheezing disorders: a systematic review and meta-analysis. PLoS Med. 2014;11(1):e1001596.
10. Adil E, Rager T, Carr M. Location of airway obstruction in term and preterm infants with laryngomalacia. Am J Otolaryngol. 2012;33(4):437–40.
11. Roksund OD, Clemm H, Heimdal JH, Aukland SM, Sandvik L, Markestad T, et al. Left vocal cord paralysis after extreme preterm birth, a new clinical scenario in adults. Pediatrics. 2010;126(6):e1569–77.
12. Van Marter LJ. Epidemiology of bronchopulmonary dysplasia. Semin Fetal Neonatal Med. 2009;14(6):358–66.
13. Patel RM, Kandefer S, Walsh MC, Bell EF, Carlo WA, Laptook AR, et al. Causes and timing of death in extremely premature infants from 2000 through 2011. N Engl J Med. 2015;372(4):331–40.
14. Northway Jr WH, Rosan RC, Porter DY. Pulmonary disease following respirator therapy of hyaline-membrane disease. Bronchopulmonary dysplasia. N Engl J Med. 1967;276(0028–4793; 7):357–68.
15. Jobe AJ. The new BPD: an arrest of lung development. Pediatr Res. 1999;46(0031–3998; 6):641–3.
16. Bancalari E, Claure N, Sosenko IR. Bronchopulmonary dysplasia: changes in pathogenesis, epidemiology and definition. Semin Neonatol. 2003;8(1):63–71.
17. Northway Jr WH, Moss RB, Carlisle KB, Parker BR, Popp RL, Pitlick PT, et al. Late pulmonary sequelae of bronchopulmonary dysplasia. N Engl J Med. 1990;323(0028–4793; 26):1793–9.

18. Doyle LW, Faber B, Callanan C, Freezer N, Ford GW, Davis NM. Bronchopulmonary dysplasia in very low birth weight subjects and lung function in late adolescence. Pediatrics. 2006;118(1098–4275; 1):108–13.
19. Vrijlandt EJ, Gerritsen J, Boezen HM, Grevink RG, Duiverman EJ. Lung function and exercise capacity in young adults born prematurely. Am J Respir Crit Care Med. 2006;173(8):890–6.
20. Watts JL, Ariagno RL, Brady JP. Chronic pulmonary disease in neonates after artificial ventilation: distribution of ventilation and pulmonary interstitial emphysema. Pediatrics. 1977;60(3):273–81.
21. Hofhuis W, Huysman MW, van der Wiel EC, Holland WP, Hop WC, Brinkhorst G, et al. Worsening of V'maxFRC in infants with chronic lung disease in the first year of life: a more favorable outcome after high-frequency oscillation ventilation. Am J Respir Crit Care Med. 2002;166(12):1539–43.
22. Kinsella JP, Greenough A, Abman SH. Bronchopulmonary dysplasia. Lancet. 2006;367(9520):1421–31.
23. Khemani E, McElhinney DB, Rhein L, Andrade O, Lacro RV, Thomas KC, et al. Pulmonary artery hypertension in formerly premature infants with bronchopulmonary dysplasia: clinical features and outcomes in the surfactant era. Pediatrics. 2007;120(6):1260–9.
24. Lenfant C. Lung biology in health and disease. New York: Marcel Dekker Inc.; 2000.
25. Saigal S, Doyle LW. An overview of mortality and sequelae of preterm birth from infancy to adulthood. Lancet. 2008;371(9608):261–9.
26. Vrijlandt EJ, Boezen HM, Gerritsen J, Stremmelaar EF, Duiverman EJ. Respiratory health in prematurely born preschool children with and without bronchopulmonary dysplasia. J Pediatr. 2007;150(3):256–61.
27. Vrijlandt EJ, Gerritsen J, Boezen HM, Duiverman EJ. Gender differences in respiratory symptoms in 19-year-old adults born preterm. Respir Res. 2005;6:117.
28. Kugelman A, Colin AA. Late preterm infants: near term but still in a critical developmental time period. Pediatrics. 2013;132(4):741–51.
29. Vrijlandt EJ, Kerstjens JM, Duiverman EJ, Bos AF, Reijneveld SA. Moderately preterm children have more respiratory problems during their first 5 years of life than children born full term. Am J Respir Crit Care Med. 2013;187(11):1234–40.
30. Abe K, Shapiro-Mendoza CK, Hall LR, Satten GA. Late preterm birth and risk of developing asthma. J Pediatr. 2010;157(1):74–8.
31. Voge GA, Katusic SK, Qin R, Juhn YJ. Risk of asthma in late preterm infants: a propensity score approach. J Allergy Clin Immunol Pract. 2015;3(6):905–10.
32. Fawke J, Lum S, Kirkby J, Hennessy E, Marlow N, Rowell V, et al. Lung function and respiratory symptoms at 11 years in children born extremely preterm: the EPICure study. Am J Respir Crit Care Med. 2010;182(2):237–45.
33. Wong PM, Lees AN, Louw J, Lee FY, French N, Gain K, et al. Emphysema in young adult survivors of moderate-to-severe bronchopulmonary dysplasia. Eur Respir J. 2008;32(1399–3003; 2):321–8.
34. Narang I. Review series: What goes around, comes around: childhood influences on later lung health? Long-term follow-up of infants with lung disease of prematurity. Chron Respir Dis. 2010;7(4):259–69.
35. Bader D, Ramos AD, Lew CD, Platzker AC, Stabile MW, Keens TG. Childhood sequelae of infant lung disease: exercise and pulmonary function abnormalities after bronchopulmonary dysplasia. J Pediatr. 1987;110(0022–3476; 5):693–9.
36. Smith VC, Zupancic JA, McCormick MC, Croen LA, Greene J, Escobar GJ, et al. Trends in severe bronchopulmonary dysplasia rates between 1994 and 2002. J Pediatr. 2005;146(4):469–73.
37. Fanta CH. Asthma. N Engl J Med. 2009;360(10):1002–14.
38. Quanjer PH, Stanojevic S, Cole TJ, Baur X, Hall GL, Culver BH, et al. Multi-ethnic reference values for spirometry for the 3-95-yr age range: the global lung function 2012 equations. Eur Respir J. 2012;40(6):1324–43.

39. Kallapur SG, Ikegami M. Physiological consequences of intrauterine insults. Paediatr Respir Rev. 2006;7(2):110–6.
40. Sonnenschein-van der Voort AM, Jaddoe VW, Raat H, Moll HA, Hofman A, de Jongste JC, et al. Fetal and infant growth and asthma symptoms in preschool children: the Generation R Study. Am J Respir Crit Care Med. 2012;185(7):731–7.
41. Vollsaeter M, Roksund OD, Eide GE, Markestad T, Halvorsen T. Lung function after preterm birth: development from mid-childhood to adulthood. Thorax. 2013;68(8):767–76.
42. Coalson JJ. Pathology of bronchopulmonary dysplasia. Semin Perinatol. 2006;30(0146–0005; 4):179–84.
43. Narayanan M, Beardsmore CS, Owers-Bradley J, Dogaru CM, Mada M, Ball I, et al. Catch-up alveolarization in ex-preterm children: evidence from (3)He magnetic resonance. Am J Respir Crit Care Med. 2013;187(10):1104–9.
44. Kotecha SJ, Edwards MO, Watkins WJ, Henderson AJ, Paranjothy S, Dunstan FD, et al. Effect of preterm birth on later FEV1: a systematic review and meta-analysis. Thorax. 2013;68(8):760–6.
45. Baraldi E, Bonetto G, Zacchello F, Filippone M. Low exhaled nitric oxide in school-age children with bronchopulmonary dysplasia and airflow limitation. Am J Respir Crit Care Med. 2005;171(1):68–72.
46. Carraro S, Piacentini G, Lusiani M, Uyan ZS, Filippone M, Schiavon M, et al. Exhaled air temperature in children with bronchopulmonary dysplasia. Pediatr Pulmonol. 2010;45(12):1240–5.
47. Clouse BJ, Jadcherla SR, Slaughter JL. Systematic review of inhaled bronchodilator and corticosteroid therapies in infants with bronchopulmonary dysplasia: implications and future directions. PLoS One. 2016;11(2):e0148188.
48. Kotecha SJ, Edwards MO, Watkins WJ, Lowe J, Henderson AJ, Kotecha S. Effect of bronchodilators on forced expiratory volume in 1 s in preterm-born participants aged 5 and over: a systematic review. Neonatology. 2015;107(3):231–40.
49. Chan KN, Silverman M. Increased airway responsiveness in children of low birth weight at school age: effect of topical corticosteroids. Arch Dis Child. 1993;69(1468–2044; 1):120–4.
50. Bolton CE, Bush A, Hurst JR, Kotecha S, McGarvey L. Republished: lung consequences in adults born prematurely. Postgrad Med J. 2015;91(1082):712–8.
51. Blanken MO, Rovers MM, Molenaar JM, Winkler-Seinstra PL, Meijer A, Kimpen JL, et al. Respiratory syncytial virus and recurrent wheeze in healthy preterm infants. N Engl J Med. 2013;368(19):1791–9.
52. Madurga A, Mizikova I, Ruiz-Camp J, Morty RE. Recent advances in late lung development and the pathogenesis of bronchopulmonary dysplasia. Am J Physiol Lung Cell Mol Physiol. 2013;305(12):L893–905.
53. Colin AA, McEvoy C, Castile RG. Respiratory morbidity and lung function in preterm infants of 32 to 36 weeks' gestational age. Pediatrics. 2010;126(1):115–28.
54. Henschen M, Stocks J, Brookes I, Frey U. New aspects of airway mechanics in pre-term infants. Eur Respir J. 2006;27(5):913–20.
55. Plopper CG, Nishio SJ, Schelegle ES. Tethering tracheobronchial airways within the lungs. Am J Respir Crit Care Med. 2003;167(1):2–3.
56. Wong P, Murray C, Louw J, French N, Chambers D. Adult bronchopulmonary dysplasia: computed tomography pulmonary findings. J Med Imaging Radiat Oncol. 2011;55(4):373–8.
57. Aquino SL, Schechter MS, Chiles C, Ablin DS, Chipps B, Webb WR. High-resolution inspiratory and expiratory CT in older children and adults with bronchopulmonary dysplasia. AJR Am J Roentgenol. 1999;173(4):963–7.
58. Boyce TG, Mellen BG, Mitchel Jr EF, Wright PF, Griffin MR. Rates of hospitalization for respiratory syncytial virus infection among children in medicaid. J Pediatr. 2000;137(6):865–70.

59. Gijtenbeek RG, Kerstjens JM, Reijneveld SA, Duiverman EJ, Bos AF, Vrijlandt EJ. RSV infection among children born moderately preterm in a community-based cohort. Eur J Pediatr. 2015;174(4):435–42.
60. Simoes EA, Groothuis JR, Carbonell-Estrany X, Rieger CH, Mitchell I, Fredrick LM, et al. Palivizumab prophylaxis, respiratory syncytial virus, and subsequent recurrent wheezing. J Pediatr. 2007;151(1):34–42. 42.e1.
61. Simoes EA, Carbonell-Estrany X, Rieger CH, Mitchell I, Fredrick L, Groothuis JR, et al. The effect of respiratory syncytial virus on subsequent recurrent wheezing in atopic and nonatopic children. J Allergy Clin Immunol. 2010;126(2):256–62.

Why Do Former Preterm Infants Wheeze? Clues from the Laboratory

Richard J. Martin and Thomas M. Raffay

Introduction

There is now considerable epidemiologic evidence that preterm infants, especially those of very low birth weight, are at heightened risk of later airway hyperreactivity [1–3]. This is clearly aggravated by the interventions that predispose these infants to developing bronchopulmonary dysplasia (BPD). Unfortunately, the biologic basis for this problem is less well understood and lagging behind the clinical data [4]. For example, how much is attributable to hyperoxic exposure, barotrauma to an immature airway, or the prenatal and postnatal proinflammatory exposure of preterm lungs? It is, therefore, important to gain greater understanding of the normal and abnormal changes that occur, not only in airway smooth muscle but also surrounding elements such as epithelium, alveolar structures, and neural elements that may modulate airway reactivity in early postnatal life [5].

Maturational Changes in Airway Reactivity

During early development, airway smooth muscle differentiates from the mesenchyme of the primordial lung and envelops the emerging bronchial tree. Airway smooth muscle at this early stage provides phasic rhythmic contractility that is thought to propel lung fluid distally and enhance lung development. Neural structures emerge in parallel to airway muscle, and their functional roles are rapidly

R.J. Martin, MD (✉) • T.M. Raffay
Case Western Reserve University School of Medicine, Cleveland, OH, USA

Rainbow Babies & Children's Hospital, Cleveland, OH, USA
e-mail: rxm6@case.edu

© Springer International Publishing AG 2017
A.M. Hibbs, M. S. Muhlebach (eds.), *Respiratory Outcomes in Preterm Infants*,
Respiratory Medicine, DOI 10.1007/978-3-319-48835-6_3

integrated such that during postnatal life tonic, rather than phasic, contractile, and relaxant functions dominate. Immunohistochemical studies of developing human and porcine fetal airways have revealed the development of an airway smooth muscle layer by the end of the human embryonic period extending from the trachea to terminal lung sacs, as well as an extensive nerve plexus comprising nerve trunks and ganglia investing the airways and innervating smooth muscle. This layer of airway smooth muscle is functional in the first trimester as evidenced by the phasic spontaneous narrowing and relaxation of airways with back-and-forth movement of lung fluid that might stimulate lung growth by providing positive intraluminal pressure. These data are consistent with human autopsy findings that airway smooth muscle is present at 23 weeks' gestation at all levels of the conducting airways and increased in amount during the earliest signs of developing chronic lung disease as early as 10 days of life [6].

The effect of postnatal maturation on airway contractile responses is somewhat controversial. Physiologic studies using isolated tracheal smooth muscle strips from several species have demonstrated that under normal maturational conditions, there is decreased cholinergic responsiveness in early postnatal life [7, 8]. These in vitro studies are complicated by the need to carefully normalize the airway contractile response for smooth muscle mass and myosin content [9]. Maturational changes in airway reactivity may also be influenced by immature lung parenchymal structures and a relatively compliant airway which may contribute to altered airway narrowing in immature animal models as discussed later [10, 11]. Nonetheless, the weight of evidence appears to point to an anatomically intact airway smooth muscle layer superimposed on highly compliant airway structures in early postnatal life.

Cholinergic Efferent Output

At any given age, neural control of airway function involves integrated networks along the neural axis that funnel information to tracheobronchopulmonary effector units via airway-related vagal preganglionic neurons (AVPNs) in the medulla oblongata (Fig. 1). The AVPNs are the final common pathway from the brain to the airways. The AVPNs innervating airways, from the extrathoracic trachea to the most distal bronchiole, arise mainly within the brain stem from the rostral nucleus ambiguus (Rna) and to a lesser degree from the rostral portion of the dorsal motor nucleus of the vagus (DMV). These cholinergic cells in the brainstem transmit signals to intrinsic tracheobronchial ganglia via the vagus nerve and give rise to postganglionic fibers distributed around airway smooth muscle cells, submucosal glands, and arterial blood vessels. In the postnatal period, neuronal innervation is already well developed and choline acetyltransferase, a specific marker for cholinergic neurons that synthesizes acetylcholine, appears in vagal preganglionic neurons,

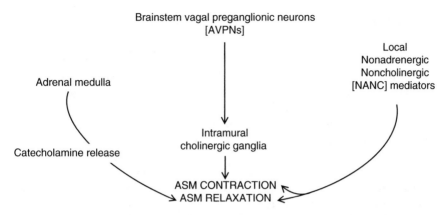

Fig. 1 Neural and nonneural pathways that contribute to airway reactivity. *AVPNs* airway-related vagal preganglionic neurons, *ASM* airway smooth muscle

postganglionic neurons, and postganglionic fibers. Postnatally, cholinergic innervation is the principal tonic input to airway smooth muscle bundles and may serve to protect the compliant, immature airways from collapsing during expiration-induced compressive narrowing.

Muscarinic receptors mediate the responsiveness of airway smooth muscle to acetylcholine during early development and adult life. Studies in the developing airways and porcine lung from birth to adulthood reveal maturational changes in muscarinic receptor subtypes (M_1, M_2, M_3) that may explain pharmacologic changes during development [12]. These muscarinic receptor subtypes, coupled to the family of G proteins, mediate airway contractile responses and their modulation, although there are considerable interspecies differences in their roles. M_1 receptors are largely present on neuronal tissue and ganglia and enhance contractile response to vagal stimulation in newborn animals [7, 13]. M_2 receptors are located on prejunctional postganglionic cholinergic fibers in airway smooth muscle in some species and exhibit an autoinhibitory action whereby the quantal release of Ach in response to nerve stimulation is reduced due to feedback inhibition. M_3 receptors are present on smooth muscle and mucus glands and airway epithelial cells, where they initiate the events leading to smooth muscle contraction, airway narrowing, and mucus secretion. In the newborn, the density of M_3 receptors has been reported to be similar to that in the adult; however, they do not appear to be tightly coupled to G-protein signal transduction mechanisms that lead to smooth muscle contraction [7]. Among the many unanswered questions in the newborn are the extent of receptor subtype differentiation in human neonates, investigation of G-protein signal transduction, the role of M_2 autoinhibitory receptors in modulating airway tone, and the possible effect of inflammatory lung injury on muscarinic receptor regulation and its pharmacologic manipulation.

Sympathetic Control of the Lower Airways

Extrinsic sympathetic innervation of airway smooth muscle is highly species specific, and in airway smooth muscle in humans, direct sympathetic innervation appears to be lacking. Nevertheless, circulating catecholamines activate airway adrenoreceptors to exert specific actions that affect smooth muscle contractile function. Beta$_2$-adrenergic responses in airway smooth muscle are composed of two inhibitory actions: first, relaxation of airway smooth muscle mediated by airway beta$_2$-receptors that are coupled to the stimulatory G-protein (Gs) and adenylate cyclase and second, inhibition of ACh release from postganglionic vagal axons through prejunctional alpha$_2$-adrenergic and beta$_1$ receptors in some species. Activation of beta-adrenergic receptors is the pharmacologic basis for neonatal bronchodilator therapy. Maturational studies have demonstrated that beta-adrenergic receptors in lung tissue increase with advancing gestation and subsequent postnatal development, but this may be more important for their role in surfactant synthesis and release. The airway relaxant response to beta-adrenoreceptor stimulation has been reported to decrease with advancing maturation, and several mechanisms including greater muscarinic antagonism of beta-receptor responses and attenuated expression of M$_2$ muscarinic receptors have been proposed [14]. A potential role for adrenergic receptors in the control of airway smooth muscle in newborn infants with bronchopulmonary dysplasia is supported by observations in preterm infants with chronic lung disease in whom ophthalmic application of the alpha$_1$-adrenergic agonist phenylephrine resulted in an increase in total pulmonary resistance and a decrease in compliance [15]. The deterioration in lung mechanics was attributed to alpha$_1$-receptor-mediated activation of airway smooth muscle contraction.

Nonadrenergic Noncholinergic Control of the Lower Airways

Rather than representing a separate pathway for modulation of airway caliber, the nonadrenergic noncholinergic (NANC) system comprises both inhibitory and excitatory components modulated by several neurotransmitters located in intrinsic ganglia and their fibers. Reference to noncholinergic (i.e., NANC) innervations reflects the neurotransmitters known *not* to mediate cholinergic or adrenergic effects. The system is highly species-specific but has been identified in human airways. The NANC inhibitory component of vagal innervations is demonstrated in vivo and in vitro by measuring the response to vagal stimulation or to electrical field stimulation, after muscarinic and beta-adrenergic effects on airway smooth muscle are blocked by atropine and propranolol; then airway tone is elevated by an infusion of contractile agonist (e.g., serotonin or histamine). Under these conditions, stimulation of vagal preganglionic axons causes bronchodilation. Vasoactive   intestinal   peptide   was   initially   proposed   as   the   primary neurotransmitter of the NANC system. Subsequently, nitric oxide was also shown to act as a NANC neurotransmitter, suggesting involvement of multiple substances and molecules in airway smooth muscle relaxation with considerable interspecies variation [16].

Limited information is available about the ontogeny of this system in the airways. Activation of vagal preganglionic axons results in a NANC-mediated bronchodilation in newborn feline airways, a response that is eliminated by ganglionic blockade with hexamethonium, confirming the efferent nature of the response [17]. Comparison with the mature response is confounded by the necessity of infusing an agonist to measure a response, and the possibility that neonatal and adult airways may possess different sensitivities to the contractile agonist. NANC inhibitory innervation also appears to be functional in young guinea pigs and rat pups. In some species, NANC inhibitory responses undergo significant developmental changes; for example, NANC relaxation responses are not present in rabbits until 2 weeks of age [18]. Interestingly, allergen sensitization significantly reduced the NANC response at 2, 4, and 12 weeks of age [18], suggesting that host or environmental factors may alter the maturation of the inhibitory NANC system and predispose to airway reactivity. The NANC inhibitory system has not been adequately explored in human neonatal airways.

NANC excitatory mechanisms also play a role in modulating airway smooth muscle. Within this system, the tachykinin peptides, such as substance P and neurokinin A, have undergone some study during early postnatal development. These tachykinins are synthesized in sensory neurons and transported to sensory nerve endings from which they are released and have the ability to elicit airway contractile responses by several interrelated mechanisms. Tachykinin release from afferent C-fiber nerve endings in the airway may directly or reflexly elicit smooth muscle contraction, modulate cholinergic responses through muscarinic receptors, and induce histamine release from mast cells. In young rabbits, substance P-induced modulation of ACh release increases with advancing postnatal age [19], and in newborn piglets, exogenously administered substance P elicits weak contractile responses of tracheal smooth muscle when compared with older animals [20].

There is some debate about whether increased expression of substance P or other neuropeptides contributes to lung or airway pathophysiology. In mature animal models, chronic exposure to irritant gas increases substance P content; however, it is controversial whether this serves to aggravate airway hyperactivity or serves a protective role for airway and lung structures. Furthermore, in addition to elicit airway smooth muscle constriction, substance P may induce relaxation of preconstricted neonatal tracheal tissue by release of NO and relaxant prostaglandins [21]. Newborn and 3-week-old rats exposed to hyperoxia exhibit increased tachykinin precursor expression, increased substance P content in the lung, and increased cholinergic responsiveness, as discussed later, although the relationship of the latter to the increased substance P content is not clear [22]. Ongoing developmental studies should focus on these neuropeptide-mediated signaling pathways that modulate airway smooth muscle contractile and relaxant responses in health and disease.

Contributors to Abnormal Airway Function

Hyperoxic Exposure

The airways of preterm infants are frequently exposed to increased supplemental oxygen. This is a likely predisposing factor to the development of airway injury (Fig. 2). In newborn animal models, most notably the guinea pig and rat pup, hyperoxic exposure has been associated with development of airway hyperreactivity [22–24]. Although hyperoxic exposure may increase smooth muscle area, this effect is variable and does not, of itself, explain the development of hyperoxia-induced airway hyperresponsiveness [25].

Many factors may contribute to the increased airway reactivity that is seen after neonatal hyperoxic exposure. Therefore, studies have focused on neonatal rodent models exposed to only moderate (e.g., 40–60 %) hyperoxic exposure as this more closely simulates the clinical condition. Recent data demonstrate that 40 % oxygen exposure elicited a greater increase in airway reactivity than 70 % oxygen exposure, associated with greater airway smooth muscle thickness [26]. This might be attributed to a dominant proliferative effect of 40 % oxygen on airway smooth muscle versus a predominantly apoptotic effect at the higher oxygen level [27, 28]. An intriguing recent observation is that in a neonatal mouse model, the increase in airway reactivity after 40 % oxygen exposure during the first week was delayed until the pups were 3 weeks old [29]. These studies employed an in vitro living lung slice preparation. Alveolar morphology was comparably diminished at 1 and 3 weeks, suggesting a selective and delayed effect of modest hyperoxic exposure on the trajectory of airway smooth muscle structure or function. These findings are consistent with the clinical observation that bronchodilator therapy is of limited use in the

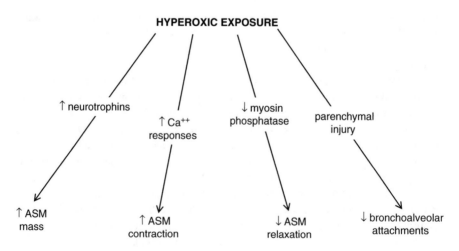

Fig. 2 Proposed mechanisms whereby neonatal hyperoxic exposure predisposes to wheezing disorders in former preterm infants. *ASM* airway smooth muscle

neonatal intensive care unit (NICU) at a time when hyperoxia-induced airway smooth proliferation has not been achieved [30]. It is also possible that the benefits of bronchodilator therapy may not be sustained in the neonatal period as evident in the hyperoxia-exposed neonatal mouse model. In a model of chronic lung disease, hyperoxia-exposed newborn mice displayed decreased lung $beta_2$-adrenergic receptor expression and were at risk for further down regulation with repeated agonist stimulation, resulting in increased airway hypersensitivity and attenuation of rescue bronchodilation [31].

Lung parenchymal injury is a well-recognized complication of neonatal intensive care and is characterized by the development of enlarged, simplified alveolar structures. This may result in decreased tethering of intraparenchymal airways; the accompanying decrease in airway lumen would increase baseline airway resistance [11]. A related observation is that lung parenchymal injury elicited by hyperoxic exposure is associated with fewer bronchiolar-alveolar attachments in a rodent model of neonatal lung injury [32]. Smaller diameter, untethered airways may well contribute to the wheezing disorders former preterm infants experience; however, altered airway smooth muscle properties are likely contributors.

Epithelial injury with loss of airway relaxant factors may also contribute to the hyperoxia-induced increase in airway contractile responses. This is supported by data from tracheal strips in preterm sheep, in which epithelium removal was associated with greater cholinergic responsiveness [33]. A similar phenomenon is observed in rat pups in which the response of lung resistance induced by vagal stimulation was increased after nonspecific blockade of NOS in normoxic animals. However, after hyperoxic exposure, NOS blockade no longer affected the contractile response induced by vagal stimulation [34]. These findings indicate that NO, released by stimulation of vagal preganglionic fibers, modulates bronchopulmonary contractile responses to endogenously released ACh in rat pups. This effect appears to be lost after prolonged hyperoxic exposure and may contribute to airway hyperreactivity under these conditions. Impairment of the prostaglandin/cyclic adenosine monophosphate (cAMP) signaling pathway may also contribute to hyperoxia-induced airway hyperreactivity [35]. These findings are somewhat analogous to observations made in young ferrets infected with human respiratory syncytial virus (RSV) in which nonadrenergic noncholinergic inhibitory responses of tracheal smooth muscle were significantly decreased for a prolonged period [36]. Of course, it is important to recognize that these animal data may not translate to the human condition.

The neurotrophins belong to a protein family essential for vertebrate nervous system development. They are also expressed in epithelial smooth muscle and immune components of the lung [37]. The neurotrophin family includes brain-derived neurotrophic factor (BDNF), nerve growth factor (NGF), neurotrophins 3, and neurotrophin 4. They share common structural features and act through their corresponding high-affinity tyrosine kinase (Trk) receptor subtypes. The rapid excitatory activity of BDNF is via activation of the TrkB receptor. BDNF appears to stabilize excitatory (e.g., cholinergic) postsynaptic receptors and/or enhance quantal excitatory neurotransmitter release probably via postsynaptic calcium signaling. During development, regulation of the lower airway appears to be influenced by neurotrophins. Data show the presence of neurotrophins and their corresponding receptor on airway smooth muscle cells in developing rat pups and upregulation of the BDNF system after hyperoxic exposure [38, 39]. Consistent with these findings, neurotrophins are overexpressed in the lower airways of RSV-infected human infants known to be at great risk for increased airway reactivity [40].

Airway smooth muscle contraction is elicited when phosphorylation of the 20-kDa regulatory light chain of myosin (MLC_{20}) allows crossbridge formation of actin and myosin. This process of phosphorylation is regulated by calcium/calmodulin-dependent myosin light chain kinase (MLCK) isoforms. Conversely, MLC_{20} dephosphorylation by myosin phosphatase (MYPT) leads to relaxation. Studies in rat pups have demonstrated that hyperoxic exposure inhibited MYPT, and the resultant prolongation of MLC_{20} phosphorylation may have contributed to hyperoxia-induced enhanced airway contractility [41]. Both plasma membrane calcium influx mechanisms, as well as intracellular calcium release and reuptake, are involved in the contractile responses of airway smooth muscle to agonist. Even in the first trimester, immature airway smooth muscle contains many of the calcium-regulating mechanisms that are present in adult tissue, contributing to spontaneous and acetylcholine-induced calcium oscillations [42]. However, there is currently limited information on which of the calcium regulatory mechanisms are involved in mediating bronchoconstriction in the normal and injured developing airway. In this regard, in human fetal airway smooth muscle, many calcium influx pathways appear to be present, as are intracellular calcium release pathways. However, compared to adult airway smooth muscle, calcium responses to agonist appear to be smaller and slower in developing fetal airway smooth muscle cells, likely reflecting differences in the kinetics of regulatory mechanisms [28]. Importantly, exposure of fetal airway smooth muscle cells to even moderate levels of hyperoxia causes enhanced calcium responses to agonist, and this may contribute to the increased airway reactivity observed in vivo following hyperoxia.

Pressure Effects

The high deformability or compliance of the trachea in the preterm period appears to be a consequence of decreased airway smooth muscle contractility and diminished cartilaginous support. The obvious result is that tracheas, and possibly lower airways, are vulnerable to deformation during positive pressure ventilation. Greater understanding of the detrimental effects of positive pressure ventilation at high inflating pressures has decreased the risk of deformation injury to the immature airway by limiting the use of excessive ventilatory pressures. Data in rat pups indicate that enhancement of airway reactivity occurs even after short-term mechanical ventilation [43]. Abnormal mechanical stress and its effect on smooth muscle contractility serve as a useful model for characterizing one aspect of neonatal lung and airway injury [44]. Cultured airway smooth muscle cells exposed to such stress eliminate the confounding effects of deformational strain on surrounding tissues.

Such studies have demonstrated strain-induced increases in cell myosin light-chain kinase (MLCK) accompanied by increased phosphorylation of the myosin light chain, all key steps in the smooth muscle contractile response [45].

In recent years, there has been a shift in NICU practice from the use of intubation and mechanical ventilation toward less invasive treatments, such as continuous positive airway pressure (CPAP), largely because of the baro- or volutrauma imposed on the lung by the former mode of respiratory support. Indeed, CPAP has the potential to mitigate the adverse pathophysiological effects on lung development that would otherwise be observed with mechanical ventilation. Most recently, animal studies have investigated the effects of neonatal CPAP on airway reactivity. This has required development of a custom-made mask to fit snugly around the head of newborn mice for CPAP (or control) delivery over several hours for the first postnatal week. Delivery of CPAP at 6 cm H_2O resulted in an increase in airway reactivity in living lung slice preparations obtained at day 21. Airway hyperreactivity after CPAP was largely limited to smaller airways. This was associated with only minimal evidence of lung parenchymal injury as assessed by alveolar morphology [46]. Interestingly, this increase in airway reactivity was less evident when CPAP was combined with hyperoxic exposure and tested in neonatal mice under in vivo conditions [47]. From these initial data, it is tempting to speculate that long-term CPAP exposure of smaller immature airways may predispose to later airway hyperreactivity. In fact, this is common practice in the NICU for infants with impaired respiratory drive and relatively uninjured lungs. Appropriate mechanistic studies are clearly needed.

Infectious/Inflammatory Contribution

Chorioamnionitis predisposes to both preterm birth and later wheezing disorders. A logical approach to understanding underlying mechanisms is to expose an immature animal model to antenatal lipopolysaccharide (LPS). This has been shown to increase airway reactivity at postnatal day 21, including a thickened airway smooth muscle layer [48]. Of interest is the observation that postnatal caffeine reverses this LPS-induced increase in airway reactivity [49].

These findings somewhat parallel the response of the immature lung and airway to hyperoxic exposure. Prior studies in neonatal rodents have combined antenatal inflammation with postnatal hyperoxia and have suggested a synergistic effect of these interventions on airway resistance, although the focus was more on lung parenchyma than airway function [50, 51]. The most recent data indicate that the combination of antenatal LPS and postnatal hyperoxia (50 % O_2 for 7 days) does not have a synergistic effect in aggravating later airway structure or function [52]. While both insults appear to upregulate growth factors such as connective tissue growth factor and transforming growth factor beta, the absence of a synergistic effect clearly requires further mechanistic study. Somewhat conflicting results may also be explained by the variable techniques for inducing antenatal chorioamnionitis and the vastly different concentrations of supplemental oxygen and their duration that have been employed. Finally, it is widely known that preterm infants are predisposed to wheezing in response to postnatal infection with a variety of viral pathogens. Neonatal mice exposed to postnatal hyperoxia have subsequently been infected with influenza A virus; this model has demonstrated a reprogramming of key immunoregulatory pathways that may aggravate later airway function [53]. Greater mechanistic understanding may lead to protective strategies during infancy for vulnerable preterm infants.

Conclusion/Speculation

While there is still much to be learned about the contributors to normal and abnormal maturations of airway function, many lessons have been learned from a host of laboratory studies. In infants with BPD, it is likely that parenchymal lung injury in the form of alveolar simplification may contribute to poorly tethered airways and increased baseline resistance. In such infants, it is, however, highly likely that airway smooth muscle hypertrophy is an important contributor. From a functional standpoint, neural and epithelial elements may contribute to both enhanced contractile and decreased relaxant regulation of airway smooth muscle. What about the preterm infant who is predisposed to later wheezing, even though neonatal lung injury is minimal or modest, and none of the criteria for BPD are met? Neonatal rodent data would suggest that exposure to low supplemental oxygen and/or the pressure effects of CPAP predispose to later airway reactivity. Such studies need to address mechanistic pathways that, hopefully, can be translated to pathophysiology and therapy for the future respiratory well-being of former preterm infants.

References

1. Been JV, Lugtenberg MJ, Smets E, van Schayck CP, Kramer BW, Mommers M, et al. Preterm birth and childhood wheezing disorders: a systematic review and meta-analysis. PLoS Med. 2014;11(1):e1001596.
2. Fawke J, Lum S, Kirkby J, Hennessy E, Marlow N, Rowell V, et al. Lung function and respiratory symptoms at 11 years in children born extremely preterm: the EPICure study. Am J Respir Crit Care Med. 2010;182(2):237–45.
3. Hack M, Schluchter M, Andreias L, Margevicius S, Taylor HG, Drotar D, et al. Change in prevalence of chronic conditions between childhood and adolescence among extremely low-birth-weight children. JAMA. 2011;306(4):394–401.
4. Reyburn B, Martin RJ, Prakash YS, MacFarlane PM. Mechanisms of injury to the preterm lung and airway: Implications for long-term pulmonary outcome. Neonatology. 2012;101:345–52.
5. Martin RJ, Raffay TM, Faksh A, Prakash YS. Regulation of lower airway function. In: Polin RA, Abman S, Benitz W, Rowitch D, editors. Fetal & neonatal physiology. 5th ed. Philadelphia: Elsevier; 2016.

6. Sward-Comunelli SL, Mabry SM, Truog WE, Thibeault DW. Airway muscle in preterm infants: changes during development. J Pediatr. 1997;130:570–6.
7. Haxhiu-Poskurica B, Ernsberger P, Haxhiu M, Miller M, Cattarossi L, Martin RJ. Development of cholinergic innervation and muscarinic receptor subtypes in piglet trachea. Am J Phys. 1993;264:L606–14.
8. Panitch HB, Allen JL, Ryan JP, Wolfson MR, Shaffer TH. A comparison of preterm and adult airway smooth muscle mechanics. J Appl Physiol. 1989;66:1760–5.
9. Murphy TM, Mitchell RW, Halayko A, Roach J, Roy L, Kelly EA, et al. Effect of maturational changes in myosin content and morphometry on airway smooth muscle contraction. Am J Physiol Lung Cell Mol Physiol. 1991;260:L471–80.
10. Ramchandani R, Shen X, Elmsley CL, Ambrosius WT, Gunst SJ, Tepper RS. Differences in airway structure in immature and mature rabbits. J Appl Physiol. 2000;89:1310–6.
11. Colin AA, McEvoy C, Castile RG. Respiratory morbidity and lung function in preterm infants of 32 to 36 weeks' gestational age. Pediatrics. 2010;126:115–28.
12. Hislop AA, Mak JC, Reader JA, Barnes PJ, Haworth SG. Muscarinic receptor subtypes in the porcine lung during postnatal development. Eur J Pharmacol. 1998;359:211–21.
13. Fisher JT, Brundage KL, Anderson JW. Cardiopulmonary actions of muscarinic receptor subtypes in the newborn dog. Can J Physiol Pharmacol. 1996;74:603–13.
14. Fayon M, de la Roque ED, Berger P, Begueret H, Ousova O, Molimard M, et al. Increased relaxation of immature airways to β₂-adrenoceptor agonists is related to attenuated expression of postjunctional smooth muscle muscarinic M₂ receptors. J Appl Physiol. 2005;98:1526–33.
15. Mirmanesh SJ, Abbasi S, Bhutani VK. Alpha-adrenergic bronchoprovocation in neonates with bronchopulmonary dysplasia. J Pediatr. 1992;121:622–5.
16. Said SI, Rattan S. The multiple mediators of neurogenic smooth muscle relaxation. Trends Endocrinol Metab. 2004;15:189–91. Review.
17. Waldron MA, Connelly BJ, Fisher JT. Nonadrenergic inhibitory innervation to the airways of the newborn cat. J Appl Physiol. 1989;66:1999–2000.
18. Colasurdo GN, Loader JE, Graves JP, Larsen GL. Maturation of nonadrenergic noncholinergic inhibitory system in normal and allergen-sensitized rabbits. Am J Physiol Lung Cell Mol Physiol. 1994;267:L739–44.
19. Tanaka DT, Grunstein MM. Maturation of neuromodulatory effect of substance P in rabbit airways. J Clin Invest. 1990;83:345–50.
20. Haxhiu-Poskurica B, Haxhiu MA, Kumar GK, Miller MJ, Martin RJ. Tracheal smooth muscle responses to substance P and neurokinin A in the piglet. J Appl Physiol. 1992;72:1090–5.
21. Mhanna MJ, Dreshaj IA, Haxhiu MA, Martin RJ. Mechanism for substance P-induced relaxation of precontracted airway smooth muscle during development. Am J Physiol Lung Cell Mol Physiol. 1999;276:L51–6.
22. Agani FH, Kuo NT, Chang CH, Dreshaj IA, Farver CF, Krause JE, et al. Effect of hyperoxia on substance P expression and airway reactivity in the developing lung. Am J Physiol Lung Cell Mol Physiol. 1997;273(17):40–5.
23. Uyehara CFT, Pichoff BE, Sim HH, Uemura HS, Nakamura KT. Hyperoxic exposure enhances airway reactivity of newborn guinea pigs. J Appl Physiol. 1993;74:2649–54.
24. Belik J, Jankov RP, Pan J, Tanswell AK. Chronic O₂ exposure enhances vascular and airway smooth muscle contraction in the newborn but not adult rat. J Appl Physiol. 2003;94:2303–12.
25. Hershenson MB, Wylam ME, Punjabi N, Umans JG, Schumacker PT, Mitchell RW, et al. Exposure of immature rats to hyperoxia increases tracheal smooth muscle stress generation in vitro. J Appl Physiol. 1994;76:743–9.
26. Wang H, Jafri A, Martin RJ, Nnanabu J, Farver C, Prakash YS, et al. Severity of neonatal hyperoxia determines structural and functional changes in developing mouse airway. Am J Physiol Lung Cell Mol Physiol. 2014;307:L295–301.

27. Yi M, Masood A, Ziino A, Johnson BH, Belcastro R, Li J, et al. Inhibition of apoptosis by 60 % oxygen: a novel pathway contributing to lung injury in neonatal rats. Am J Physiol Lung Cell Mol Physiol. 2011;300:L319–29.
28. Hartman WR, Smelter DF, Sathish V, Karass M, Kim S, Aravamudan B, et al. Oxygen dose responsiveness of human fetal airway smooth muscle cells. Am J Physiol Lung Cell Mol Physiol. 2012;303:L711–9.
29. Onugha H, MacFarlane PM, Mayer CA, Abrah A, Jafri A, Martin RJ. Airway hyperreactivity is delayed after mild neonatal hyperoxic exposure. Neonatology. 2015;108:65–72.
30. Ng G, da Silva O, Ohlsson A. Bronchodilators for the prevention and treatment of chronic lung disease in preterm infants. Cochrane Database Syst Rev. 2012;6:CD003214. doi:10.1002/14651858.CD003214.pub2.
31. Raffay T, Kc P, Reynolds J, Di Fiore J, MacFarlane P, Martin RJ. Repeated β_2-adrenergic receptor agonist therapy attenuates the response to rescue bronchodilation in a hyperoxic newborn mouse model. Neonatology. 2014;106:126–32.
32. O'Reilly M, Harding R, Sozo F. Altered small airways in aged mice following neonatal exposure to hyperoxic gas. Neonatology. 2014;105(1):39–45.
33. Panitch HB, Wolfson MR, Shaffer TH. Epithelial modulation of preterm airway smooth muscle contraction. J Appl Physiol. 1993;74:1437–43.
34. Iben SC, Dreshaj IA, Farver CF, Haxhiu MA, Martin RJ. Role of endogenous nitric oxide in hyperoxia-induced airway hyperreactivity in maturing rats. J Appl Physiol. 2000;89:1205–12.
35. Mhanna MJ, Haxhiu MA, Jaber MA, Walenga RW, Chang C-H, Liu S, et al. Hyperoxia impairs airway relaxation in immature rats via a cAMP-mediated mechanism. J Appl Physiol. 2004;96:1854–60.
36. Colasurdo GN, Hemming VG, Prince GA, Gelfand AS, Loader JE, Larsen GL. Human respiratory syncytial virus produces prolonged alterations of neural control in airways of developing ferrets. Am J Respir Crit Care Med. 1998;157:1506–11.
37. Prakash YS, Pabelick CM, Martin RJ. Regulation of contractility in immature airway smooth muscle. In: Wang YS, editor. Calcium signaling in airway smooth muscle cells. Cham: Springer International Publishing; 2014. p. 333–40.
38. Yao Q, Haxhiu MA, Zaidi SI, Liu S, Jafri A, Martin RJ. Hyperoxia enhances brain-derived neurotrophic factor and tyrosine kinase B receptor expression in peribronchial smooth muscle of neonatal rats. Am J Physiol Lung Cell Mol Physiol. 2005;289:307–14.
39. Prakash YS, Iyanoye A, Ay B, Mantilla CB, Pabelick CM. Neurotrophin effects on intracellular Ca^{2+} and force in airway smooth muscle. Am J Physiol Lung Cell Mol Physiol. 2006;291:L447–56.
40. Tortorolo L, Langer A, Polidori G, Vento G, Stampachiacchere B, Aloe L, et al. Neurotrophin overexpression in lower airways of infants with respiratory syncytial virus infection. Am J Respir Crit Care Med. 2005;172:233–7.
41. Smith PG, Dreshaj A, Chaudhuri S, Onder BM, Mhanna MJ, Martin RJ. Hyperoxic conditions inhibit airway smooth muscle myosin phosphatase in rat pups. Am J Physiol Lung Cell Mol Physiol. 2007;292:L68–73.
42. Sieck GC, Han YS, Pabelick CM, Prakash YS. Temporal aspects of excitation-contraction coupling in airway smooth muscle. J Appl Physiol. 2001;91:2266–74.
43. Iben SC, Haxhiu MA, Farver CF, Miller MJ, Martin RJ. Short-term mechanical ventilation increases airway reactivity in rat pups. Pediatr Res. 2006;60:136–40.
44. Tepper RS, Ramchandani R, Agay E, Zhang L, Xue Z, Liu Y, et al. Chronic strain alters the passive and contractile properties of rabbit airways. J Appl Physiol. 2005;98:1949–54.
45. Smith PG, Tokui T, Ikebe M. Mechanical strain increases contractile enzyme activity in cultured airway smooth muscle cells. Am J Physiol Lung Cell Mol Physiol. 1995;268:L999–1005.
46. Mayer CA, Martin RJ, MacFarlane PM. Increased airway reactivity in a neonatal mouse model of continuous positive airway pressure [CPAP]. Pediatr Res. 2015;78:145–51.

47. Reyburn B, Di Fiore JM, Raffay T, Martin RJ, Prakash YS, Jafri A, et al. The effect of continuous positive airway pressure in a mouse model of hyperoxic neonatal lung injury. Neonatology. 2016;109:6–13.
48. Faksh A, Britt RD, Vogel ER, Kuipers I, Thompson MA, Sieck GC, et al. Effects of antenatal lipopolysaccharide and postnatal hyperoxia on airway reactivity and remodeling in a neonatal mouse model. Pediatr Res. 2015;79(3):391–400. doi:10.1038/pr.2015.232.
49. Köroğlu OA, MacFarlane PM, Balan KV, Zenebe WJ, Jafri A, Martin RJ, et al. Anti-inflammatory effect of caffeine is associated with improved lung function after lipopolysaccharide-induced amnionitis. Neonatology. 2014;106:235–40.
50. Velten M, Heyob KM, Rogers LK, Welty SE. Deficits in lung alveolarization and function after systemic maternal inflammation and neonatal hyperoxia exposure. J Appl Physiol. 2010;108:1347–56.
51. Choi CW, Kim BI, Mason SN, Potts-Kant EN, Brahmajothi MV, Auten RL. Intra-amniotic LPS amplifies hyperoxia-induced airway hyperreactivity in neonatal rats. Pediatr Res. 2013;1:11–8.
52. Faksh A, Britt Jr RD, Vogel ER, Thompson MA, Pandya HC, Martin RJ, et al. TLR3 activation increases chemokine expression in human fetal airway smooth muscle cells. Am J Physiol Lung Cell Mol Physiol. 2015;310:L202–11.
53. O'Reilly MA, Marr SH, Yee M, McGrath-Morrow SA, Lawrence BP. Neonatal hyperoxia enhances the inflammatory response in adult mice infected with influenza A virus. Am J Respir Crit Care Med. 2008;177:1103–10.

The Bronchopulmonary Dysplasia Diagnosis: Definitions, Utility, Limitations

Roberta L. Keller

Abbreviations

BPD   Bronchopulmonary dysplasia
FRC   Functional residual capacity
HHFNC   Humidified high flow nasal cannula

Bronchopulmonary Dysplasia: Description and Clinical Definitions

Bronchopulmonary dysplasia (BPD) was initially described as a condition characterized by clinical, radiographic, and pathological findings in preterm infants who had prolonged exposure to high airway pressures and hyperoxic gas mixtures for support of neonatal respiratory distress syndrome (hyaline membrane disease), secondary to insufficient surfactant production [1]. Lung parenchymal changes included thickening of the alveolar septae, fibrosis, and emphysema, with associated abnormal lymphatic vessels. Pronounced changes in the bronchial and bronchiolar mucosa, including necrosis and inflammation, and fibrosis and increased musculature in the bronchial walls were noted [1–3]. Infants with radiographic cardiomegaly ultimately died from right heart failure and pulmonary hypertension (with supportive pathological findings) [2], and those who survived with persistent need for supplemental oxygen usually had only mild hyperinflation as residual radiographic sequelae. Thus, the persistent need for supplemental oxygen (FiO_2 >0.21) with accompanying radiographic changes was defined as bronchopulmonary dysplasia in surviving preterm infants, with Tooley and others choosing 28–30 days of age as the timing for determination of this diagnosis [4, 5].

However, the affected infants described by Northway were predominantly >30 weeks' gestational age (and >1500 g at birth), a population that has since been

R.L. Keller, MD
Department of Pediatrics/Neonatology, UCSF Benioff Children's Hospital,
550 16th Street, 5th Floor, UCSF Box 0748, San Francisco, CA 94143, USA
e-mail: kellerr@peds.ucsf.edu

© Springer International Publishing AG 2017
A.M. Hibbs, M. S. Muhlebach (eds.), *Respiratory Outcomes in Preterm Infants*,
Respiratory Medicine, DOI 10.1007/978-3-319-48835-6_4

at low risk for these severe prolonged respiratory complications [5]. In fact, in describing evolving practices in neonatal intensive care, including early application of positive end expiratory pressure as a strategy to decrease exposure to hyperoxia, Tooley noted no mortality and a very low incidence of BPD in infants with birth weight >1500 g [4]. Thus, extremely preterm infants who were and currently are surviving at 28 days of age remain very immature, with many not yet in the alveolar stage of lung development [6]. Shennan et al. retrospectively evaluated the utility of the timing of weaning off supplemental oxygen as a predictor for later respiratory outcomes in infants ≤1500 g [7]. Poor respiratory outcome was defined as mortality, persistent oxygen therapy at 40 weeks' postmenstrual age, respiratory tract surgery, recurrent hospitalizations for respiratory indication, or medication for wheeze by 2 years of age, or radiographic changes, wheeze or respiratory distress with growth failure or neurodevelopmental consequences at 1 year of age. Twenty percent of infants (119/605) had abnormal respiratory outcome, and, regardless of gestational age at birth, infants who did not meet criteria for abnormal respiratory outcome weaned off supplemental oxygen at similar postmenstrual age. In fact, in assessing the persistent use of supplemental oxygen therapy for prediction of outcome, sensitivity decreased and specificity increased with advancing postmenstrual age. At 36 weeks' postmenstrual age, oxygen therapy demonstrated moderate sensitivity and strong specificity for outcome prediction, with improved accuracy compared to 28 days of age. Thus, from this cohort that included less mature infants (~220 infants were ≤1000 g at birth), BPD was explicitly offered as a predictor of later respiratory outcomes, with a proposal to delay its determination until near-term corrected age. As the increasing use of antenatal steroids and the approval of exogenous surfactant for treatment of respiratory distress syndrome further improved survival among the most preterm infants in the early 1990s, BPD determined at 36 weeks' postmenstrual age was increasingly reported as a neonatal respiratory outcome [8, 9].

Similar to the findings of Shennan et al., a secondary analysis of infants enrolled in the Trial of Indomethacin Prophylaxis (TIPP, birth weight 500–999 g, born 1996–1998) demonstrated that, with advancing postmenstrual age at persistence of oxygen supplementation, sensitivity decreased and specificity increased for prediction of pulmonary outcome at 18 months corrected age [10]. The majority of these infants were exposed to antenatal steroids and were treated with surfactant replacement therapy. Criteria for poor pulmonary outcome were similar to those of Shennan and colleagues: mortality, any home respiratory support, respiratory medication administration (bronchodilators or inhaled or systemic steroids) for >2 months, or any hospitalization for respiratory indication. Fifty-four percent (506/945) of these extremely low gestational age newborns met criteria for poor outcome. Persistence of oxygen supplementation had equivalent predictive accuracy for pulmonary outcome regardless of the timing of assessment (28 days, or 32, 34, 36, 38, or 40 weeks' postmenstrual age). Based on these results, the investigators recommended no change to the current state of the field, with assessment and diagnosis of BPD at 36 weeks' postmenstrual age; some publications have referred to these criteria for the definition of BPD, the "traditional" criteria. However, it is interesting to note that the positive and negative predictive values (PPV and NPV) do change over the two study eras and with advancing postmenstrual age. In data from Shennan and colleagues, PPV and NPV at 36 weeks' postmenstrual age are 63 % and 90 %, respectively, whereas they are 75 % and 57 % at 36 weeks in the later study and 90 % and 55 % at 40 weeks [7, 10]. Thus, in the current era, assessment at term (40 weeks' postmenstrual age) likely improves specificity and positive predictive value, and could improve overall predictive accuracy for pulmonary outcome at follow-up at 1–2 years corrected age, depending on characteristics of the patient population under evaluation and the outcome of interest (Table 2).

Along with increased survival for the most immature infants, lung pathology of infants dying with BPD was changing. Husain et al. examined lung parenchymal changes in infants dying with and without surfactant [11]. They demonstrated that the degree of alveolar hypoplasia and enlargement (alveolar simplification) was similar regardless of surfactant administration, but fibrosis was more universal and severe in infants who were not treated with surfactant. Bhatt and colleagues further noted that infants dying with BPD had a decreased alveolar capillary network present within the thickened alveolar septae [12]. Commentaries focused on these findings proposed a "new" BPD, characterized by an arrest of alveolar and microvascular development in these extremely preterm infants (born in the late canalicular/early saccular phases of lung development), in whom the usual signals for alveolarization and angiogenesis became disrupted through premature exposure to the extrauterine environment, including inflammatory stimuli and ambient or supplemental oxygen [6, 13–15].

In considering this evolving clinical entity, participants in an NIH-sponsored workshop in 2000 proposed a severity scale for the diagnosis of BPD. Their recommendations were based on the utility of BPD as a predictor of later respiratory morbidity, without regard for radiographic findings [16]. BPD was to be assessed at 36 weeks' postmenstrual age, and infants without 28 days of supplemental oxygen exposure (for >12 h per day) up to that point were classified as no BPD. Of those infants with at least 28 days of exposure to supplemental oxygen, infants on assisted ventilation (positive pressure ventilation or nasal continuous positive airway pressure), or with $FiO_2 \geq 0.30$, were classified as severe BPD. Infants supported with FiO_2 0.22–0.29 were classified as moderate BPD, and those without supplemental FiO_2 were classified as mild BPD. These recommendations also stated that the level of support used for the determination of severity of BPD at 36 weeks should be representative of the support the infant was receiving (e.g., an infant usually on low flow nasal cannula support with FiO_2 0.25, who was intubated for a procedure should not be classified as severe BPD). This severity scale was validated by Ehrenkranz et al. in retrospective data from 3848 infants ≤ 1000 g born from 1995 to 1999, with minor modifications due to discharge or transfer at <36 weeks' postmenstrual age, lack of data on duration of daily oxygen supplementation, and classification of all infants receiving nasal cannula support with FiO_2 >0.22 as moderate [17]. Increasing severity of BPD was associated with higher rates of respiratory morbidity at 18–22 months corrected (for prematurity) age, although sensitivity and specificity were modest (Table 2). In further support of the proposed NIH Workshop definition, the requirement for an abnormal chest radiograph did not substantially impact the utility of the dichotomous BPD definitions at 28 days and 36 weeks' postmenstrual age.

Bronchopulmonary Dysplasia: Physiologic Definitions and Considerations

Ultimately, BPD status for any infant based on these definitions of BPD hinges upon the clinical prescription of supplemental oxygen, which is known to vary by center, and will depend on oxygen saturation targets [18, 19]. In evaluation of this clinical variability, Walsh and colleagues proposed the use of a "physiologic challenge," at 36 ± 1 weeks' in which infants who are not on assisted ventilation but are receiving supplemental oxygen, undergo a protocolized reduction of oxygen and flow (if on nasal cannula support) [20, 21]. Additional eligibility for the challenge includes an FiO_2 <0.30, which is further clarified to be "effective" FiO_2 by some investigators and clinicians (since delivered FiO_2 by nasal cannula will vary based on the flow and its relationship to the infant's size, in addition to the FiO_2 set from the gas source) [18, 22–26]. Infants who are unable to maintain a prespecified oxygen saturation either during the pretest observation period, in the course of the oxygen and flow reduction stage, or in the postreduction observation period (in room air off respiratory support), are classified as BPD. In an initial multicenter experience with the physiologic challenge in 17 academic centers, the diagnosis of BPD fell from 35 to 25 % in 1598 infants, with considerable variability in rates of BPD persisting across the centers [21]. However, more recent data suggest that lesser differences may be present in comparing the clinical and physiologic definitions; Stoll et al. describe incidences of BPD of 42 % and 40 % with the clinical and physiologic definitions, respectively, in a cohort of 9575 infants from 20 academic centers with birth weight $\leq$1500 g [27]. Clinical and physiologic definitions of BPD are summarized in Table 1.

As the impact of the physiologic challenge test on rates of BPD has decreased, failure rates for the physiologic challenge test have increased. In the initial multicenter experience, 44 % (101/227) of infants passed the physiologic challenge [21]. In contrast, only 30 % (80/266) of infants in the recent Prematurity and Respiratory Outcomes Program (PROP) study passed the challenge [28]. It is important to note that these studies both used the same oxygen saturation cutoff for failure (<90 %) [21, 29]. Higher oxygen saturation cutoffs will result in lower rates of passing the physiologic challenge; therefore, overall rates of BPD by physiologic definitions will vary based on oxygen saturation targets [20]. In practice, lower clinical oxygen saturation targets result in fewer infants remaining on supplemental oxygen and eligible for the challenge, while lower test saturation targets result in fewer infants failing the physiologic challenge, together resulting in lower rates of BPD.

Given consistency in oxygen saturation criteria, the results of the physiologic challenge have been validated with respect to baseline level of support. Infants on low flow nasal cannula (0.02–2.00 LPM) with effective FiO_2 0.21–0.49 who underwent physiologic challenge were more likely to pass the challenge with a lower baseline effective FiO_2 (0.23 ± 0.03 versus 0.26 ± 0.05) [23].

An additional potential benefit of the physiologic challenge is for the classification of infants receiving respiratory support without supplemental oxygen. This scenario

Table 1 Definitions of bronchopulmonary dysplasia, based on ongoing use of supplemental oxygen and/or level of respiratory support (see text for detail)

Definition	Comments
Clinical	
28 days of age [4, 5]	Only receipt of supplemental oxygen required, without specification for level of respiratory support
	May be specified to require supplemental oxygen for each of the first 28 days
36 weeks' PMA [7]	Only receipt of supplemental oxygen required, without specification for level of respiratory support
	May be modified to classify all infants on assisted ventilation as BPD (similar to physiologic definitions), but this is not specified in most publications
	May be modified to include status at discharge to home or transfer to another hospital prior to 36 weeks' PMA
NIH Workshop ("severity" definition of none, mild, moderate, severe) [16, 17]	Should reflect infant's usual level of support at 36 weeks' PMA
	28 days of FiO_2 >0.21 for at least 12 h per day prior to 36 weeks' PMA required, but some have modified the definition to require FiO_2 >0.21 at 28 days of age (rather than 28 days of supplemental oxygen), or to drop this requirement (infants without supplemental oxygen at 36 weeks' PMA are No BPD)
	Infants on assisted ventilation are classified as severe
	"Effective FiO_2" may be used in some cases to determine severe versus moderate classification
	Categories may be collapsed to moderate-to-severe versus none
Physiologic	
"Severity" definition (none, mild, moderate, severe) [16, 24]	Determined at 36 ± 1 weeks' PMA with ongoing need for supplemental oxygen determined by physiologic challenge
	"Effective FiO_2" <0.30 may be used to determine eligibility for challenge
	Categories may be collapsed to moderate-to-severe versus none
36 weeks' PMA [20, 21]	Determined at 36 ± 1 weeks' PMA as ongoing assisted ventilation or ongoing need for supplemental oxygen (FiO_2 >0.21)

PMA postmenstrual age

is not explicitly addressed by any of the clinical definitions for BPD, with the exception of the use of assisted ventilation for support in infants with severe BPD. Walsh and colleagues described infants on low flow nasal cannula (0.13–2.00 LPM) with FiO_2 0.21; 15/22 (68 %) of infants passed the challenge [23]. Similarly, in PROP, 55/81 (68 %) of infants on nasal cannula support without supplemental oxygen passed the physiologic challenge [28]. Use of newer respiratory support strategies, such as humidified high flow nasal cannula (HHFNC), which provides variable degrees of positive pressure respiratory support (that are not measured in most clinical settings), is particularly challenging to classify (with or without supplemental oxygen) [30]. In addition to the inability to assess its contribution to stabilizing an infant's respiratory status due to inconsistent provision of positive pressure, the use of HHFNC adds further variability to a clinical diagnosis of BPD as it is not currently employed in a consistent manner within and across centers [31–33].

Another aspect of the respiratory status of former preterm newborns to be considered when evaluating the need for ongoing respiratory support is dysmaturity of control of breathing. Infants born more preterm are more likely to have persistent episodes of periodic breathing and/or desaturation at and beyond 36 weeks' postmenstrual age and term [34–37]. Coste et al. demonstrated that control of breathing was an important factor in passing the physiologic challenge test for BPD at 36 weeks' postmenstrual age [38]. Sixteen of 17 preterm infants who experienced increased periodic breathing during the challenge subsequently failed the challenge due to desaturation. This does not preclude the coexistence of lung disease, however. In healthy former preterm infants off respiratory support, both frequency of apnea and proportion of apneic events with desaturation were inversely related to functional residual capacity (FRC), and desaturations were also inversely related to minute ventilation [39]. Consistent with these findings, Coste and colleagues found that infants failing the physiologic challenge averaged higher baseline nasal cannula flows than those passing the test (1.1 LPM versus 0.4 LPM), whereas FiO_2 was not a significant discriminator of the challenge result [38]. Thus, positive pressure provided by nasal cannula support could stabilize an infant's FRC, decreasing periodic breathing and desaturation, and account for the ongoing prescription of respiratory support in the clinical setting, as well as failure to maintain oxygenation during the physiologic challenge [30, 40]. This could be true even in the absence of supplemental oxygen, which would explain why approximately one third of infants on nasal cannula flow without supplemental oxygen are reported to have failed the challenge test [23, 28].

Interestingly, with respect to the variable physiology of BPD that is reflected in the persistence of respiratory support with or without oxygen supplementation in extremely premature newborns, Ballard and colleagues prospectively planned for repeat clinical or physiologic assessments at 40 weeks' postmenstrual age (term) in two trials of investigative therapies to prevent BPD [24, 26, 41]. Both of these studies showed substantial decreases in the diagnosis of BPD in survivors between 36 and 40 weeks (66 % versus 38 % in the more recent Trial of Late Surfactant) [26].

Validation of the Diagnosis of BPD: Respiratory Morbidity Outcomes

Although there are multiple studies demonstrating that various definitions of BPD are significantly associated with respiratory morbidity at follow-up, there are few studies that explicitly evaluate validity of the BPD diagnosis for prediction of later pulmonary outcomes [42–44]. As previously noted, Shennan and Davis and their colleagues evaluated evolving clinical definitions of BPD for accuracy in predicting various pulmonary outcomes at 1–2 years corrected age, while Ehrenkranz et al. also provided important validation data [7, 10, 17]. Findings are summarized in

Table 2. Parad et al. evaluated the utility of BPD diagnoses at 28 days and 36 weeks' postmenstrual age for respiratory morbidity outcomes defined at 2 years corrected age (cough, wheeze, respiratory medication use, and hospitalization for respiratory indication) [45]. They found poor utility for both BPD definitions (area under the receiver-operator curve 0.50–0.62) in both development and validation cohorts. They also compared the performance of the BPD classifications to prevalence of respiratory symptoms or medications use at 1 year corrected age, demonstrating that 1-year respiratory morbidity was significantly better at predicting 2-year outcomes than BPD (area under the receiver-operator curve 0.64–0.78) [45]. Taken together, these studies suggest that sensitivity is higher than specificity at 28 days, while the reverse is true at 36 weeks' postmenstrual age, although this does not necessarily translate into greater accuracy for outcome prediction. Also, BPD may be a better predictor of composite morbidity outcomes (which incorporate home respiratory support and respiratory medications and hospitalizations, with or without symptoms) than it is of individual respiratory morbidity domains (home support, medications, hospitalization, or symptoms).

Ehrenkranz also demonstrated significant increases in rates of use of respiratory medications (diuretics and bronchodilators) and hospitalization for respiratory indication with increasing severity of BPD, by the NIH Workshop definition [17]. I have been unable to identify published reports of the relationship of the physiologic definitions of BPD and later pulmonary outcomes.

Validation of the Diagnosis of BPD: Pulmonary Function

The classification of BPD based on physiologic definitions demonstrates that, at least for brief observation periods, infants without BPD do not require respiratory support (with or without supplemental oxygen) to maintain adequate oxygen saturations. The differences leading to the ongoing need for respiratory support are likely related to lung structure and function, with some contribution of variable maturation of control of breathing. Kaempf and colleagues demonstrated that infants with BPD (as classified by both clinical and physiologic definitions) have higher capillary PCO_2 at 36 weeks' postmenstrual age than infants without BPD, indicating poorer respiratory system function at the time of the diagnosis of BPD [46]. We have recently reviewed pulmonary function in former preterm infants in infancy and childhood [47]. Generally, pulmonary function tests demonstrate that lung function in infants and young children is decreased following a diagnosis of BPD (by various definitions, although most commonly a clinical diagnosis at 36 weeks' postmenstrual age) compared to full-term controls. Former preterm infants without BPD also often demonstrate lower lung function than controls but better function than infants with BPD. Airway obstruction, with or without differences in lung volumes, is the most common abnormality in lung function. Former preterm children with

Table 2 Sensitivity, specificity, and utility of clinical definitions of bronchopulmonary dysplasia for various respiratory morbidity outcomes at 1–2 years corrected age

Study	Patient population	Corrected age at assessment	Outcome	Outcome incidence	BPD definition	Sensitivity	Specificity	Accuracy/ discrimination
Shennan (1988)	≤1500 g, born 1981–1985, $n = 605$	2 years	Composite of various respiratory morbidities (including medication use and hospitalizations)	20 %	28 days	79 %	69 %	71 % correctly classified
					36 weeks' PMA	63 %	91 %	85 % correctly classified
Davis (2002)	500–999 g, born 1996–1998, $n = 945$	18 months	Composite of various respiratory morbidities (including medication use and hospitalizations)	54 %	28 days	67 %	54 %	61 % correctly classified
					36 weeks' PMA	46 %	82 %	63 % correctly classified
					40 weeks' PMA	33 %	96 %	62 % correctly classified
Ehrenkranz (2005)	≤1000 g, <32 weeks', born 1995–1999, $n = 3848$	18–22 months	Bronchodilators or diuretics	35 %	36 weeks' PMA	54 %	62 %	NA
			Hospitalization for respiratory indication	30 %	36 weeks' PMA	52 %	60 %	NA

Stevens (2014)	24–27 weeks', born 2005–2009, n = 918	6–22 months	Persistent cough or wheeze	61 %	36 weeks' PMA	44 %	64 %	NA
			Inhaled steroids	26 %		56 %	64 %	NA
			Hospitalization for respiratory indication	31 %		51 %	64 %	NA
Parad (2015)	23–28 weeks', ventilated on first day of life, born 1998–2001, n = 76 (development cohort) and n = 227 (validation cohort)	2 years	Respiratory symptoms and/or medications	NA	28 days	NA	NA	AUROC 0.53
					36 weeks' PMA	NA	NA	AUROC 0.53–0.62
			Hospitalization for respiratory indication	NA	28 days	NA	NA	AUROC 0.50–0.55
					36 weeks' PMA	NA	NA	AUROC 0.54–0.55

AUROC area under the receiver-operator curve, *BPD* bronchopulmonary dysplasia, *NA* not available, *PMA* postmenstrual age and without BPD may have evidence of relative decline in lung growth, before compensatory growth is seen, although there can be a persistence of decreased lung function at school age and beyond. Filbrun and colleagues demonstrated that one factor associated with improving lung function in children with a diagnosis of BPD is "catch-up" growth, which exceeds expected growth rates [48]. Other work has shown that children with a diagnosis of BPD experience less compensatory lung growth than children without BPD [49].

Balinotti and colleagues have shown that infants with BPD have decreased alveolar-capillary surface area, relative to lung volume, compared to full-term controls [50]. Follow-up work showed this difference is due to proportional decreases in both the pulmonary diffusion membrane and capillary blood volume components [51]. These data are consistent with enlarged alveoli with decreased septation. In addition, both of the components (capillary membrane and capillary bed) were directly related to body length, providing a pathway by which enhanced somatic growth in former preterm infants could result in improved lung structure and normalization of lung function, as well as an explanation for increasing or persistent decrements in lung function in childhood, particularly in children with a diagnosis of BPD.

Validation of the Diagnosis of BPD: Nonpulmonary Outcomes

Generally, the diagnosis of BPD correlates with other neonatal morbidities of prematurity. This convergent validity has been demonstrated for both clinical and physiologic definitions of BPD [17, 25, 28]. Ehrenkranz et al. evaluated a modification of the NIH Workshop definition, demonstrating increased rates of severe intraventricular/intracranial hemorrhage, sepsis, and necrotizing enterocolitis with increasing severity of BPD [17]. Similarly, Poindexter and colleagues evaluated two clinical definitions of BPD determined at 36 weeks' postmenstrual age—modified versions of the definition proposed by Shennan et al. and the NIH workshop definition. Infants with BPD by either definition were significantly more likely to have severe intraventricular/intracranial hemorrhage, sepsis, and severe retinopathy of prematurity [28]. With respect to the binary physiologic definition of BPD at 36 weeks' postmenstrual age, Natarajan et al. showed that BPD was significantly associated with increased rates of severe intraventricular/intracranial hemorrhage, sepsis, necrotizing enterocolitis requiring surgery, and severe retinopathy of prematurity [25]. Thus, the level of illness and immaturity that lead to the diagnosis of BPD, also carry risks of these other morbidities, which, in some cases, may directly increase the risk of BPD due to associated inflammation (particularly sepsis and necrotizing enterocolitis) [52]. Similarly, neurologic injury is associated with delayed brain development, which may influence maturation of respiratory control [53–55].

The diagnosis of BPD has also been associated with poor somatic growth. Poindexter and colleagues showed increased rates of growth failure (weight <10th percentile) at 36 weeks' postmenstrual age with both of their clinical definitions of BPD [28]. In infants with severe BPD, the prevalence of growth failure increased with advancing postmenstrual age (36–48 weeks') among infants who remained hospitalized [56]. Rates of growth failure (<10th percentile) at 18–22 months corrected age also increased with increasing severity of BPD by the NIH Workshop definition and the diagnosis of BPD by the physiologic definition, with length and head circumference more variably affected [17, 25].

Multiple neonatal morbidities are associated with adverse neurodevelopmental outcomes in extremely preterm infants [57–59]. Among the nonneurologic morbidities, the diagnosis of BPD has been consistently associated with poorer neurodevelopmental status, at least doubling the odds of developmental disability [57, 59]. Schmidt and colleagues used a clinical definition of ongoing receipt of supplemental oxygen at 36 weeks' postmenstrual age for these analyses. Other investigators have also shown associations between clinical diagnoses of BPD and neurological outcomes, although some studies have focused on more severe definitions of BPD (e.g., including only those infants discharged on supplemental oxygen) [10, 60, 61]. However, Laughon and colleagues were unable to show a significant relationship between BPD and neurodevelopmental outcome at 2 years corrected age after adjusting for various antenatal factors considered to be antecedents of BPD [62]. Ehrenkranz and colleagues did show a significant association with severity of BPD using the clinical NIH Workshop definition and various neurodevelopmental outcomes [17]. And, Davis et al. showed similar utility of both 36- and 40-week clinical definitions of BPD for neurodevelopmental outcomes at 18 months corrected age [10]. Finally, Natarajan and colleagues demonstrated significant associations between the binary physiologic definition of BPD and various cognitive and motor outcomes at 18–22 months corrected age [25].

Implications of BPD Definitions: Clinical Practice and Clinical Trials

There is considerable variability in rates of BPD between centers, which persists even after adjustment for important infant characteristics [63]. Thus, there are both research and clinical implications to the selection of a definition for BPD. Beam and colleagues performed a systematic review of clinical drug trials for the prevention of BPD published from 1992–2014 [64]. The majority of these trials used clinical definitions of BPD as outcomes, two thirds determined BPD at 36 weeks' postmenstrual age and one third at 28 days; only two trials used a physiologic definition of BPD. Therefore, the variability in rates of BPD between centers is problematic in the conduct and interpretation of clinical trials, a challenge which is only partially ameliorated by use of the physiologic definition of BPD [21, 65, 66]. However, this variability also increases concern for the generalizability of data from single center studies.

Multicenter collaborations focused on benchmarking and quality improvement, such as the Vermont Oxford Network and the California Perinatal Quality Control Collaborative primarily focus on clinical definitions of BPD, which are the most straightforward for staff to collect and report [46, 66]. However, in benchmarking clinical outcomes within these collaborations, differences in infant baseline characteristics, clinical management strategies, and the application of respiratory support strategies near term (including oxygen saturation targets) may not be accounted for, despite their importance.

One of the major limitations of both the clinical and physiologic definitions of BPD is that they convey little information about those infants who do not carry that diagnosis from the neonatal period. Many of these infants have abnormal lung function near-term corrected age. And, as previously noted, up to 25–30 % of these infants have later respiratory morbidity by a variety of measures, with increased risks of wheezing illness compared to term-born children, regardless of the extent of prematurity or diagnosis of BPD [17, 67]. Thus, various observational and interventional studies focused on BPD as an outcome, regardless of the definition used, fail to fully evaluate the relationship of various clinical and biological factors to important respiratory outcomes.

However, the use of later respiratory outcomes (e.g., at 1–2 years corrected age) for both clinical trials and benchmarking has not been widely adopted, although various outcomes have been investigated [68, 69]. It is likely these later outcomes are influenced by a variety of socioeconomic and genetic factors, some of which may also effect lung growth and function over time, complicating their application in neonatal practice and investigation [70, 71]. Yet, neurodevelopmental status at 18 months – 2 years corrected age is commonly used as an outcome in neonatal clinical trials; assessment of respiratory outcomes should not be considered differently, particularly as later respiratory morbidity may be more predictive of lifetime respiratory outcomes than BPD.

Conclusion

BPD remains an important early marker of later pulmonary outcomes, but the patient population of interest, the specific definition of BPD, and any later respiratory outcomes under evaluation must be considered in the interpretation of any findings. In investigation of strategies to improve respiratory outcomes in preterm infant, particularly in those born extremely preterm, it is important to measure outcomes beyond the diagnosis of BPD alone, as it may not fully represent the degree of underlying lung dysplasia and remains an imperfect predictor of later respiratory morbidity.

References

1. Northway WH, Rosan RC, Porter DY. Pulmonary disease following respiratory therapy of hyaline-membrane disease. Bronchopulmonary dysplasia. N Engl J Med. 1967;276:357–68.

2. Bonikos DS, Bensch KG, Northway WH, Edwards DK. Bronchopulmonary dysplasia: the pulmonary pathologic sequel of necrotizing bronchiolitis and pulmonary fibrosis. Hum Pathol. 1976;7:643–66.

3. Taghizadeh A, Reynolds EO. Pathogenesis of bronchopulmonary dysplasia following hyaline membrane disease. Am J Pathol. 1976;82:241–64.

4. Tooley WH. Epidemiology of bronchopulmonary dysplasia. J Pediatr. 1979;95(5 Pt 2):851–8.

5. Avery ME, Tooley WH, Keller JB, Hurd SS, Bryan H, Cotton RB, et al. Is chronic lung disease in low birth weight infants preventable? A survey of eight centers. Pediatrics. 1987;79(1):26–30.

6. Hislop AA, Wigglesworth JS, Desai R. Alveolar development in the human fetus and infant. Early Hum Dev. 1986;13:1–11.

7. Shennan AT, Dunn MS, Ohlsson A, Lennox K, Hoskins EM. Abnormal pulmonary outcomes in premature infants: prediction from oxygen requirement in the neonatal period. Pediatrics. 1988;82:527–32.

8. Fanaroff AA, Wright LL, Stevenson DK, Shankaran S, Donovan EF, Ehrenkranz RA, et al. Very-low-birth-weight outcomes of the National Institute of Child Health and Human Development Neonatal Research Network, May 1991 through December 1992. Am J Obstet Gynecol. 1995;173:1423–31.

9. Wright LL, Verter J, Younes N, Stevenson D, Fanaroff AA, Shankaran S, et al. Antenatal corticosteroid administration and neonatal outcome in very low birth weight infants: the NICHD Neonatal Research Network. Am J Obstet Gynecol. 1995;173:269–74.

10. Davis PG, Thorpe K, Roberts R, Schmidt B, Doyle LW, Kirpalani H, et al. Evaluating "old" definitions for the "new" bronchopulmonary dysplasia. J Pediatr. 2002;140:555–60.

11. Husain AN, Siddiqui NH, Stocker JT. Pathology of arrested acinar development in postsurfactant bronchopulmonary dysplasia. Hum Pathol. 1998;29(7):710–7.

12. Bhatt AJ, Pryhuber GS, Huyck H, Watkins RH, Metlay LA, Maniscalco WM. Disrupted pulmonary vasculature and decreased vascular endothelial growth factor, Flt-1, and TIE-2 in human infants dying with bronchopulmonary dysplasia. Am J Respir Crit Care Med. 2001;164(10 Pt 1):1971–80.

13. Jobe AH. The new BPD: an arrest of lung development. Pediatr Res. 1999;46:641–3.

14. Abman S. Bronchopulmonary dysplasia: "a vascular hypothesis". Am J Respir Crit Care Med. 2001;164:1755–6.

15. Hislop AA. Airway and blood vessel interaction during lung development. J Anat. 2002;201:325–34.

16. Jobe AH, Bancalari E. Bronchopulmonary dysplasia. Am J Respir Crit Care Med. 2001;163(7):1723–9.

17. Ehrenkranz RA, Walsh MC, Vohr BR, Jobe AH, Wright LL, Fanaroff AA, et al. Validation of the National Institutes of Health consensus definition of bronchopulmonary dysplasia. Pediatrics. 2005;116:1353–60.

18. The STOP-ROP Multicenter Study Group. Supplemental Therapeutic Oxygen for Prethreshold Retinopathy Of Prematurity (STOP-ROP), a randomized, controlled trial. I: primary outcomes. Pediatrics. 2000;105(2):295–310.

19. Lagatta J, Clark R, Spitzer A. Clinical predictors and institutional variation in home oxygen use in preterm infants. J Pediatr. 2012;160:232–8.

20. Walsh MC, Wilson-Costello D, Zadell A, Newman N, Fanaroff A. Safety, reliability and valididty of a physiological definition of bronchopulmoanry dysplasia. J Perinatol. 2003;23:451–6.

21. Walsh MC, Yao Q, Gettner P, Hale E, Collins M, Hensman A, et al. Impact of a physiologic definition on bronchopulmonary dysplasia rates. Pediatrics. 2004;114:1305–11.

22. Benaron D, Benitz W. Maximizing the stability of oxygen delivered by nasal cannula. Arch Pediatr Adolesc Med. 1994;148:294–300.

23. Walsh M, Engle W, Laptook A, Kazzi SN, Buchter S, Rasmussen M, et al. Oxygen delivery through nasal cannulae to preterm infants: can practice be improved? Pediatrics. 2005;116:857–61.

24. Ballard RA, Truog WE, Cnaan A, Martin RJ, Ballard PL, Merrill JD, et al. Inhaled nitric oxide in preterm infants undergoing mechanical ventilation. N Engl J Med. 2006;355(4):343–53.

25. Natarajan G, Pappas A, Shankaran S, Kendrick DE, Das A, Higgins RD, et al. Outcomes of extremely low birth weight infants with bronchopulmonary dysplasia: impact of the physiologic definition. Early Hum Dev. 2012;88:509–15.
26. Ballard RA, Keller RL, Black DM, Ballard PL, Merrill JD, Eichenwald EC, et al. Randomized trial of late surfactant treatment in ventilated preterm infants receiving inhaled nitric oxide. J Pediatr. 2016;168:23–9. e4.
27. Stoll BJ, Hansen NI, Bell EF, Shankaran S, Laptook AR, Walsh MC, et al. Neonatal outcomes of extremely preterm infants from the NICHD Neonatal Research Network. Pediatrics. 2010;126:443–56.
28. Poindexter BB, Feng R, Schmidt B, Aschner JL, Ballard RA, Hamvas A, et al. Comparisons and limitations of current definitions of bronchopulmonary dysplasia for the Prematurity and Respiratory Outcomes Program. Ann Am Thorac Soc. 2015;12:1822–30.
29. Pryhuber GS, Maitre NL, Ballard RA, Cifelli D, Davis SD, Ellenberg JH, et al. Prematurity and Respiratory Outcomes Program (PROP): study protocol of a prospective multicenter study of respiratory outcomes of preterm infants in the United States. BMC Pediatr. 2015;15:37.
30. Dani C, Pratesi S, Migliori C, Bertini G. High flow nasal cannula therapy as respiratory support in the preterm infant. Pediatr Pulmonol. 2009;44:629–34.
31. Hough JL, Shearman AD, Jardine LA, Davies MW. Humidified high flow nasal cannulae: current practice in Australasian nurseries, a survey. J Paediatr Child Health. 2012;48:106–13.
32. Ojha S, Gridley E, Dorling J. Use of heated humidified high-flow nasal cannula oxygen in neonates: a UK wide survey. Acta Paediatr. 2013;102:249–53.
33. Lavizzari A, Veneroni C, Colnaghi M, Ciuffini F, Zannin E, Fumagalli M, et al. Respiratory mechanics during NCPAP and HHHFNC at equal distending pressures. Arch Dis Child Fetal Neonatal Ed. 2014;99:F315–20.
34. Eichenwald EC, Aina A, Stark AR. Apnea frequently persists beyond term gestation in infants delivered at 24 to 28 weeks. Pediatrics. 1997;100(3 Pt 1):354–9.
35. Hunt CE, Corwin MJ, Weese-Mayer DE, Ward SL, Ramanathan R, Lister G, et al. Longitudinal assessment of hemoglobin oxygen saturation in preterm and term infants in the first six months of life. J Pediatr. 2011;159:377–83. e1.
36. Naulaers G, Daniels H, Allegaert K, Rayyan M, Debeer A, Devlieger H. Cardiorespiratory events recorded on home monitors: the effect of prematurity on later serious events. Acta Paediatr. 2007;96:195–8.
37. Ramanathan R, Corwin MJ, Hunt CE, Lister G, Tinsley LR, Baird T, et al. Cardiorespiratory events recorded on home monitors: Comparison of healthy infants with those at increased risk for SIDS. JAMA. 2001;285:2199–207.
38. Coste F, Ferkol T, Hamvas A, Cleveland C, Linneman L, Hoffman J, et al. Ventilatory control and supplemental oxygen in premature infants with apparent chronic lung disease. Arch Dis Child Fetal Neonatal Ed. 2015;100:F233–7.
39. Tourneux P, Léké A, Kongolo G, Cardot V, Dégrugilliers L, Chardon K, et al. Relationship between functional residual capacity and oxygen desaturation during short central apneic events during sleep in "late preterm" infants. Pediatr Res. 2008;64:171–6.
40. Sreenan C, Lemke RP, Hudson-Mason A, Osiovich H. High-flow nasal cannulae in the management of apnea of prematurity: a comparison with conventional nasal continuous positive airway pressure. Pediatrics. 2001;107:1081–3.
41. Ballard RA. Inhaled nitric oxide in preterm infants – correction. N Engl J Med. 2007;357:1444–5.
42. Greenough A, Limb E, Marston L, Marlow N, Calvert S, Peacock J. Risk factors for respiratory morbidity in infancy after very premature birth. Arch Dis Child Fetal Neonatal Ed. 2005;90:F320–F3.
43. Hennessy EM, Bracewell MA, Wood N, Wolke D, Costeloe K, Gibson A, et al. Respiratory health in pre-school and school age children following extremely preterm birth. Arch Dis Child. 2008;93:1037–43.

44. Stevens TP, Finer NN, Carlo WA, Szilagyi PG, Phelps DL, Walsh MC, et al. Respiratory outcomes of the surfactant positive pressure and oximetry randomized trial (SUPPORT). J Pediatr. 2014;165:240–9. e4.
45. Parad RB, Davis JM, Lo J, Thomas M, Marlow N, Calvert S, et al. Prediction of respiratory outcome in extremely low gestational age infants. Neonatology. 2015;107:241–8.
46. Kaempf JW, Campbell B, Brown A, Bowers K, Gallegos R, Goldsmith JP. PCO2 and room air saturation values in premature infants at risk for bronchopulmonary dysplasia. J Perinatol. 2008;28:48–54.
47. Islam JY, Keller RL, Aschner JL, Hartert TV, Moore PE. Understanding the short and long-term respiratory outcomes of prematurity and bronchopulmonary dysplasia. Am J Respir Crit Care Med. 2015;192(2):134–56.
48. Filbrun AG, Popova AP, Linn MJ, McIntosh NA, Hershenson MB. Longitudinal measures of lung function in infants with bronchopulmonary dysplasia. Pediatr Pulmonol. 2011;46:369–75.
49. Fortuna M, Carraro S, Temporin E, Berardi M, Zanconato S, Salvadori S, et al. Mid-childhood lung function in a cohort of children with "new bronchopulmonary dysplasia". Pediatr Pulmonol. 2016;51(10):1057–64.
50. Balinotti JE, Chakr VC, Tiller C, Kimmel R, Coates C, Kisling J, et al. Growth of lung parenchyma in infants and toddlers with chronic lung disease of infancy. Am J Respir Crit Care Med. 2010;181:1093–7.
51. Chang DV, Assaf SJ, Tiller CJ, Kisling JA, Tepper RS. Membrane and Capillary Components of Lung Diffusion in Infants with Bronchopulmonary Dysplasia. Am J Respir Crit Care Med. 2016;193:767–71.
52. Ambalavanan N, Carlo WA, D'Angio CT, McDonald SA, Das A, Schendel D, et al. Cytokines associated with bronchopulmonary dysplasia or death in extremely low birth weight infants. Pediatrics. 2009;123:1132–41.
53. Cheung PY, Barrington KJ, Finer NN, Robertson CM. Early childhood neurodevelopment in very low birth weight infants with predischarge apnea. Pediatr Pulmonol. 1999;27:14–20.
54. Bonifacio SL, Glass HC, Chau V, Berman JI, Xu D, Brant R, et al. Extreme premature birth is not associated with impaired development of brain microstructure. J Pediatr. 2010;157:726–32. e1.
55. Kidokoro H, Anderson PJ, Doyle LW, Woodward LJ, Neil JJ, Inder TE. Brain injury and altered brain growth in preterm infants: predictors and prognosis. Pediatrics. 2014;134:e444–53.
56. Natarajan G, Johnson YR, Brozanski B, Farrow KN, Zaniletti I, Padula MA, et al. Postnatal weight gain in preterm infants with severe bronchopulmonary dysplasia. Am J Perinatol. 2014;31:223–30.
57. Schmidt B, Asztalos EV, Roberts RS, Robertson CM, Sauve RS, Whitfield MF, et al. Impact of bronchopulmonary dysplasia, brain injury, and severe retinopathy on the outcome of extremely low-birth-weight infants at 18 months: results from the trial of indomethacin prophylaxis in preterms. JAMA. 2003;289:1124–9.
58. Ambalavanan N, Carlo WA, Tyson JE, Langer JC, Walsh MC, Parikh NA, et al. Outcome trajectories in extremely preterm infants. Pediatrics. 2012;130:e115–25.
59. Schmidt B, Roberts RS, Davis PG, Doyle LW, Asztalos EV, Opie G, et al. rediction of late death or disability at age 5 years using a count of 3 neonatal morbidities in very low birth weight infants. J Pediatr. 2015;167:982–6. e2.
60. Majnemer A, Riley P, Shevell M, Birnbaum R, Greenstone H, Coates AL. Severe bronchopulmonary dysplasia increases risk for later neurological and motor sequelae in preterm survivors. Dev Med Child Neurol. 2000;42:53–60.
61. Van Marter LJ, Kuban KC, Allred E, Bose C, Dammann O, O'Shea M, et al. Does bronchopulmonary dysplasia contribute to the occurrence of cerebral palsy among infants born before 28 weeks of gestation? Arch Dis Child Fetal Neonatal Ed. 2011;96:F20–9.

62. Laughon M, O'Shea MT, Allred EN, Bose C, Kuban K, Van Marter LJ, et al. Chronic lung disease and developmental delay at 2 years of age in children born before 28 weeks' gestation. Pediatrics. 2009;124:637–48.
63. Ambalavanan N, Walsh M, Bobashev G, Das A, Levine B, Carlo WA, et al. Intercenter differences in bronchopulmonary dysplasia or death among very low birth weight infants. Pediatrics. 2011;127:e106–16.
64. Beam KS, Aliaga S, Ahlfeld SK, Cohen-Wolkowiez M, Smith PB, Laughon MM. A systematic review of randomized controlled trials for the prevention of bronchopulmonary dysplasia in infants. J Perinatol. 2014;34:705–10.
65. Walsh M, Laptook A, Kazzi SN, Engle WA, Yao Q, Rasmussen M, et al. A cluster-randomized trial of benchmarking and multimodal quality improvement to improve rates of survival free of bronchopulmonary dysplasia for infants with birth weights of less than 1250 grams. Pediatrics. 2007;119:876–90.
66. Lapcharoensap W, Gage SC, Kan P, Profit J, Shaw GM, Gould JB, et al. Hospital variation and risk factors for bronchopulmonary dysplasia in a population-based cohort. JAMA Pediatr. 2015;169:e143676.
67. Been JV, Lugtenberg MJ, Smets E, van Schayck CP, Kramer BW, Mommers M, et al. Preterm birth and childhood wheezing disorders: a systematic review and meta-analysis. PLoS Med. 2014;11:e1001596.
68. Hibbs AM, Walsh MC, Martin RJ, Truog WE, Lorch SA, Alessandrini E, et al. One-year respiratory outcomes of preterm infants enrolled in the Nitric Oxide (to prevent) Chronic Lung Disease trial. J Pediatr. 2008;153(4):525–9.
69. Gage S, Kan P, Oehlert J, Gould JB, Stevenson DK, Shaw GM, et al. Determinants of chronic lung disease severity in the first year of life; a population based study. Pediatr Pulmonol. 2015;50:878–88.
70. Hoo AF, Gupta A, Lum S, Costeloe KL, Huertas-Ceballos A, Marlow N, et al. Impact of ethnicity and extreme prematurity on infant pulmonary function. Pediatr Pulmonol. 2014;49:679–87.
71. Doyle LW, Cheong JL, Burnett A, Roberts G, Lee KJ, Anderson PJ, et al. Biological and social influences on outcomes of extreme-preterm/low-birth weight adolescents. Pediatrics. 2015;136:e1513–20.

Structural and Functional Changes in the Preterm Lung

Shu Wu and Eduardo Bancalari

Abbreviations

BPD	Bronchopulmonary dysplasia
CPAP	Continuous positive airway pressure
CTGF	Connective tissue growth factor
COPD	Chronic obstructive pulmonary disease
DLco	Carbon monoxide diffusing capacity
FEV_1	Forced expiratory volume in 1 s
FEV_{75}	FEV at 75 % of expired FVC
FRC	Functional residual capacity
FVC	Forced vital capacity
HRCT	High-resolution computed tomography
IL-1β	Interleukin-1beta
IL-1RA	IL-1 receptor antagonist
RSV	Respiratory syncytial virus
RV	Residual volume
TGF-β	Transforming growth factor beta
Th1	T-helper cytokines 1
TTN	Transient tachypnea of newborn
VA	Alveolar volume
VO_{2max}	Oxygen uptake at maximal exercise
VEGF	Vascular endothelial growth factor

S. Wu, MD (✉)
Department of Pediatrics/Division of Neonatology, University of Miami School of Medicine,
Batchelor Children's Research Institute, Room 346, 1580 NW 10th Ave,
Miami, FL 33136, USA
e-mail: Swu2@med.miami.edu

E. Bancalari, MD
Department of Pediatrics/Division of Neonatology, University of Miami School of Medicine,
Mail Box R-131, Miami, FL 33136, USA
e-mail: ebancalari@miami.edu

© Springer International Publishing AG 2017
A.M. Hibbs, M. S. Muhlebach (eds.), *Respiratory Outcomes in Preterm Infants*,
Respiratory Medicine, DOI 10.1007/978-3-319-48835-6_5

Introduction

Over the last few decades, the survival of preterm infants has significantly increased with the improvements in neonatal intensive care and respiratory support [1–3]. The preterm infants, and particularly those born before 28 week of gestation, are at significant risk for developing bronchopulmonary dysplasia (BPD) [1–4]. BPD is the most common chronic pulmonary complication causing significant morbidity and mortality in this population. Multiple factors, such as lung immaturity, oxygen toxicity, mechanical ventilation, and prenatal or postnatal infections, contribute to the pathogenesis of BPD. Insults to an immature lung induced by these factors produce lung injury that is associated with inflammation, including accumulation of inflammatory cells with elevation of pro-inflammatory cytokines, production of reactive oxygen species, and edema, all of which may damage the alveolar/capillary unit [5]. Injury at early stages of development can disrupt alveolar and vascular development and induce tissue remodeling with interstitial fibrosis, all of which results in the pathological hallmarks of BPD [4]. Severe BPD is often complicated by vascular remodeling leading to pulmonary hypertension and right ventricular hypertrophy [6, 7].

Many BPD survivors are now well into their adulthood providing a better understanding on these long-term respiratory outcomes. Evidence from clinical data and research studies indicate that these BPD survivors can have persistent abnormalities in their lung structure, imaging results, and lung function [8, 9]. This population is at a greater risk for rehospitalizations due to respiratory illnesses, often being admitted into pediatric intensive care units [10]. It is also possible that BPD survivors may have a reduced ability to reach their peak potential in lung function that occurs at around 20 years of age and may have an accelerated decline in function with aging [8, 11].

This chapter provides a brief overview of normal lung developmental processes, BPD pathogenesis, and long-term respiratory outcomes including structural, radiographic, and functional perspectives, in preterm infants, particularly in those with BPD.

Part I: Stages of Lung Development

Because BPD is primarily a derangement of lung development, it is important to consider the normal processes of lung development to better understand the pathogenesis of BPD.

Human lung development begins as formation of airway primordia in the embryonic period and subsequently undergoes branching morphogenesis to form the conducting airway. This is followed by expansion of the terminal airways in combination with epithelial cell differentiation and vascular development to form the alveoli. Based on the histological appearances, lung development is classically divided into five overlapping stages: embryonic, pseudoglandular, cannalicular, saccular, and alveolar [12, 13].

Embryonic Stage

The embryonic stage of human lung development is from 4 to 7 weeks of gestation. At the beginning of this stage, the lung originates as the laryngotracheal groove from the ventral surface of the primitive foregut. The proximal portion of the laryngotracheal groove separates dorsoventrally from the primitive esophagus to form the tracheal rudiment, which gives rise to the left and right main stem bronchi by branching into the ventrolateral mesenchyme derived from the splanchnic mesoderm. Subsequently, the right main bronchus branches to form three lobar bronchi, and the left main bronchus branches to form two lobar bronchi, giving rise to the three lobar right lung and two lobar left lung [12, 13].

Pseudoglandular Stage

During the pseudoglandular stage (5–17 weeks of gestation), the airway epithelial tubules undergo reproducible, bilaterally asymmetrical, and stereotypical branching to form a tree-like structure which gives rise to 16 generations of conducting airways up to the level of terminal bronchioles. There is also proximal airway epithelial differentiation with the appearance of basal cells, goblet cells, pulmonary neuroendocrine cells, ciliated cells, and nonciliated columnar (Clara) cells. The surrounding mesenchymal cells differentiate into fibroblasts, myofibroblasts, smooth muscle cells, and chondrocytes to form muscle and cartilage around the proximal airways. The vascular growth is in close proximity to the airway branching during this stage. By the end of the pseudoglandular stage, the conducting airways and their accompanying pulmonary and bronchial arteries are developed into the pattern corresponding to that found in the adult lung [12, 13].

Cannalicular Stage

During the cannalicular stage (16–26 weeks of gestation), the terminal bronchioles continue to branch to form the final 7 generations of the respiratory tree that supply gas to the distal airspaces. The respiratory bronchioles branch out from the terminal bronchioles to form the acini, a process that is accompanied by increasing development of the capillary bed, the beginning of alveolar type II epithelial (AT II) cell differentiation to synthesize surfactant proteins, and the thinning of the surrounding mesenchymal tissues. The lung appears "canalized" as capillaries begin to arrange themselves around the airspaces and come into close apposition with the overlying epithelium. At sites of apposition, thinning of the epithelium occurs to form the first sites of the air-blood barrier. Thus, if a fetus is born at around 24 weeks of gestation, the end of the cannalicular stage, these primitive acini have the capacity to perform some degree of gas exchange with or without respiratory support [12, 13].

Saccular Stage

The saccular stage is from 24 to 36 weeks of gestation. During this stage, clusters of thin-walled saccules appear in the distal lung to form the alveolar ducts, the last generation of airways prior to the development of alveoli. Small mesenchymal ridges are developed on the saccule walls to form the initial stage of alveolar septation. The capillaries form a bilayer "double capillary network" within the relatively broad and cellular intersaccular septae. The AT II cells are further differentiated and become functionally mature with the ability to produce surfactant. Also, the alveolar type I epithelial (AT I) cells are differentiated from the AT II cells at sites apposing the capillaries for gas exchange. The interstitium between the air spaces becomes thinner as the result of decreased collagen fiber deposition. Furthermore, elastic fibers are deposited in the interstitium, which lays the foundation for subsequent septation and formation of alveoli [12, 13].

Alveolar Stage

During the alveolar stage (36 weeks of gestation to childhood), the saccules are subdivided by the ingrowth of ridges or crests known as secondary septae. The AT II and AT I cells continue to differentiate. Postnatally, the alveoli continue to multiply by increasing secondary septae. Between birth and adulthood, the alveolar surface area expands nearly 20-fold. Early in this stage, the capillary network is in a double pattern in the alveolar septae. Postnatally, with the process of alveolar septation and thinning of the primary septae, the matching capillary network undergoes a maturational process with the double capillary network fusing into a single layer to assume the form present in the adult lung. Thus, the capillary volume is increased by 35-fold from birth to adulthood [12, 13].

Part II: Pathogenesis of BPD

With its vast airway and alveolar epithelium open to the atmosphere, the newborn lung is at great risk for harmful environmental insults such as oxidative stress, physical forces, and infective agents. These environmental challenges place the lung under constant threat of injury, repair, and remodeling processes. The lungs of full-term neonates have a great ability to overcome various injuries, to mount the needed repair and remodeling processes, and ultimately to maintain and/or restore normal lung architecture and normal lung function. When premature delivery occurs, particularly between 24 and 28 weeks of gestation, the lungs of these preterm infants are in the late canalicular to early saccular stage. Alveolarization has not yet begun and surfactant production is minimal. These lungs are at great risk for injury and altered development leading to BPD.

Over the past four decades, due to the significant improvement of neonatal intensive care, introduction of exogenous surfactant therapy and advanced ventilator strategies, survival rates among extremely premature infants have markedly improved. Along with this, the incidence of BPD has also increased. The current definition of BPD is based on oxygen dependency or respiratory support at 36 weeks postmenstrual corrected age [4]. The present form of BPD is increasingly being recognized as a developmental arrest of the immature lung secondary to multiple antenatal and postnatal factors. Larger and simplified alveoli and decreased vascular growth are the key pathological features observed in the lungs of infants dying of BPD at present [14]. The combination of decreased vascular growth and excessive pulmonary vascular remodeling frequently leads to pulmonary hypertension which significantly contributes to the morbidity and mortality of these infants [6, 7].

Inflammatory injury triggered by prenatal and postnatal infections, oxygen toxicity or mechanical ventilation is recognized as central to the pathogenesis of BPD. Numerous clinical and experimental studies have demonstrated the critical role of inflammatory cytokines and chemokines in BPD development and progression [5, 15, 16]. There is an increasing recognition of the role of interleukin-1beta (IL-1β) in the pathogenesis of BPD. In clinical studies, increased levels of IL-1β in lung lavage of preterm infants correlate with increased BPD risk [17]. In experimental models of BPD, treatment with an IL-1 receptor antagonist (IL-1RA) prevents lung inflammation and injury in newborn mice that are exposed to perinatal inflammation and moderate postnatal hyperoxia similar to the double hit that is commonly experienced by preterm infants who are at risk for developing BPD [18]. Activated IL-1β is the end product of the assembly and activation of the inflammasome, a large molecular platform that triggers the activation of inflammatory caspases and processing of prointerleukin-1β [19]. It is now well established that these inflammasomes act as signaling platforms that can respond to a plethora of microbial products, as well as endogenous host products associated with cellular stress and damage, and they play a pivotal role in innate immunity. These multiprotein complexes contain a sensor protein (NLR) which upon activation by pathogen-associated molecular patterns or damage-associated molecular patterns, oligomerize, and recruit the adaptor protein ASC (apoptosis-related speck-like protein containing a caspase recruitment domain) and the cysteine protease procaspase-1, leading to the autocatalysis and activation of caspase-1. Active caspase-1 ultimately cleaves the precursor pro-inflammatory cytokines pro-IL-1β and pro-IL-8 into their mature secreted forms. Activation of inflammasome pathway also plays a critical role in the pathogenesis of adult pulmonary diseases [20]. A recent study has demonstrated a critical role of NLRP3 in the development of BPD by demonstrating that hyperoxia activates caspase-1 and IL-1β and induces lung inflammation in newborn mice, and blocking NLRP3 inflammasome or knockout of NLRP3 gene prevents these responses [21].

Experimental data also indicate that alterations of growth factors signaling pathways that regulate normal lung development may also play an important role in BPD pathogenesis. Although many growth factors have been shown to be involved in neonatal lung injury, transforming growth factor beta (TGF-β) and vascular endothelial growth factor (VEGF) are probably the two most important growth factors. Clinical studies have found that increased TGF-β concentrations in bronchoalveolar lavage fluid (BAL) of preterm infants or amniotic fluid of preterm deliveries are correlated with subsequent development of BPD [22, 23]. Preterm infants who subsequently developed BPD have lower VEGF concentration in their tracheal aspirates compared to those who did not develop BPD [24]. Expression of VEGF and VEGF receptor 1 is decreased in lung autopsy specimens from preterm infants dying with BPD, and this was correlated with decreased PECAM expression in alveolar capillary endothelial cells [25].

Recently, some of the newer growth factors have been shown to also play an important role in lung development and BPD. One of these factors is connective tissue growth factor (CTGF), a member of CCN family of multimodular and matricellular proteins [26]. Historically, CTGF is best known for its fibroproliferative effect and is implicated in various forms of adult lung fibrosis [27, 28]. Increasing evidence indicates that CTGF also plays an important role in BPD pathogenesis. The clinical association of CTGF with BPD is best established by studies demonstrating increased CTGF concentrations in bronchoalveolar lavage fluid from preterm infants developing BPD and increased CTGF expression in lung tissues of infants who died of BPD [29, 30]. Several studies have examined the potential role of CTGF in experimental BPD and demonstrated that increased CTGF expression is associated with chronic hyperoxia as well as mechanical ventilation induced lung injury in neonatal rodents [31–33]. Recent studies utilizing genetic gain of function have demonstrated that targeted overexpression of CTGF in AT II cells induces the pathological hallmarks of severe BPD, including decreased alveolar and vascular development, and increased vascular remodeling and pulmonary hypertension [34]. In contrast, in a hyperoxia-induced newborn rat model of BPD, administration of a CTGF neutralizing antibody improved alveolar and vascular development and decreased pulmonary vascular remodeling and pulmonary hypertension (Fig. 1) [30].

Part III: Long-Term Respiratory Outcomes of BPD Survivors

There is clear evidence that infants surviving with BPD have prolonged respiratory symptoms and persistent abnormalities in their lung structure and function that can persist into adulthood. While respiratory disease in adults is discussed in chapter "Sequelae of Prematurity: The Adolescent and Young Adult Patient", and the options for diagnostic modalities are discussed in chapter "Diagnostic Modalities: Pulmonary Function Testing and Imaging", this chapter will provide an overview of the respiratory symptomes, structural changes and functional abnormalities of patients born preterm.

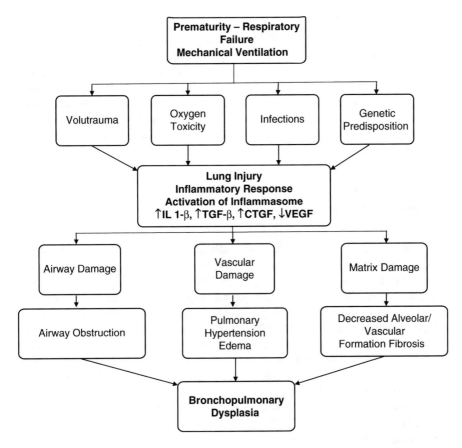

Fig. 1 Pathogenesis of BPD

Respiratory Symptoms

Many of the premature infants with severe BPD are oxygen dependent for months prior to being discharged home, although this oxygen dependency is rarely seen after 2 years of age [35, 36]. Preterm infants are at a greater risk for being rehospitalized over the first few years of life, secondary to respiratory illnesses such as airway obstruction and respiratory tract infections [10, 37]. Early preterm infants (<32 weeks of gestation) require significantly more chronic oxygen therapy, tracheostomy, and treatment for pulmonary hypertension as compared to late-preterm (32–35 weeks of gestation) and full-term infants while being admitted to pediatric intensive care units [10]. Throughout childhood, adolescence, and young adulthood, BPD survivors have persistent respiratory symptoms. A recent study showed that at school age, children with BPD have more respiratory symptoms including coughing, shortness of breath, wheezing, and activity restriction when compared to children born preterm without BPD and children born at term [38]. In addition, children in the BPD group are significantly more likely to be treated with asthma medications. Some of these respiratory symptoms persist into adulthood. In a systematic review that included 14 cohort studies on the respiratory outcome in adult BPD survivors, increased respiratory symptoms were reported in this population compared with their peers [39]. Adult BPD survivors are twice as likely to report wheezing and three times more likely to use asthma medication than preterm-born adults without BPD and term-born adult controls [40].

Structural Abnormalities

There is increasing evidence that BPD survivors have persistent lung structural abnormalities. Although the exact mechanisms contributing to these observations are not well established, early developmental disturbance and a sustained inflammatory process secondary to early insults such as oxygen toxicity and mechanical ventilation, as well as increased susceptibility to later infections or cigarette exposure are postulated as some of the underlying pathological causes.

Inflammation caused by mechanical forces, oxygen therapy and infections plays a key role in the development and progression of BPD. Some studies have indicated that the inflammatory process persists in BPD survivors. Increased levels of chemokines (interferon-gamma inducible protein-10, macrophage inflammatory protein-1α, Eotaxin, monocyte chemoattractant protein-1), growth factors (platelet-derived growth factor-bb, VEGF, fibroblast growth factor-basic, granulocyte macrophage colony-stimulating factor), T-helper cytokines 1 (Th1) (IL-12, interferon-γ), Th2 (IL-9, IL-13), Th17 (IL-6, IL-17) cytokines, and immunomodulatory mediators (IL-1RA and granulocyte colony-stimulating factor) were detected in nasopharyngeal aspirate of preterm infants at 1 year of age [41]. Increased neutrophils and IL-8 concentrations are also found in the sputum of school children who were born before 32 weeks of gestation [42]. These results suggest that there is a possible ongoing airway inflammatory process in infants with BPD that could contribute to long-lasting respiratory symptoms and functional disturbance.

Another marker of ongoing airway disease is increased oxidative stress that is linked to airway inflammation and remodeling. Evidence of increased oxidative stress in former preterm infants with or without BPD is also emerging. 8-isoprostane is a prostaglandin F2α isomer formed by arachidonic acid peroxidation, catalyzed by free radicals, i.e., a biomarker of lipid peroxidation and oxidative stress. In one particular study with adolescents born before 32 weeks of gestation with or without history of BPD and control subjects who were born at term, increased exhaled breath condensate 8-isoprostane concentrations were detected in the preterm groups with or without BPD [43]. In adult lung diseases, increased oxidative stress in the airways is associated with chronic obstructive pulmonary disease (COPD) [44].

This persistence of increased oxidative stress well into the adolescence of former premature infants may place them at a greater risk for future development of COPD.

The pathological hallmarks of BPD include decreased alveolarization and vascular growth that can lead to inhibition of alveolar–capillary membrane structural development and function (Fig. 2) [45]. Much of our understanding of BPD pathology is from histopathological studies in lung autopsy specimens from infants who died of BPD. In the presurfactant era, generalized emphysematous changes were found in mechanically ventilated preterm infants and particularly the extremely premature infants [46]. Studies in the postsurfactant era demonstrated similar emphysematous changes in preterm infants who died of BPD in infancy [14]. In addition, alveolar enlargement with blunted secondary septa, thickened alveolar–capillary membrane, and poor alveolar growth were also found in lungs of mechanical ventilated preterm infants [47].

Given the limited availability of such lung autopsy specimens in later BPD survivors, it is unclear whether these structural abnormalities of alveolar–capillary membrane persist into childhood, adolescence, and adulthood. However, studies assessing pulmonary gas exchange strongly support that there is a decreased alveolar–capillary membrane function in older BPD survivors. Multiple studies have

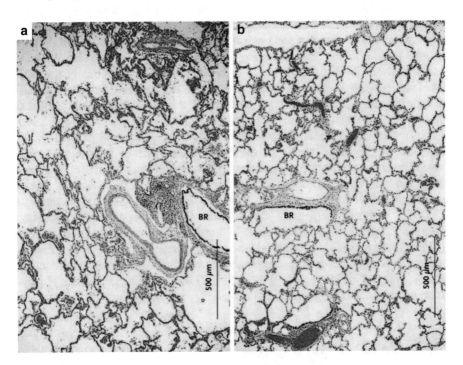

Fig. 2 (a) Lung autopsy from a 12-year-old with BPD who was born at 26 weeks shows abnormally large air spaces (*asterisk*) with simplified alveoli. A small bronchiole (BR) shows mild, chronic peribronchitis. (b) Lung section from an age-matched control shows normal alveolarization with numerous alveoli and a normal small bronchiole (BR) [45]

used carbon monoxide diffusing capacity (DLco) to assess alveolar–capillary membrane function in preterm survivors at childhood, adolescence, and adulthood [48–52]. These studies consistently demonstrated a lower diffusing capacity in the subjects with a history of BPD. Furthermore, in the EPICure study with 11-year pulmonary outcomes, it was found that children with a history of BPD not only had a decreased DLco but they also had a reduced exercise capacity, even though these children were clinically well [53]. Taken together, these evidence highlight the complexity and persistence of lung structural abnormalities that last well into the later life of preterm infants, particularly those survivors who had BPD. Furthermore, these structural alterations provide a pathological basis for the persistent respiratory symptoms and functional disturbance observed in this population.

Radiographic Abnormalities

Persistent radiographic abnormalities including multifocal hypoattenuated areas, linear and subpleural opacities, bronchial wall thickening, bullae, and bronchiectasis are commonly reported in BPD survivors [50, 54–57]. High-resolution computed tomography (HRCT) of the chest is a sensitive tool for assessing lung parenchyma abnormalities in survivors of preterm infants [50, 54, 55]. A population-based study showed that linear opacities and triangular subpleural opacities are the two most common chest CT abnormalities in BPD survivors at 10 and 18 years of age [57]. The hypoattenuated areas may reflect "obstructive emphysema," whereas the well-defined linear densities may reflect areas of atelectasis, all of which are radiographic abnormalities that correlate with the pathological hallmarks of the "Old" BPD. These results further support that there is persistent lung structural damage in the survivors of BPD. The clinical relevance of these chest CT abnormalities was investigated in several studies. A retrospective study reported that the presence of areas of decreased attenuation significantly correlated with the BPD severity [54]. Chest CT abnormalities are also associated with decreased lung function in long-term survivors of BPD. The increased subpleural opacities and limited linear opacities are associated with low functional residual capacity (FRC) and longer duration of oxygen therapy [58]. The linear/triangular opacities and hypoattenuated areas were significantly associated with decreased forced expiratory volume at 1 s (FEV_1) in BPD survivors at a mean age of 10–18 years [59]. In adult BPD survivors, the presence of emphysema on chest CT is inversely related to the FEV_1 z-score [50].

Abnormal Pulmonary Function

Children, adolescents, and adults born extremely or very preterm, with or without BPD tend to have persistent lung function abnormalities. Measurements of forced flows and volumes, respiratory system mechanics, lung volumes and ventilation homogeneity, and pulmonary gas exchange studies have been performed in these subjects. Common findings are airway obstruction, increased resistance and decreased compliance of the respiratory system, decreased alveolar–capillary diffusion capacity, and decreased exercise capacity.

Persistent airway obstruction is one of the most common pulmonary function abnormalities associated with preterm birth at various ages. In early childhood, studies have uniformly demonstrated that BPD survivors have decreased airflow [60–62]. A longitudinal study assessing pulmonary function in infants with BPD up to 3 years of age demonstrated significant airflow obstruction and modest restriction that tends to persist with time [63]. These abnormal findings were detected by spirometry using the raised volume rapid thoracoabdominal compression technique and by assessment of lung volume using plethysmography. Spirometry showed significant reductions in FEV in 0.5 s ($FEV_{0.5}$), FEV at 75 % of expired FVC (FEV_{75}), and FEV_{25-75}. Lung volume measurements demonstrated a mild elevation of residual volume (RV)/total lung capacity (TLC). These lung function abnormalities persisted at a mean postnatal age of almost 2 years. Other studies have also showed similar findings in infants with history of BPD [59–61]. In addition, infants with the most severe obstruction also demonstrate increased bronchodilator responsiveness [63]. These abnormal findings may be attributed to persistent airway injury and remodeling resulting from a combination of lung immaturity and injury caused by mechanical ventilation, oxygen therapy, and infection. Multiple studies have assessed pulmonary function at early infancy in healthy premature infants born at 30–34 weeks of gestation without neonatal respiratory complications and found persistently reduced airflow in the presence of normal lung volumes [64, 65]. These data suggest that prematurity alone could result in persistent airway obstruction in early infancy.

At school age, preterm-born infants, particularly those who had history of BPD, continue to have airway obstruction on pulmonary function tests [38, 53, 66–71]. The EPICure study assessed children's lung function at 11 years after extremely preterm birth (<25 weeks of gestation) and compared them to their full-term born classmates [53]. Even after correction for height, age, and sex using standardized z-scores, the premature born children have significantly worse baseline lung function, including FEV_1, FVC, FEV_1/FVC, and FEV_{25-75}. These differences are most prevalent in those with history of BPD. Children who were born with very low birth weight (≤1500 g) and without history of BPD also have lower FEV_1, high residual volume to TLC, high flow resistance, and higher rate of bronchial hyperreactivity as compared to the cohort of term controls [51, 66, 67]. These abnormalities are associated with low birth weight, long duration of oxygen therapy, low socioeconomic status, and exposure to animal dander [68]. In addition, prematurely born children also have a more frequent response to bronchodilator and lower post bronchodilator FEV_1, indicating some degree of fixed airway obstruction [38, 69, 70]. It is important to note that airway obstruction persists into adulthood in those born preterm as well [71]. A recent controlled population-based study assessed lung function from mid-childhood to adulthood after extreme preterm birth [72]. Two cohorts that represent the presurfactant era (born at 1982–1985) and the postsurfactant era (born at

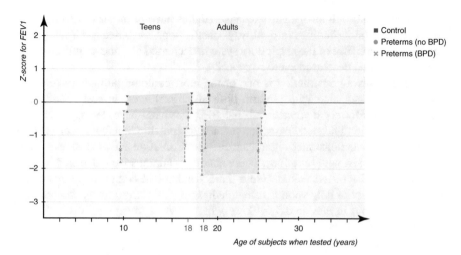

Fig. 3 Measurements of forced expiratory volume in 1 s (FEV1) in two birth cohorts born in 1991–1992 (Teens) and 1982–1985 (Adults) [72]

1991–1992) were included in this study. It was found that preterm-born cohorts, particularly those with history of BPD, have significantly lower FEV_1 and FEV_{25-75} at 10 and 18 and at 18 and 25 years of age, respectively. In addition, in subjects with moderate/severe BPD, the predicted FEV_1 barely exceeded 80 % that is considered a cut-off level required for the diagnosis of COPD (Fig. 3).

Besides airway obstruction and increased respiratory system resistance, preterm infants have decreased respiratory system compliance, particularly in those with moderate/severe BPD [73, 74]. This low compliance tends to normalize at 2 years of age, which may be related to increased alveolar formation. As discussed in the lung structural abnormalities section, children with history of BPD have reduced alveolar–capillary gas exchange as assessed by DLco and DLco to alveolar volume (DLco/VA). At 11 months of age, preterm infants with BPD exhibit lower DLco and DLco/VA, despite unchanged VA [75]. In older children, around 8 years of age, those born very preterm (≤32 weeks of gestation) also have lower DLco and DLco/VA compared to age-matched controls born at term [68]. Increasing length of oxygen therapy, but not gestational age or birth weight, is the strongest risk factor correlating negatively with the z-DLco/VA measurement [51].

Both normal and abnormal exercise capacities, reflected by oxygen uptake at maximal exercise (VO_{2max}) and 6-min walking distance, were reported in children, adolescents, and young adults born preterm [39, 71, 76–83]. Studies showed that adults who were born extremely premature in 1980s had reduced peak VO_2 [78, 84], while adolescents who were born in 1991–1992 had modestly reduced peak VO_2 and treadmill distance compared to a term-born control group [81]. However, the values were within normal range in most subjects. Children with history of BPD have a reduced 6-min walking distance as compared to preterm children without BPD and term controls [80]. However, this difference was not significant after adjusting for confounding factors including gender, body height, and weight. A study reported that at 10 years of age, children who were born extreme preterm have significantly lower peak VO_2 but normal 6 min walking distance when compared to full-term born subjects [77]. A systematic review and meta-analysis concluded that preterm-born subjects with or without BPD have lower exercise capacity than term-born control subjects [85]. The differences are small, and the BPD subjects are able to achieve near normal exercise capacity, but this may be at the expense of using more of their ventilatory reserve.

Taken together, the evidence is that long-term survivors of prematurity, particularly those born very premature and those with BPD, have chronic pulmonary function impairment, particularly airway obstruction and gas trapping in childhood, adolescence, and young adulthood. Those who had BPD have more compromised lung function, alveolar–capillary gas exchange, and excise capacity than those who did not have BPD early in life. The long-term functional impairment may be related to persistent structural abnormalities in the small airways and alveoli. These findings support the hypothesis that adults born preterm may be at increased risk for premature onset COPD.

Long-Term Respiratory Outcomes in Late-Preterm-Born Infants

Most of the studies of long-term respiratory outcomes have been conducted in extremely and very preterm-born infants. Late-preterm infants born between 34 and 36 weeks of gestation account for over 70 % of all preterm births and about 8 % of all birth in the United States [86, 87]. These infants were previously referred to as near-term infants, and until recently, they have been considered mature enough to be treated as term infants. The lungs of late-preterm infants are at the late saccular and beginning of alveolar stage. The surfactant production may still be relatively insufficient, and the antioxidant systems are not optimal. The alveolar structures are also immature with fewer alveoli and thicker alveolar septa. Delivery at this period can interrupt the critical developmental processes of alveolar formation and maturation and contribute to both short-term and long-term respiratory morbidities.

It is quite clear that infants born late preterm have increased short-term respiratory complications compared to term-born infants [88–90]. Late-preterm infants have an increased need for resuscitation at birth due to respiratory insufficiency [90]. A systematic review in 2011 demonstrated that they are more likely to need mechanical ventilation (RR, 4.9; 95 % CI, 2.8–8.6), nasal continuous positive airway pressure (RR, 9.8; 95 % CI, 5.1–18.8), and oxygen therapy (RR, 24.4; 95 % CI, 5.1–116.1) [91]. They also have a significant increase in respiratory distress syndrome (RR, 17.3; 95 % CI, 3.3–17.3), transient tachypnea of the newborn (RR, 7.5; 95 % CI, 5.0–11.2), and pneumonia (RR, 3.5; 95 % CI, 1.4–8.9). These respiratory complications are inversely associated with gestational age [90, 92]. Given that mechanical ventilation and oxygen therapy are important risk factors for lung injury in preterm infants, the increased need for these methods of support in the late-preterm infants may also put their relative immature lungs at a great risk for short-term injury and perhaps long-term injury. Furthermore, respiratory infections, whether acquired prenatally or postnatally, are recognized to be a risk factor in the pathogenesis of BPD. The increased rate of pneumonia in late-preterm infants not only highlights the risk for early lung disease but also indicates a risk factor for long-term lung injury.

Persistent respiratory symptoms are being recognized in children born late preterm. During infancy and early childhood, these children are at an increased risk for respiratory tract infections, particularly from respiratory syncytial virus (RSV) [93–97]. A retrospective study showed that infants <6 months of age who were born at 33–35 weeks of gestation have increased rates of hospitalization due to RSV infection compared to term-born infants [97]. The late-preterm infants with proven or probable RSV infection also have significant increases in all hospital utilization parameters and a mortality rate of 8.1 % compared to 1.6 % in the control cohort [98]. Exposure to smoke is recognized to be an important risk factor for severe RSV infection requiring hospitalization in late-preterm infants from smoking families [99]. In addition, outpatient RSV respiratory tract infection is higher, ranging from 183.3 to 245.7/1000 among late-preterm infants than in full-term infants (128.8 to 171.3/1000) [97]. There are also reports that infants and children who were born at 34–36 weeks of gestation, may be at increased risk for developing wheezing and asthma compared to those born at term [100, 101]. Persistent asthma and corticosteroids usage were found to be associated with late-preterm birth by 18 months of age [100]. At near school age, late-preterm-born children also experienced more wheezing and nocturnal cough, and received more inhaled steroids than term-born children [102]. A recent study reported that children at 3–5 years of age who were born late preterm have increased risks for asthma (18.4 %) and bronchitis (10.2 %) as compared to those born at term (asthma, 12.8 %; bronchitis, 8.3 %) [103]. It also found that needing oxygen therapy or mechanical ventilation during the neonatal period, or RSV infection, was associated with higher rates of asthma and bronchitis. There is little information on respiratory complications in adults who were born late preterm. A Swedish national cohort study reported no association between late-preterm birth and using asthma medication in young adults, age 25–35 years [104].

Some studies have assessed pulmonary function by spirometry in children born late preterm and found increased incidence of airway obstruction. One of the these studies showed that at around 11 years of age, children who were born at 34–36 weeks of gestation had a significantly higher increased residual volume and residual volume/TLC as compared to their siblings who were born at term [105]. In the Avon Longitudinal Study, reduced FEV_1/FVC and FEV_{25-75} were found at 8–9 years of age in children who were born at 33–34 weeks of gestation compared to term-born controls [106]. However, in follow-up studies at 14–17 years of age, measures of airway function were similar between late-preterm-born subjects and term-born subjects with the exception of FEV_{25-75}, suggesting that there are improvements in lung function during this period. Data are lacking in regard to whether late-preterm infants have other pulmonary function abnormalities, such as airway hyper responsiveness and decreased alveolar–capillary gas diffusion that are frequently observed in very preterm infants.

Conclusions

Significant progress has been made in the understanding of basic lung developmental processes, mechanisms of injury, and repair of the immature lung, as well as in the pathogenesis of BPD. In contrast, long-term respiratory outcomes in preterm infant survivors, particularly those with a history of BPD, who are now well into their adulthood, are less clear. There are still many unanswered questions as to why early injury to an immature lung has long-lasting negative impact on its structure and function. It is also unknown what the impact of early lung injury on lung function and overall health will be as these BPD survivors age to late adulthood. Thus, additional studies of these BPD survivors are needed to better understand the mechanisms contributing to the prolonged disruption of lung structure and respiratory dysfunction seen in these patients. It is also important that long-term follow-up and care by pulmonary specialists are provided to enhance the overall lung health of these survivors.

References

1. Bhandari A, Bhandari V. Pitfalls, problems, and progress in bronchopulmonary dysplasia. Pediatrics. 2009;123(6):1562–73.
2. Patel RM, Kandefer S, Walsh MC, Bell EF, Carlo WA, Laptook AR, et al. Causes and timing of death in extremely premature infants from 2000 through 2011. N Engl J Med. 2015;372(4):331–40.
3. Van Marter LJ. Epidemiology of bronchopulmonary dysplasia. Semin Fetal Neonatal Med. 2009;14(6):358–66.
4. Jobe AH, Bancalari E. Bronchopulmonary dysplasia. Am J Respir Crit Care Med. 2001;163(7):1723–9.
5. Wright CJ, Kirpalani H. Targeting inflammation to prevent bronchopulmonary dysplasia: can new insights be translated into therapies? Pediatrics. 2011;128(1):111–26.
6. Stenmark KR, Abman SH. Lung vascular development: implications for the pathogenesis of bronchopulmonary dysplasia. Annu Rev Physiol. 2005;67:623–61.
7. Thebaud B, Abman SH. Bronchopulmonary dysplasia: where have all the vessels gone? Roles of angiogenic growth factors in chronic lung disease. Am J Respir Crit Care Med. 2007;175(10):978–85.
8. Gibson A-M, Doyle LW. Respiratory outcomes for the tiniest or most immature infants. Semin Fetal Neonatal Med. 2014;19(2):105–11.
9. Greenough A. Long term respiratory outcomes of very premature birth (<32 weeks). Semin Fetal Neonatal Med. 2012;17(2):73–6.
10. Gunville CF, Sontag MK, Stratton KA, Ranade DJ, Abman SH, Mourani PM. Scope and impact of early and late preterm infants admitted to the PICU with respiratory illness. J Pediatr. 2010;157(2):209–14. e1.
11. Tager IB, Weiss ST, Rosner B, Speizer FE. Effect of parental cigarette smoking on the pulmonary function of children. Am J Epidemiol. 1979;110(1):15–26.
12. Wu S. Chapter 1 – Molecular bases for lung development, injury, and repair A2. In: Bancalari E, editor. The newborn lung: neonatology questions and controversies. 2 ed. Philadelphia: W.B. Saunders; 2012. p. 3–27.
13. Copland I, Post M. Lung development and fetal lung growth. Paediatr Respir Rev. 2004;5(Suppl A):S259–64.

14. Husain AN, Siddiqui NH, Stocker JT. Pathology of arrested acinar development in postsurfactant bronchopulmonary dysplasia. Hum Pathol. 1998;29(7):710–7.
15. Bose CL, Dammann CE, Laughon MM. Bronchopulmonary dysplasia and inflammatory biomarkers in the premature neonate. Arch Dis Child Fetal Neonatal Ed. 2008;93(6):F455–61.
16. Ambalavanan N, Carlo WA, D'Angio CT, McDonald SA, Das A, Schendel D, et al. Cytokines associated with bronchopulmonary dysplasia or death in extremely low birth weight infants. Pediatrics. 2009;123(4):1132–41.
17. Cayabyab RG, Jones CA, Kwong KY, Hendershott C, Lecart C, Minoo P, et al. Interleukin-1beta in the bronchoalveolar lavage fluid of premature neonates: a marker for maternal chorioamnionitis and predictor of adverse neonatal outcome. J Matern Fetal Neonatal Med. 2003;14(3):205–11.
18. Nold MF, Mangan NE, Rudloff I, Cho SX, Shariatian N, Samarasinghe TD, et al. Interleukin-1 receptor antagonist prevents murine bronchopulmonary dysplasia induced by perinatal inflammation and hyperoxia. Proc Natl Acad Sci U S A. 2013;110(35):14384–9.
19. Martinon F, Burns K, Tschopp J. The inflammasome: a molecular platform triggering activation of inflammatory caspases and processing of proIL-beta. Mol Cell. 2002;10(2):417–26.
20. Hosseinian N, Cho Y, Lockey RF, Kolliputi N. The role of the NLRP3 inflammasome in pulmonary diseases. Ther Adv Respir Dis. 2015;9(4):188–97.
21. Liao J, Kapadia VS, Brown LS, Cheong N, Longoria C, Mija D, et al. The NLRP3 inflammasome is critically involved in the development of bronchopulmonary dysplasia. Nat Commun. 2015;6:8977.
22. Kotecha S, Wangoo A, Silverman M, Shaw RJ. Increase in the concentration of transforming growth factor beta-1 in bronchoalveolar lavage fluid before development of chronic lung disease of prematurity. J Pediatr. 1996;128(4):464–9.
23. Ichiba H, Saito M, Yamano T. Amniotic fluid transforming growth factor-beta1 and the risk for the development of neonatal bronchopulmonary dysplasia. Neonatology. 2009;96(3):156–61.
24. Lassus P, Ristimaki A, Ylikorkala O, Viinikka L, Andersson S. Vascular endothelial growth factor in human preterm lung. Am J Respir Crit Care Med. 1999;159(5 Pt 1):1429–33.
25. Bhatt AJ, Pryhuber GS, Huyck H, Watkins RH, Metlay LA, Maniscalco WM. Disrupted pulmonary vasculature and decreased vascular endothelial growth factor, Flt-1, and TIE-2 in human infants dying with bronchopulmonary dysplasia. Am J Respir Crit Care Med. 2001;164(10 Pt 1):1971–80.
26. de Winter P, Leoni P, Abraham D. Connective tissue growth factor: structure-function relationships of a mosaic, multifunctional protein. Growth Factors. 2008;26(2):80–91.
27. Howell DC, Goldsack NR, Marshall RP, McAnulty RJ, Starke R, Purdy G, et al. Direct thrombin inhibition reduces lung collagen, accumulation, and connective tissue growth factor mRNA levels in bleomycin-induced pulmonary fibrosis. Am J Pathol. 2001;159(4):1383–95.
28. Bonniaud P, Martin G, Margetts PJ, Ask K, Robertson J, Gauldie J, et al. Connective tissue growth factor is crucial to inducing a profibrotic environment in "fibrosis-resistant" BALB/c mouse lungs. Am J Respir Cell Mol Biol. 2004;31(5):510–6.
29. Kambas K, Chrysanthopoulou A, Kourtzelis I, Skordala M, Mitroulis I, Rafail S, et al. Endothelin-1 signaling promotes fibrosis in vitro in a bronchopulmonary dysplasia model by activating the extrinsic coagulation cascade. J Immunol. 2011;186(11):6568–75.
30. Alapati D, Rong M, Chen S, Hehre D, Rodriguez MM, Lipson KE, et al. Connective tissue growth factor antibody therapy attenuates hyperoxia-induced lung injury in neonatal rats. Am J Respir Cell Mol Biol. 2011;45(6):1169–77.
31. Chen CM, Wang LF, Chou HC, Lang YD, Lai YP. Up-regulation of connective tissue growth factor in hyperoxia-induced lung fibrosis. Pediatr Res. 2007;62(2):128–33.
32. Wu S, Capasso L, Lessa A, Peng J, Kasisomayajula K, Rodriguez M, et al. High tidal volume ventilation activates Smad2 and upregulates expression of connective tissue growth factor in newborn rat lung. Pediatr Res. 2008;63(3):245–50.

33. Wallace MJ, Probyn ME, Zahra VA, Crossley K, Cole TJ, Davis PG, et al. Early biomarkers and potential mediators of ventilation-induced lung injury in very preterm lambs. Respir Res. 2009;10:19.

34. Chen S, Rong M, Platteau A, Hehre D, Smith H, Ruiz P, et al. CTGF disrupts alveolarization and induces pulmonary hypertension in neonatal mice: implication in the pathogenesis of severe bronchopulmonary dysplasia. Am J Physiol Lung Cell Mol Physiol. 2011;300(3):L330–40.

35. Greenough A, Alexander J, Burgess S, Chetcuti PA, Cox S, Lenney W, et al. Home oxygen status and rehospitalisation and primary care requirements of infants with chronic lung disease. Arch Dis Child. 2002;86(1):40–3.

36. Greenough A, Alexander J, Burgess S, Bytham J, Chetcuti PA, Hagan J, et al. Preschool healthcare utilisation related to home oxygen status. Arch Dis Child Fetal Neonatal Ed. 2006;91(5):F337–41.

37. Greenough A, Cox S, Alexander J, Lenney W, Turnbull F, Burgess S, et al. Health care utilisation of infants with chronic lung disease, related to hospitalisation for RSV infection. Arch Dis Child. 2001;85(6):463–8.

38. Vom Hove M, Prenzel F, Uhlig HH, Robel-Tillig E. Pulmonary outcome in former preterm, very low birth weight children with bronchopulmonary dysplasia: a case-control follow-up at school age. J Pediatr. 2014;164(1):40–5. e4.

39. Gough A, Spence D, Linden M, Halliday HL, McGarvey LP. General and respiratory health outcomes in adult survivors of bronchopulmonary dysplasia: a systematic review. Chest. 2012;141(6):1554–67.

40. Gough A, Linden MA, Spence D, Halliday HL, Patterson CC, McGarvey L. Executive functioning deficits in young adult survivors of bronchopulmonary dysplasia. Disabil Rehabil. 2015;37(21):1940–5.

41. Matias V, San Feliciano L, Fernandez JE, Lapena S, Garrido E, Ardura J, et al. Host and environmental factors influencing respiratory secretion of pro-wheezing biomarkers in preterm children. Pediatr Allergy Immunol. 2012;23(5):441–7.

42. Teig N, Allali M, Rieger C, Hamelmann E. Inflammatory markers in induced sputum of school children born before 32 completed weeks of gestation. J Pediatr. 2012;161(6):1085–90.

43. Filippone M, Bonetto G, Corradi M, Frigo AC, Baraldi E. Evidence of unexpected oxidative stress in airways of adolescents born very pre-term. Euro Respir J. 2012;40(5):1253–9.

44. Wiegman CH, Michaeloudes C, Haji G, Narang P, Clarke CJ, Russell KE, et al. Oxidative stress-induced mitochondrial dysfunction drives inflammation and airway smooth muscle remodeling in patients with chronic obstructive pulmonary disease. J Allergy Clin Immunol. 2015;136(3):769–80.

45. Cutz E, Chiasson D. Chronic Lung Disease after Premature Birth. Engl J Med. 2008;358:743–6.

46. Hislop AA, Wigglesworth JS, Desai R, Aber V. The effects of preterm delivery and mechanical ventilation on human lung growth. Early Hum Dev. 1987;15(3):147–64.

47. Thibeault DW, Mabry SM, Norberg M, Truog WE, Ekekezie II. Lung microvascular adaptation in infants with chronic lung disease. Biol Neonate. 2004;85(4):273–82.

48. Hakulinen AL, Jarvenpaa AL, Turpeinen M, Sovijarvi A. Diffusing capacity of the lung in school-aged children born very preterm, with and without bronchopulmonary dysplasia. Pediatr Pulmonol. 1996;21(6):353–60.

49. Satrell E, Roksund O, Thorsen E, Halvorsen T. Pulmonary gas transfer in children and adolescents born extremely preterm. Eur Respir J. 2013;42(6):1536–44.

50. Wong PM, Lees AN, Louw J, Lee FY, French N, Gain K, et al. Emphysema in young adult survivors of moderate-to-severe bronchopulmonary dysplasia. Eur Respor J. 2008;32(2):321–8.

51. Cazzato S, Ridolfi L, Bernardi F, Faldella G, Bertelli L. Lung function outcome at school age in very low birth weight children. Pediatr Pulmonol. 2013;48(8):830–7.

52. Ahlfeld SK, Conway SJ. Assessment of inhibited alveolar-capillary membrane structural development and function in bronchopulmonary dysplasia. Birth Defects Res A Clin Mol Teratol. 2014;100(3):168–79.
53. Bolton CE, Stocks J, Hennessy E, Cockcroft JR, Fawke J, Lum S, et al. The EPICure study: association between hemodynamics and lung function at 11 years after extremely preterm birth. J Pediatr. 2012;161(4):595–601. e2.
54. Tonson la Tour A, Spadola L, Sayegh Y, Combescure C, Pfister R, Argiroffo CB, et al. Chest CT in bronchopulmonary dysplasia: clinical and radiological correlations. Pediatr Pulmonol. 2013;48(7):693–8.
55. Wilson AC. What does imaging the chest tell us about bronchopulmonary dysplasia? Paediatr Respir Rev. 2010;11(3):158–61.
56. Oppenheim C, Mamou-Mani T, Sayegh N, de Blic J, Scheinmann P, Lallemand D. Bronchopulmonary dysplasia: value of CT in identifying pulmonary sequelae. AJR Am J Roentgenol. 1994;163(1):169–72.
57. Aukland SM, Halvorsen T, Fosse KR, Daltveit AK, Rosendahl K. High-resolution CT of the chest in children and young adults who were born prematurely: findings in a population-based study. Am J Roentgenol. 2006;187(4):1012–8.
58. Mahut B, De Blic J, Emond S, Benoist MR, Jarreau PH, Lacaze-Masmonteil T, et al. Chest computed tomography findings in bronchopulmonary dysplasia and correlation with lung function. Arch Dis Child Fetal Neonatal Ed. 2007;92(6):F459–64.
59. Aukland SM, Rosendahl K, Owens CM, Fosse KR, Eide GE, Halvorsen T. Neonatal bronchopulmonary dysplasia predicts abnormal pulmonary HRCT scans in long-term survivors of extreme preterm birth. Thorax. 2009;64(5):405–10.
60. Vrijlandt EJ, Boezen HM, Gerritsen J, Stremmelaar EF, Duiverman EJ. Respiratory health in prematurely born preschool children with and without bronchopulmonary dysplasia. J Pediatr. 2007;150(3):256–61.
61. Talmaciu I, Ren CL, Kolb SM, Hickey E, Panitch HB. Pulmonary function in technology-dependent children 2 years and older with bronchopulmonary dysplasia. Pediatr Pulmonol. 2002;33(3):181–8.
62. Kairamkonda VR, Richardson J, Subhedar N, Bridge PD, Shaw NJ. Lung function measurement in prematurely born preschool children with and without chronic lung disease. J Perinatol. 2008;28(3):199–204.
63. Filbrun AG, Popova AP, Linn MJ, McIntosh NA, Hershenson MB. Longitudinal measures of lung function in infants with bronchopulmonary dysplasia. Pediatr Pulmonol. 2011;46(4):369–75.
64. Friedrich L, Pitrez PM, Stein RT, Goldani M, Tepper R, Jones MH. Growth rate of lung function in healthy preterm infants. Am J Respir Crit Care Med. 2007;176(12):1269–73.
65. Hoo AF, Dezateux C, Henschen M, Costeloe K, Stocks J. Development of airway function in infancy after preterm delivery. J Pediatr. 2002;141(5):652–8.
66. Kotecha SJ, Edwards MO, Watkins WJ, Henderson AJ, Paranjothy S, Dunstan FD, et al. Effect of preterm birth on later FEV1: a systematic review and meta-analysis. Thorax. 2013;68(8):760–6.
67. Pelkonen AS, Hakulinen AL, Turpeinen M. Bronchial lability and responsiveness in school children born very preterm. Am J Respir Crit Care Med. 1997;156(4 Pt 1):1178–84.
68. Korhonen P, Laitinen J, Hyodynmaa E, Tammela O. Respiratory outcome in school-aged, very-low-birth-weight children in the surfactant era. Acta Paediatr. 2004;93(3):316–21.
69. Brostrom EB, Thunqvist P, Adenfelt G, Borling E, Katz-Salamon M. Obstructive lung disease in children with mild to severe BPD. Respir Med. 2010;104(3):362–70.
70. Baraldi E, Bonetto G, Zacchello F, Filippone M. Low exhaled nitric oxide in school-age children with bronchopulmonary dysplasia and airflow limitation. Am J Respir Crit Care Med. 2005;171(1):68–72.

71. Vrijlandt EJ, Gerritsen J, Boezen HM, Grevink RG, Duiverman EJ. Lung function and exercise capacity in young adults born prematurely. Am J Respir Crit Care Med. 2006;173(8):890–6.
72. Vollsaeter M, Roksund OD, Eide GE, Markestad T, Halvorsen T. Lung function after preterm birth: development from mid-childhood to adulthood. Thorax. 2013;68(8):767–76.
73. Baraldi E, Filippone M, Trevisanuto D, Zanardo V, Zacchello F. Pulmonary function until two years of life in infants with bronchopulmonary dysplasia. Am J Respir Crit Care Med. 1997;155 (1):149–55.
74. Thunqvist P, Gustafsson P, Norman M, Wickman M, Hallberg J. Lung function at 6 and 18 months after preterm birth in relation to severity of bronchopulmonary dysplasia. Pediatr Pulmonol. 2015;50(10):978–86.
75. Balinotti JE, Chakr VC, Tiller C, Kimmel R, Coates C, Kisling J, et al. Growth of lung parenchyma in infants and toddlers with chronic lung disease of infancy. Am J Respir Crit Care Med. 2010;181(10):1093–7.
76. Kilbride HW, Gelatt MC, Sabath RJ. Pulmonary function and exercise capacity for ELBW survivors in preadolescence: effect of neonatal chronic lung disease. J Pediatr. 2003;143(4):488–93.
77. Smith LJ, van Asperen PP, McKay KO, Selvadurai H, Fitzgerald DA. Reduced exercise capacity in children born very preterm. Pediatrics. 2008;122(2):e287–93.
78. Clemm H, Roksund O, Thorsen E, Eide GE, Markestad T, Halvorsen T. Aerobic capacity and exercise performance in young people born extremely preterm. Pediatrics. 2012;129(1):e97–e105.
79. Kathegesu E, Beucher J, Daniel V, Guillot S, Lefeuvre S, Deneuville E, et al. Respiratory outcome of bronchopulmonary dysplasia in school-age children. Arch Pediatr. 2016;23(4):325–32.
80. Praprotnik M, Stucin Gantar I, Lucovnik M, Avcin T, Krivec U. Respiratory morbidity, lung function and fitness assessment after bronchopulmonary dysplasia. J Perinatol. 2015;35(12):1037–42.
81. Clemm HH, Vollsaeter M, Roksund OD, Markestad T, Halvorsen T. Adolescents who were born extremely preterm demonstrate modest decreases in exercise capacity. Acta Paediatr. 2015;104(11):1174–81.
82. Farrell ET, Bates ML, Pegelow DF, Palta M, Eickhoff JC, O'Brien MJ, et al. Pulmonary Gas Exchange and Exercise Capacity in Adults Born Preterm. Ann Am Thorac Soc. 2015;12(8):1130–7.
83. Tsopanoglou SP, Davidson J, Goulart AL, Barros MC, dos Santos AM. Functional capacity during exercise in very-low-birth-weight premature children. Pediatr Pulmonol. 2014;49(1):91–8.
84. Clemm HH, Vollsaeter M, Roksund OD, Eide GE, Markestad T, Halvorsen T. Exercise capacity after extremely preterm birth. Development from adolescence to adulthood. Ann Am Thorac Soc. 2014;11(4):537–45.
85. Edwards MO, Kotecha SJ, Lowe J, Watkins WJ, Henderson AJ, Kotecha S. Effect of preterm birth on exercise capacity: a systematic review and meta-analysis. Pediatr Pulmonol. 2015;50(3):293–301.
86. Davidoff MJ, Dias T, Damus K, Russell R, Bettegowda VR, Dolan S, et al. Changes in the gestational age distribution among U.S. singleton births: impact on rates of late preterm birth, 1992 to 2002. Semin Perinatol. 2006;30(1):8–15.
87. Martin JA, Hamilton BE, Sutton PD, Ventura SJ, Menacker F, Munson ML. Births: final data for 2002. Natl Vital Stat Rep. 2003;52(10):1–113.
88. Pike KC, Lucas JS. Respiratory consequences of late preterm birth. Paediatr Respir Rev. 2015;16(3):182–8.
89. Kotecha SJ, Dunstan FD, Kotecha S. Long term respiratory outcomes of late preterm-born infants. Semin Fetal Neonatal Med. 2012;17(2):77–81.

90. Hibbard JU, Wilkins I, Sun L, Gregory K, Haberman S, Hoffman M, et al. Respiratory morbidity in late preterm births. JAMA. 2010;304(4):419–25.
91. Teune MJ, Bakhuizen S, Gyamfi Bannerman C, Opmeer BC, van Kaam AH, van Wassenaer AG, et al. A systematic review of severe morbidity in infants born late preterm. Am J Obstet Gyn. 2011;205(4):374. e1-9.
92. Celik IH, Demirel G, Canpolat FE, Dilmen U. A common problem for neonatal intensive care units: late preterm infants, a prospective study with term controls in a large perinatal center. J Matern Fetal Neonatal Med. 2013;26(5):459–62.
93. Resch B, Paes B. Are late preterm infants as susceptible to RSV infection as full term infants? Early Hum Dev. 2011;87(Suppl 1):S47–9.
94. Carbonell-Estrany X, Bont L, Doering G, Gouyon JB, Lanari M. Clinical relevance of prevention of respiratory syncytial virus lower respiratory tract infection in preterm infants born between 33 and 35 weeks gestational age. Eur J Clin Microbiol Infect Dis Off Publ Eur Soc Clin Microbiol. 2008;27(10):891–9.
95. Colin AA, McEvoy C, Castile RG. Respiratory morbidity and lung function in preterm infants of 32 to 36 weeks' gestational age. Pediatrics. 2010;126(1):115–28.
96. Meert K, Heidemann S, Abella B, Sarnaik A. Does prematurity alter the course of respiratory syncytial virus infection? Crit Care Med. 1990;18(12):1357–9.
97. Boyce TG, Mellen BG, Mitchel Jr EF, Wright PF, Griffin MR. Rates of hospitalization for respiratory syncytial virus infection among children in medicaid. J Pediatr. 2000;137(6):865–70.
98. Sampalis JS. Morbidity and mortality after RSV-associated hospitalizations among premature Canadian infants. J Pediatr. 2003;143(5 Suppl):S150–6.
99. Carbonell-Estrany X, Fullarton JR, Gooch KL, Vo PG, Figueras-Aloy J, Lanari M, et al. Effects of parental and household smoking on the risk of respiratory syncytial virus (RSV) hospitalisation in late-preterm infants and the potential impact of RSV prophylaxis. J Matern Fetal Neonatal Med. 2013;26(9):926–31.
100. Goyal NK, Fiks AG, Lorch SA. Association of late-preterm birth with asthma in young children: practice-based study. Pediatrics. 2011;128(4):e830–8.
101. Kugelman A, Colin AA. Late preterm infants: near term but still in a critical developmental time period. Pediatrics. 2013;132(4):741–51.
102. Vrijlandt EJ, Kerstjens JM, Duiverman EJ, Bos AF, Reijneveld SA. Moderately preterm children have more respiratory problems during their first 5 years of life than children born full term. Am J Respir Crit Care Med. 2013;187(11):1234–40.
103. Odibo IN, Bird TM, McKelvey SS, Sandlin A, Lowery C, Magann EF. Childhood respiratory morbidity after late preterm and early term delivery: a study of medicaid patients in South Carolina. Pediatr Perinat Epidemiol. 2016;30(1):67–75.
104. Crump C, Winkleby MA, Sundquist J, Sundquist K. Risk of asthma in young adults who were born preterm: a Swedish national cohort study. Pediatrics. 2011;127(4):e913–20.
105. Todisco T, de Benedictis FM, Iannacci L, Baglioni S, Eslami A, Todisco E, et al. Mild prematurity and respiratory functions. Eur J Pediatr. 1993;152(1):55–8.
106. Kotecha SJ, Watkins WJ, Paranjothy S, Dunstan FD, Henderson AJ, Kotecha S. Effect of late preterm birth on longitudinal lung spirometry in school age children and adolescents. Thorax. 2012;67(1):54–61.

Diagnostic Modalities: Pulmonary Function Testing and Imaging

A. Ioana Cristea, Clement L. Ren, and Stephanie D. Davis

Introduction

Premature birth is associated with adverse late pulmonary outcomes, most commonly manifested as reduced pulmonary function, recurrent wheeze, exercise limitation, and chronic cough [1–3]. The realization that insults to the developing lung may have lifelong effects, with respiratory disease burden noted later in life, has led to the need to develop sensitive methods of assessing respiratory function and structural disease during infancy as well as the preschool and school-age years.

Infant PFT Findings

A variety of infant PFT methods have been applied to the study of lung function in premature infants. Different techniques provide complementary information about lung function in this group of infants. However, some consistent findings have been reported regardless of the infant PFT method. In general, lung compliance is reduced in preterm infants, but improves over time, probably as a result of decreased chest wall compliance and lung growth and repair as the child ages. Airflow obstruction is the most consistent finding. Since development of the conducting airways is completed at the end of the pseudoglandular stage (16 weeks gestation), this finding suggests that premature birth affects future airway growth and development in later childhood.

A.I. Cristea (✉) • C.L. Ren • S.D. Davis
Department of Pediatrics, Section of Pediatric Pulmonology, Allergy and Sleep Medicine,
Riley Hospital for Children at Indiana University Health,
705 Riley Hospital Drive, ROC 4270, Indianapolis, IN 46202-5225, USA
e-mail: aicriste@iu.edu; sddavis3@iu.edu

© Springer International Publishing AG 2017
A.M. Hibbs, M. S. Muhlebach (eds.), *Respiratory Outcomes in Preterm Infants*,
Respiratory Medicine, DOI 10.1007/978-3-319-48835-6_6

Overview of Infant Pulmonary Function Testing

While children aged 5 years or older have been able to reliably perform pulmonary function tests via an active exhalation, assessing lung function testing during infancy has proven challenging. Despite challenges, which include the need for sedation and the lack of cooperation, infant lung function testing has been performed for more than 30 years to better understand lung development and disease. Guidelines for performing infant pulmonary function testing have been published through the American Thoracic Society and/or European Respiratory Society [4–9]. Furthermore, normative data have also been collected and reported [10–13].

Sedation typically with chloral hydrate is a requirement for most methods of measuring lung function in infants. Chloral hydrate has been shown to have an excellent safety record and has been administered to hundreds of infants worldwide for the purpose of lung function testing without serious adverse effects [14]. For the preterm infant, upper airway obstruction should be closely monitored given the risk of laryngomalacia and pharyngeal wall collapse in this population, and astute attention to oxygen saturation is indicated given the underlying lung disease.

Dynamic Measurements of Respiratory Mechanics

Dynamic respiratory mechanics can be measured during tidal breathing by placing an esophageal manometer. By using esophageal pressure as an estimate of intrapleural pressure and measuring pressure and flow at the mouth, airway resistance (sRaw) and lung compliance (C_L) are calculated. Studies performed in the 1980s (when the epidemiology of prematurity and BPD differed from today) showed that preterm infants have both increased sRaw and decreased C_L [15]. Furosemide therapy decreased resistance and increased compliance, demonstrating that short-term diuretic therapy can improve respiratory mechanics in BPD [16]. Although dynamic respiratory mechanics are abnormal in preterm infants, they did not differ in infants who required supplemental O_2 compared to those who did not [17], suggesting that hypoxemia may be more dependent upon ventilation inhomogeneity than respiratory mechanics.

Passive Expiratory Mechanics

Resistance and compliance can also be measured during passive exhalation by using a facemask with a balloon or shutter to occlude flow at the airway opening at end inspiration. This maneuver triggers the Hering-Breuer reflex in infants, leading to a passive exhalation. By measuring the pressure plateau generated by the occlusion

Table 1 Summary of respiratory function test studies in preterm infants and children by age and method (Please refer to text for details and citations)

Method	Results compared to full-term normal controls
Infants	
Dynamic and passive expiratory respiratory mechanics	Increased resistance Decreased compliance [15, 18, 19]
Tidal breathing measurements	Tpef/Te decreased [20, 21] 　Lower Tpef/Te in infants with BPD compared to those without BPD [24] Elevated PA [25, 26] 　PA not different between infants with and without BPD [26]
Forced expiratory flow measurements	Decreased VmaxFRC [27, 31–33] Decreased $FEV_{0.5}$ and FEF_{75} [28, 29]
Lung volume measurement	FRC decreased or normal in preterm infants [36–39]
Diffusion capacity	Decreased DLCO [42, 43]
Ventilation inhomogeneity	LCI – not a sensitive index to discriminate disease in preterm infants compared to term infants [24, 40]
Preschool age	
Interrupter resistance	Increased Rint 　Higher Rint in children with a history of severe BPD [49–51]
Forced oscillometry	Increased resistance Decreased low-frequency reactance Lung function is worse in children with a history of BPD [51, 53]
Older children and adults	
Spirometry	Decreased [2, 51–64] 　FVC 　FEV_1 　$FEF_{25–75}$
Lung volumes	Increased RV Increased RV/TLC [63, 65–68]
Diffusion capacity	Decreased DLCO in children and adults [64, 65, 69]

Abbreviations: BPD bronchopulmonary dysplasia, *DLCO* carbon monoxide lung diffusion capacity, $FEV_{0.5}$ forced expiratory volume in 0.5 s, FEF_{75} forced expiratory flow, 75 %, FEV_1 forced expiratory volume in 1 s, $FEF_{25–75}$ forced expiratory flow, 25–75 %, *FRC* functional residual capacity, *FVC* forced vital capacity, *LCI* lung clearance index, *PA* phase angle, *Rint* interrupter resistance, *RV* residual volume, *Tpef/Te* time to peak expiratory flow over total expiratory time, *TLC* total lung capacity, *VmaxFRC* the maximal flow at functional residual capacity

and expiratory flow and volume, the expiratory time constant, compliance, and resistance can be determined. Similar to dynamic measurements, studies of passive expiratory mechanics in preterm infants also have shown evidence of increased resistance and decreased compliance (Table 1). These measures can improve during the first year of life [18], although it remains uncertain whether normal function will be achieved in these preterm infants (Fig. 1) [19].

Fig. 1 Plethysmography maneuver being performed during infant pulmonary function testing

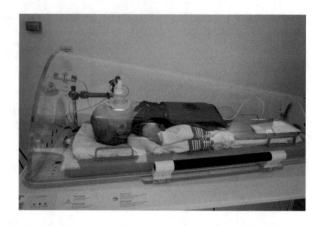

Tidal Breathing Measurements

Tidal breathing analysis can be performed using a mask with pneumotachometer or using respiratory inductance plethysmography (RIP). With the former method, the primary measure of interest has been the ratio of the time to peak expiratory flow over total expiratory time (Tpef/Te). Tpef/Te has been shown to be decreased in obstructive lung disease [20, 21]. In term infants, a low Tpef/Te is predictive of wheezing in the first year of life [22] and asthma at 10 years [23]. Preterm infants demonstrate lower Tpef/Te, and infants with BPD have lower Tpef/Te compared to those without BPD [24]. However, measurement of Tpef/Te does not add to the ability to predict respiratory disease in the first year of life [24].

RIP can be used to measure the asynchrony between thoracic and abdominal motion during tidal breathing. Healthy infants demonstrate remarkable synchrony, but in the setting of airway obstruction or decreased lung compliance, thoracoabdominal asynchrony increases. The phase angle (PA) is a quantitative measure of thoracoabdominal asynchrony that ranges from 0 (no asynchrony at all) to 180° (paradoxical breathing). Preterm infants have an elevated PA [25, 26], and PA correlates with measures of lung elastance and compliance [25]. However, PA does not differ between infants with and without BPD [26].

Forced Expiratory Flows

Early studies of forced expiratory flows (FEF) in preterm infants utilized the rapid thoracoabdominal compression (RTC) technique, where expiratory flow is generated by rapidly inflating a vest around the chest and abdomen at end inspiration of the tidal breath, and the maximal flow at functional residual capacity (VmaxFRC) is measured. Studies have shown that VmaxFRC is consistently lower in preterm infants compared to healthy term infants (Table 1). In one small study of children with moderate to severe BPD, VmaxFRC at 24 months correlated with FEV_1 and FEF_{25-75} in school-age years, indicating a lack of "catch-up" growth [27].

A major disadvantage of the RTC technique is that FRC is unstable in infants, leading to variability in VmaxFRC. With the raised volume RTC (RVRTC) technique, the infant's lungs are inflated to 30 cm H_2O, which is near total lung capacity. This allows generation of flows across a larger lung volume, replicating adult-type spirometry. Over time, the RVRTC technique has supplanted the RTC or partial flow-volume method, and most recent studies of preterm infants have employed this method. As with VmaxFRC, RVRTC measures such as the forced expiratory volume in 0.5 s ($FEV_{0.5}$) and FEF at 75 % FVC (FEF_{75}) are also reduced in preterm infants. Using the RVRTC technique, the degree of obstruction has been reported to be more severe in BPD compared to non-BPD infants; [28] however, in contrast, others have reported that BPD is not associated with decreased forced expiratory flows [29]. Furthermore, infants with better somatic growth during the first 1–2 years of life were reported to have higher forced expiratory flows compared to those with poorer growth [30].

Airway function may even deteriorate during the first year of life in infants with BPD [31, 32], probably reflecting the coupled effects of an unresolved lung injury plus the developmental interferences related to prematurity itself, at a time when the infant's respiratory system is growing rapidly [33]. Similar airway function abnormalities have also been reported in preterm infants without BPD, underscoring the important influence of prematurity on developmental changes in the lung [34, 35].

Lung Volume Measurements

Similar to adult PFTs, infant lung volumes can be measured using gas dilution techniques or body plethysmography. The former can be done using gas washout techniques with either an inert tracer gas such as helium (He) or sulfur hexafluoride (SF_6) or washing out the resident nitrogen (N_2) in the lungs. With body plethysmography, the infant tidal breathes against a closed valve or balloon, generating the pressure swings needed to apply Boyle's law. FRC is normal or even low in infants with BPD compared to healthy full-term controls during early infancy (36–42 weeks postmenstrual age), probably as a result of decreased lung compliance in the setting of a compliant chest wall [36]. However, over time, as lung repair occurs and the chest wall becomes stiffer, FRC tends to increase, consistent with an obstructive pattern [18]. Some studies did not detect any significant differences in FRC when comparing "healthy" term and preterm infants [37], or when relating results from healthy preterm infants to published reference equations for FRCHe [38]. In contrast, Hjalmarson and Sandberg reported significantly reduced FRCN2 in healthy preterm infants compared to term neonates (data only normalized for weight at test) [39]. In summary, in young preterm infants, FRC has been reported to be low or normal; these differences can be attributed to variations in methods and subject characteristics between these studies.

Measurements of Ventilation Homogeneity

The multiple breath washout technique assesses ventilation homogeneity. The lung clearance index (LCI) represents the number of tidal breaths needed to completely wash out either the resident N_2 gas or a tracer gas to 1/40th of its original concentration. In the preterm population, LCI is not a sensitive index to discriminate disease in preterm infants compared to term infants [24, 40], as opposed to other obstructive lung diseases, such as cystic fibrosis.

Diffusion Capacity

The diffusion capacity of the lung to carbon monoxide (DLCO) can be measured in infants; however, the methodology is technically challenging, not commercially available, and requires analysis of $C^{18}O$ with a mass spectrometer, which makes the measurements expensive. The two components of DLCO, the pulmonary membrane-diffusing capacity (DM) and the pulmonary capillary blood volume (VC), can be determined by measuring DLCO under conditions of room air and high inspired oxygen [41]. Infants with BPD demonstrate decreased DLCO but normal alveolar volume (VA) when compared to full-term controls, adjusting for race, gender, body length, and corrected age [42]. In addition, both DM and VC are lower in infants with BPD compared with infants born at term [43]. These in vivo physiological findings are consistent with pathological autopsy reports with impaired alveolar development with larger, but fewer alveoli and decreased pulmonary capillary density [44–47]. In contrast with infants with BPD, infants born prematurely without BPD had higher DLCO than full-term subjects, after adjusting for body length, gender, and race, suggesting that prematurity per se does not impair lung parenchymal development [48].

Lung Function in Preschool Aged Preterm Children

Recommendations for conducting preschool lung function testing have been endorsed by the American Thoracic Society and European Respiratory Society [49]. Obtaining PFT data from the preschool population (i.e., ages 3–5 years) presents a special challenge. They are too old for the RVRTC technique, but performing the voluntary breathing maneuvers needed for spirometry, body plethysmography, or DLCO requires cooperation, which proves challenging in this age group. There are some preschool PFT methods that require less cooperation (tidal breathing techniques) than spirometry that have been used to study lung function in preschool preterm children.

With the interrupter technique, children breathe through a mouthpiece or mask, and passive expiratory flow is briefly occluded with a balloon or shutter for 100 ms. By measuring flow just prior to the occlusion (V') and the resultant pressure plateau (Pplat), the interrupter resistance (Rint) can be calculated using the equation Rint = Pplat/V'. Rint reflects airway resistance, although it is not a direct measure. Rint is elevated in preterm children compared to full-term ones, and children with a history of severe BPD have higher Rint than other preterm children [49–51].

Another PFT technique that has been used in studies of preschool children is forced oscillometry (FO), which measures the total respiratory system impedance (Zrs) across a spectrum of oscillation frequencies [52]. Zrs is composed of resistance (R) and reactance (X). At lower frequencies, the latter reflects the viscoelastic forces of the lung. Several studies using FO have shown that preschool preterm children have elevated R and decreased low-frequency X, therefore demonstrating that lung function is worse in children with a history of BPD [51, 53].

Lung Function in Older Children and Adults Born Prematurely

Many studies of lung function have been conducted in older children and adults born prematurely. Most of the information on long-term lung function in survivors of BPD has been derived from preterm infants born before surfactant treatment was available, or studies are limited to selected populations of children who had severe pulmonary disease as neonates. Study results often reflect the outcome for children with "old" BPD and may not reflect physiological findings in children who received modern neonatal care or who have "new" BPD [54].

Spirometry Results

Spirometric values reflecting airflow are consistently lower in survivors of BPD at any age compared to controls born at term; those with BPD have substantial airway obstruction and alveolar hyperinflation [2, 55–58]. In most studies [2, 57, 59, 60], the mean forced expiratory volume in 1 s (FEV_1) values in those with BPD range from normal to values indicative of significant airflow limitation, reflecting the heterogeneity in the functional expression of the disease. These data should be interpreted with caution, however, since they are not generally applicable to the whole population of survivors, and especially not to those with new BPD or mild neonatal pulmonary disease. Patients who were born prematurely but did not have BPD usually fare better [61], but they too may have airflow limitation at school age [2, 58, 59, 62] and into adolescence and adulthood [3, 63, 64].

Lung Volume Measurements

Air trapping has been reported in premature children with BPD [65–67] secondary to obstructive airway disease, impaired alveolarization, and/or abnormal lung growth or injury. In contrast, normal FRC has also been reported in former preterm adolescents with BPD [63]. The presence of residual lung function abnormalities, mainly airflow obstruction and progressive static hyperinflation, raise the question as to whether chronic lung disease of infancy may ultimately affect pulmonary aging, leading to the development of chronic obstructive pulmonary disease (COPD) [68].

Diffusion Capacity

DLCO in school-age children born prematurely has been noted to be impaired in several studies [64, 65]. The decrease of DLCO/Va may reflect a deficit in the alveolar number leading to increased airspace and a reduction in the gas exchange-surface area [69]. Due to the challenges to performing DLCO during infancy, there are no longitudinal studies tracking DLCO from infancy into childhood and adulthood.

Evolution of Lung Function Over Time in Preterm Children and Adults

The degree of airflow limitation in the first years of life also predicts later pulmonary function. In a small group of infants with severe BPD who were followed from birth, VmaxFRC at 2 years of age was closely related to FEV_1 at 8 years, suggesting tracking of lung function with time and negligible "catch-up" growth of the lung [27]. This finding highlights an irreversible early airway-remodeling process.

There are limited longitudinal outcome data in preterm children born in the post-surfactant era. Most studies demonstrate that lung function deficits persist into adulthood and do not worsen over time. This finding has been reported even in those with severe BPD requiring home ventilation [70]. Two small studies reported some improvement in airway obstruction [71] or lung hyperinflation [72] in adolescents with BPD. According to a meta-analysis and follow-up study, the adverse effects of prematurity on pulmonary function were still detectable in school-aged children prematurely born in comparison to sex-matched controls born at term [73]. On the other hand, Doyle et al. [63] reported that survivors of BPD may have a substantial decline in pulmonary function over time, on the basis of data from a large cohort with a birth weight of < 1500 g who were followed from 8 to 18 years of age [63]. Overall, most studies suggest that airway growth in preterm infants is maintained with somatic growth, but does not "catch up."

Summary

In summary, prematurity has a profound impact on lung development and growth, thereby leading to lung function deficits. Early in life, respiratory compliance is low. For some infants born prematurely, especially those with BPD, substantial airway obstruction persists into adolescence and young adulthood. This pulmonary derangement remains latent in many, but a reduced respiratory reserve could increase the risk of a COPD-like phenotype later in life. Studies suggest that airway growth in preterm infants is maintained with somatic growth, but does not "catch up."

Imaging Studies

Structural defects have been noted in infants and children born preterm; these structural defects have been assessed using a number of modalities including chest radiographs, chest computed tomography (CT), ultrashort echo time magnetic resonance imaging (UTE MRI), and hyperpolarized gas MRI.

Chest Radiograph

The chest radiograph (CXR) is the simplest and most widely available method for imaging preterm children. The original case description of BPD included CXR abnormalities such as linear fibrotic opacities and hyperexpanded regions of lung parenchyma [74], thereby leading to the bronchopulmonary dysplasia terminology describing radiological changes [74]. Several scoring systems were subsequently developed [75]. These severe changes on CXR are rarely seen in today's "new" BPD, and in general, CXRs in contemporary preterm cohorts demonstrate minimal abnormalities. The modern clinical diagnosis of BPD does not incorporate a radiological component and instead focuses on the clinically assessed need for supplemental oxygen. Although chest radiographs have the advantages of accessibility and simplicity, the modality is considered only marginally useful for diagnosis. While chest films may only provide limited information to guide care, this modality is performed routinely to assess progression of disease.

Chest Computed Tomography

Chest computed tomography (CT) provides more detailed imaging of the lung parenchyma and airways compared to CXR. CT images can be obtained during quiet breathing or at full inspiration. Expiratory images are useful when identifying air trapping. This includes the interpretation of mixed attenuation, where either the area of high attenuation can represent a parenchymal abnormality or a low attenuation can be due to air trapping. There are often indications of air trapping on inspiratory images, but expiratory images may identify air trapping not seen on inspiratory images in the same patient. Young or uncooperative children may need to be sedated due to the difficulty with interpreting images due to motion artifact, which can further be decreased using a controlled ventilation technique [76, 77].

Chest CT is considered the most sensitive imaging modality to detect structural abnormalities in patients with BPD [78]. Chest CT may provide insight into BPD pathophysiology; the early neonatal course may be predictive of later impairment noted on imaging [79]. Several CT protocols and scoring methods have been described over the last 30 years to characterize and quantify the structural abnormalities of preterm patients with BPD. Most of them assessed the clinical severity of BPD (mild, moderate, severe) and reported an increase in CT abnormalities within those with more severe BPD [79–85]. CT findings of BPD patients have been compared with control patients, which were either healthy term-born [81] or preterm without BPD [79, 86, 87]. These studies report higher or worse CT scores in those with BPD. In CTs of survivors of old BPD, persistent radiological abnormalities have been reported in a majority of patients [88]. Respiratory mechanical measurements and functional residual capacity during infancy have been reported to be associated with structural disease on chest CT; [85, 89] however, diffusing capacity and forced expiratory flows were reported to not correlate with the structural disease [81]. Furthermore, chest CT has been reported to be more sensitive to identifying disease during infancy in those with chronic lung disease of infancy compared to diffusing capacity and forced flows [81]. Wong et al. [90] described a definitive appearance of emphysema in a group of young adults with a history of moderate to severe old BPD, and the extent of emphysema on CT was inversely related to their FEV_1 z-scores. Aukland et al. [79] studied two cohorts of BPD survivors, one from 1982–1985 and the other from 1991–1992, using inspiratory and expiratory high-resolution CT images. Participants were evaluated at a mean age of 10 and 18 years. Abnormalities were reported on chest CT scans in 86 % of the participants; the majority of the findings were linear/triangular opacities. Although the CT scores were higher or worse in the older cohort, the difference between the two groups was

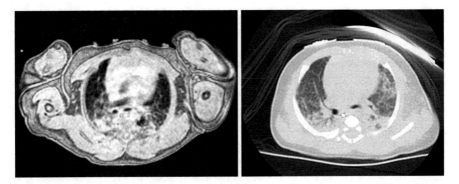

Fig. 2 Comparing magnetic resonance imaging (MRI) (*left*) and computed tomography (CT) (*right*) in a neonatal intensive care unit patient diagnosed with bronchopulmonary dysplasia (BPD) (Courtesy of Dr. Jason C. Woods, Center for Pulmonary Imaging Research, Cincinnati Children's Hospital Medical Center)

not statistically significant. A higher or worse HRCT score was associated with worse lung function as assessed through spirometric variables as well as the ratio of residual volume (RV) and total lung capacity (TLC). It is important to note that, to date, there are no validated and universally accepted CT scoring systems for quantifying structural changes [91]. Given the wide variations in the visual appearance of lung parenchyma observed in this population, the potential for imaging-based phenotyping is a possibility. These quantitative imaging biomarkers could be further refined to phenotype BPD and inform clinical care (Fig. 2) [92].

Magnetic Resonance Imaging

Magnetic resonance imaging (MRI) allows imaging to be performed without exposure to ionizing radiation. This is particularly important for imaging children who are more vulnerable to damage from radiation exposure and is appealing in those with chronic illness where longitudinal monitoring is desirable.

Traditional proton (1H) MRI of the lung has been challenging due to low parenchymal tissue density [93, 94], rapid signal decay [95, 96], and artifact from respiratory and cardiac motion [97]. However, there have been studies using proton MRI that have reported increased amount of water content in the lung tissue in infants with BPD compared to term infants [98, 99]. During fetal life, fluid is secreted into the lungs, whereas at term, secretions stop and reabsorption occurs rapidly during the latter part of labor; [100] this process is immature in the preterm, leading to higher residual lung fluid content [101]. More recently, investigators using a unique, specially designed small footprint MRI scanner with conventional MRI sequences have shown fibrosis, edema, and atelectasis in a small cohort of ($N = 6$) infants with BPD. Signal density was decreased in infants with severe BPD, which is suggestive of decreased alveolarization [102]. Another recent advance in MRI chest imaging has been the introduction of ultrashort echo time (UTE) sequences, which minimize the signal decay caused by a short transverse relaxation time in the lung, resulting in image quality that approaches that of chest CT (Fig. 2). UTE MRI has not been used to study preterm lung disease, but it has been successfully applied to the study of other lung diseases, such as chronic obstructive pulmonary disease and cystic fibrosis.

Hyperpolarized noble gases (e.g., 3He and 129Xe) have a strong MR signal, and can be used as a tracer gas to study ventilation in the lung. Furthermore, the apparent diffusion constant (ADC) of the gas can be used as a noninvasive method to estimate alveolar number, as the walls of alveoli, bronchioles, alveolar ducts, sacs, and other branches of the airway tree serve as obstacles to the path of diffusing 3He atoms and reduce 3He displacement. Altes and colleagues [103] performed 3He MRI in BPD survivors (mean age 9.7 years old) and reported that BPD survivors had more heterogeneous ADC maps than age-matched controls. In addition to focal areas of increased ADC, children with BPD had higher mean ADC values than controls, which is consistent with histological evidence of arrested lung development resulting in simplified alveoli. In another study, Narayanan and colleagues [104] reported that BPD survivors (age range of 10–14 years old) had similar alveolar size and numbers compared with full-term peers as determined with 3He ADC measurements, suggesting catch-up alveolarization in premature infants as they age, although this was limited to children who had mild to moderate BPD. This study highlights the ability of hyperpolarized gas ADC measurements to quantify lung microstructure and pediatric lung development.

Conclusions

Although chest radiograph will continue to be the first line of clinical radiological inquiry, especially for acute morbidity, the future of BPD imaging lies in nonionizing modalities, semiautomated, and fully automated quantitative techniques that allow for objective, longitudinal assessment, and the translation of these methods to predict outcomes and personalize patient care. Newer, low-dose CT protocols continue to lessen radiation burden, but for BPD survivors with chronic lung disease, balancing the benefits of longitudinal assessment with the risks of serial radiation exposure must be considered. Many of the major technological hurdles that historically limited the clinical utility of pulmonary MRI are resolving, and furthermore, these technologies are being extended to the youngest, most challenging patients to image.

References

1. Fawke J, Lum S, Kirkby J, et al. Lung function and respiratory symptoms at 11 years in children born extremely preterm: the EPICure study. Am J Respir Crit Care Med. 2010;182(2):237–45.

2. Pelkonen AS, Hakulinen AL, Turpeinen M. Bronchial lability and responsiveness in school children born very preterm. Am J Respir Crit Care Med. 1997;156(4 Pt 1):1178–84.
3. Halvorsen T, Skadberg BT, Eide GE, Roksund OD, Carlsen KH, Bakke P. Pulmonary outcome in adolescents of extreme preterm birth: a regional cohort study. Acta Paediatr. 2004;93(10):1294–300.
4. American Thoracic S, European Respiratory S. ATS/ERS statement: raised volume forced expirations in infants: guidelines for current practice. Am J Respir Crit Care Med. 2005;172(11):1463–71.
5. Sly P, Tepper R, Henschen M, Gappa M, Stocks J. Testing EATFoSfIRF. Tidal forced expirations. Eur Respir J. 2000;16(4):741–8.
6. Gappa M, Colin AA, Goetz I, Stocks J. Society EATFoSfIRFTERSAT. Passive respiratory mechanics: the occlusion techniques. Eur Respir J. 2001;17(1):141–8.
7. Stocks J, Godfrey S, Beardsmore C, Bar-Yishay E, Castile R, Society EATFoSfIRFTERSAT . Plethysmographic measurements of lung volume and airway resistance. ERS/ATS Task Force on Standards for Infant Respiratory Function Testing. European Respiratory Society/ American Thoracic Society. Eur Respir J. 2001;17(2):302–12.
8. Frey U, Stocks J, Coates A, Sly P, Bates J. Specifications for equipment used for infant pulmonary function testing. ERS/ATS task force on standards for infant respiratory function testing. European respiratory society/American thoracic society. Eur Respir J. 2000;16(4):731–40.
9. Morris MG, Gustafsson P, Tepper R, Gappa M, Stocks J. Testing EATFoSfIRF. The bias flow nitrogen washout technique for measuring the functional residual capacity in infants. ERS/ ATS Task Force on Standards for Infant Respiratory Function Testing. Eur Respir J. 2001;17(3):529–36.
10. Castile R, Filbrun D, Flucke R, Franklin W, McCoy K. Adult-type pulmonary function tests in infants without respiratory disease. Pediatr Pulmonol. 2000;30(3):215–27.
11. Jones M, Castile R, Davis S, et al. Forced expiratory flows and volumes in infants. Normative data and lung growth. Am J Respir Crit Care Med. 2000;161(2 Pt 1):353–9.
12. Lum S, Bountziouka V, Wade A, et al. New reference ranges for interpreting forced expiratory manoeuvres in infants and implications for clinical interpretation: a multicentre collaboration. Thorax. 2016;71(3):276–83.
13. Nguyen TTD, Hoo AF, Lum S, Wade A, Thia LP, Stocks J. New reference equations to improve interpretation of infant lung function. Pediatr Pulmonol. 2013;48(4):370–80.
14. Davis SD, Rosenfeld M, Kerby GS, et al. Multicenter evaluation of infant lung function tests as cystic fibrosis clinical trial endpoints. Am J Respir Crit Care Med. 2010;182(11):1387–97.
15. Kao LC, Durand DJ, Nickerson BG. Effects of inhaled metaproterenol and atropine on the pulmonary mechanics of infants with bronchopulmonary dysplasia. Pediatr Pulmonol. 1989;6(2):74–80.
16. Kao LC, Warburton D, Cheng MH, Cedeño C, Platzker AC, Keens TG. Effect of oral diuretics on pulmonary mechanics in infants with chronic bronchopulmonary dysplasia: results of a double-blind crossover sequential trial. Pediatrics. 1984;74(1):37–44.
17. Talmaciu I, Ren CL, Kolb SM, Hickey E, Panitch HB. Pulmonary function in technology-dependent children 2 years and older with bronchopulmonary dysplasia. Pediatr Pulmonol. Mar 2002;33(3):181–8.
18. Baraldi E, Filippone M, Trevisanuto D, Zanardo V, Zacchello F. Pulmonary function until two years of life in infants with bronchopulmonary dysplasia. Am J Respir Crit Care Med. 1997;155(1):149–55.
19. Mello RR, Silva KS, Costa AM, Ramos JR. Longitudinal assessment of the lung mechanics of very low birth weight preterm infants with and without bronchopulmonary dysplasia. Sao Paulo Med J. 2015;133(5):401–7.
20. Morris MJ, Lane DJ. Tidal expiratory flow patterns in airflow obstruction. Thorax. 1981;36(2):135–42.

21. Van der Ent C, Brackel H, Van der Laag J, Bogaard JM. Tidal breathing analysis as a measure of airway obstruction in children three years of age and older. Am J Respir Crit Care Med. 1996;153(4):1253–8.

22. Martinez FD, Morgan WJ, Wright AL, Holberg CJ, Taussig LM. Diminished lung function as a predisposing factor for wheezing respiratory illness in infants. N Engl J Med. 1988;319(17):1112–7.

23. Håland G, Carlsen KCL, Sandvik L, et al. Reduced lung function at birth and the risk of asthma at 10 years of age. N Engl J Med. 2006;355(16):1682–9.

24. Latzin P, Roth S, Thamrin C, et al. Lung volume, breathing pattern and ventilation inhomogeneity in preterm and term infants. PLoS One. 2009;4(2):e4635.

25. Allen JL, Wolfson MR, Mcdowell K, Shaffer TH. Thoracoabdominal asynchrony in Infants with. Am Rev Respir Dis. 1990;141:337–42.

26. Warren R, Horan S, Robertson P. Chest wall motion in preterm infants using respiratory inductive plethysmography. Eur Respir J. 1997;10(10):2295–300.

27. Filippone M, Sartor M, Zacchello F, Baraldi E. Flow limitation in infants with bronchopulmonary dysplasia and respiratory function at school age. Lancet. 2003;361(9359):753–4.

28. Sanchez-Solis M, Garcia-Marcos L, Bosch-Gimenez V, Perez-Fernandez V, Pastor-Vivero MD, Mondejar-Lopez P. Lung function among infants born preterm, with or without bronchopulmonary dysplasia. Pediatr Pulmonol. 2012;47(7):674–81.

29. Thunqvist P, Gustafsson P, Norman M, Wickman M, Hallberg J. Lung function at 6 and 18 months after preterm birth in relation to severity of bronchopulmonary dysplasia. Pediatr Pulmonol. 2015;50(10):978–86.

30. Filbrun AG, Popova AP, Linn MJ, McIntosh NA, Hershenson MB. Longitudinal measures of lung function in infants with bronchopulmonary dysplasia. Pediatr Pulmonol. 2011;46(4):369–75.

31. Hofhuis W, Huysman MWA, van der Wiel EC, et al. Worsening of V'maxFRC in infants with chronic lung disease in the first year of life: a more favorable outcome after high-frequency oscillation ventilation. Am J Respir Crit Care Med. 2002;166(12 Pt 1):1539–43.

32. Hoo A-F, Dezateux C, Henschen M, Costeloe K, Stocks J. Development of airway function in infancy after preterm delivery. J Pediatr. 2002;141(5):652–8.

33. Jobe AH. An unknown: lung growth and development after very preterm birth. Am J Respir Crit Care Med. 2002;166(12):1529–30.

34. Friedrich L, Pitrez PMC, Stein RT, Goldani M, Tepper R, Jones MH. Growth rate of lung function in healthy preterm infants. Am J Respir Crit Care Med. 2007;176(12):1269–73.

35. Friedrich L, Stein RT, Pitrez PM, Corso AL, Jones MH. Reduced lung function in healthy preterm infants in the first months of life. Am J Respir Crit Care Med. 2006;173(4):442–7.

36. Gerhardt T, Hehre D, Feller R, Reifenberg L, Bancalari E. Serial determination of pulmonary function in infants with chronic lung disease. J Pediatr. 1987;110(3):448–56.

37. Merth IT, de Winter JP, Borsboom GJ, Quanjer PH. Pulmonary function during the first year of life in healthy infants born prematurely. Eur Respir J. 1995;8(7):1141–7.

38. de Winter JP, Merth IT, Brand R, Quanjer PH. Functional residual capacity and static compliance during the first year in preterm infants treated with surfactant. Am J Perinatol. 2000;17(7):377–84.

39. Hjalmarson O, Sandberg K. Abnormal lung function in healthy preterm infants. Am J Respir Crit Care Med. 2002;165(1):83–7.

40. Hulskamp G, Lum S, Stocks J, et al. Association of prematurity, lung disease and body size with lung volume and ventilation inhomogeneity in unsedated neonates: a multicentre study. Thorax. 2009;64(3):240–5.

41. Roughton F, Forster R. Relative importance of diffusion and chemical reaction rates in determining rate of exchange of gases in the human lung, with special reference to true diffusing capacity of pulmonary membrane and volume of blood in the lung capillaries. J Appl Physiol. 1957;11(2):290–302.

42. Balinotti JE, Chakr VC, Tiller C, et al. Growth of lung parenchyma in infants and toddlers with chronic lung disease of infancy. Am J Respir Crit Care Med. 2010;181(10):1093–7.
43. Chang DV, Assaf SJ, Tiller CJ, Kisling JA, Tepper RS. Membrane and capillary components of lung diffusion in infants with bronchopulmonary dysplasia. Am J Respir Crit Care Med. 2016;193(7):767–71.
44. Husain AN, Siddiqui NH, Stocker JT. Pathology of arrested acinar development in postsurfactant bronchopulmonary dysplasia. Hum Pathol. 1998;29(7):710–7.
45. Coalson JJ. Pathology of new bronchopulmonary dysplasia. Paper presented at: seminars in neonatology 2003.
46. Sobonya RE, Logvinoff M, Taussig L, Theriault A. Morphometric analysis of the lung in prolonged bronchopulmonary dysplasia. Pediatr Res. 1982;16(11):969–72.
47. Hislop A, Wigglesworth J, Desai R, Aber V. The effects of preterm delivery and mechanical ventilation on human lung growth. Early Hum Dev. 1987;15(3):147–64.
48. Assaf SJ, Chang DV, Tiller CJ, et al. Lung parenchymal development in premature infants without bronchopulmonary dysplasia. Pediatr Pulmonol. 2015;50(12):1313–9.
49. Beydon N, Davis SD, Lombardi E, et al. An official American Thoracic Society/European Respiratory Society statement: pulmonary function testing in preschool children. Am J Respir Crit Care Med. 2007;175(12):1304–45.
50. Kairamkonda V, Richardson J, Subhedar N, Bridge P, Shaw N. Lung function measurement in prematurely born preschool children with and without chronic lung disease. J Perinatol. 2008;28(3):199–204.
51. Vrijlandt EJLE, Boezen HM, Gerritsen J, Stremmelaar EF, Duiverman EJ. Respiratory health in prematurely born preschool children with and without bronchopulmonary dysplasia. J Pediatr. 2007;150(3):256–61.
52. Udomittipong K, Sly PD, Patterson HJ, Gangell CL, Stick SM, Hall GL. Forced oscillations in the clinical setting in young children with neonatal lung disease. Eur Respir J. 2008;31(6):1292–9.
53. Malmberg L, Mieskonen S, Pelkonen A, Kari A, Sovijärvi AR, Turpeinen M. Lung function measured by the oscillometric method in prematurely born children with chronic lung disease. Eur Respir J. 2000;16(4):598–603.
54. Baraldi E, Filippone M. Chronic lung disease after premature birth. N Engl J Med. 2007;357(19):1946–55.
55. Gross SJ, Iannuzzi DM, Kveselis DA, Anbar RD. Effect of preterm birth on pulmonary function at school age: a prospective controlled study. J Pediatr. 1998;133(2):188–92.
56. Giacoia GP, Venkataraman PS, West-Wilson KI, Faulkner MJ. Follow-up of school-age children with bronchopulmonary dysplasia. J Pediatr. 1997;130(3):400–8.
57. Korhonen P, Laitinen J, HyoUdynmaa E, Tammela O. Respiratory outcome in school-aged, very-low-birth-weight children in the surfactant era. Acta Paediatr. 2004;93(3):316–21.
58. Jacob SV, Lands LC, Coates AL, et al. Exercise ability in survivors of severe bronchopulmonary dysplasia. Am J Respir Crit Care Med. 1997;155(6):1925–9.
59. Baraldi E, Bonetto G, Zacchello F, Filippone M. Low exhaled nitric oxide in school-age children with bronchopulmonary dysplasia and airflow limitation. Am J Respir Crit Care Med. 2005;171(1):68–72.
60. Doyle LW, Anderson P, Callanan C, et al. Respiratory function at age 8–9 years in extremely low birthweight/very preterm children born in Victoria in 1991–1992. Pediatr Pulmonol. 2006;41(6):570–6.
61. Doyle L, Cheung M, Ford G, Olinsky A, Davis N, Callanan C. Birth weight <1501 g and respiratory health at age 14. Arch Dis Child. 2001;84(1):40–4.
62. Kennedy JD, Edward LJ, Bates DJ, et al. Effects of birthweight and oxygen supplementation on lung function in late childhood in children of very low birth weight. Pediatr Pulmonol. 2000;30(1):32–40.

63. Doyle LW, Faber B, Callanan C, Freezer N, Ford GW, Davis NM. Bronchopulmonary dysplasia in very low birth weight subjects and lung function in late adolescence. Pediatrics. 2006;118(1):108–13.
64. Vrijlandt EJLE, Gerritsen J, Boezen HM, Grevink RG, Duiverman EJ. Lung function and exercise capacity in young adults born prematurely. Am J Respir Crit Care Med. 2006;173(8):890–6.
65. Kaplan E, Bar-Yishay E, Prais D, et al. Encouraging pulmonary outcome for surviving, neurologically intact, extremely premature infants in the postsurfactant era. Chest. 2012;142(3):725–33.
66. Lum S, Bush A, Stocks J. Clinical pulmonary function testing for children with bronchopulmonary dysplasia. Pediatr Allergy Immunol Pulmonol. 2011;24(2):77–88.
67. Cazzato S, Ridolfi L, Bernardi F, Faldella G, Bertelli L. Lung function outcome at school age in very low birth weight children. Pediatr Pulmonol. 2013;48(8):830–7.
68. Bush A. COPD: a pediatric disease. COPD: J Chron Obstruct Pulmon Dis. 2008;5(1):53–67.
69. Thébaud B, Abman SH. Bronchopulmonary dysplasia: where have all the vessels gone? Roles of angiogenic growth factors in chronic lung disease. Am J Respir Crit Care Med. 2007;175(10):978–85.
70. Cristea IA, Ackerman VL, Swigonski NL, Yu ZP, Slaven JE, Davis SD. Physiologic findings in children previously ventilator dependent at home due to bronchopulmonary dysplasia. Pediatr Pulmonol. 2015;50(11):1113–8.
71. Blayney M, Kerem E, Whyte H, O'Brodovich H. Bronchopulmonary dysplasia: improvement in lung function between 7 and 10 years of age. J Pediatr. 1991;118(2):201–6.
72. Koumbourlis AC, Motoyama EK, Mutich RL, Mallory GB, Walczak SA, Fertal K. Longitudinal follow-up of lung function from childhood to adolescence in prematurely born patients with neonatal chronic lung disease. Pediatr Pulmonol. 1996;21(1):28–34.
73. Ronkainen E, Dunder T, Peltoniemi O, Kaukola T, Marttila R, Hallman M. New BPD predicts lung function at school age: Follow-up study and meta-analysis. Pediatr Pulmonol. 2015;50(11):1090–8.
74. Northway Jr WH, Rosan RC, Porter DY. Pulmonary disease following respirator therapy of hyaline-membrane disease. Bronchopulmonary dysplasia. Engl J Med. 1967;276(7):357–68.
75. Toce SS, Farrell PM, Leavitt LA, Samuels DP, Edwards DK. Clinical and roentgenographic scoring systems for assessing bronchopulmonary dysplasia. Am J Dis Child. 1984;138(6):581–5.
76. Lucaya J, Garcia-Pena P, Herrera L, Enriquez G, Piqueras J. Expiratory chest CT in children. AJR Am J Roentgenol. 2000;174(1):235–41.
77. Long FR, Castile RG, Brody AS, et al. Lungs in infants and young children: improved thin-section CT with a noninvasive controlled-ventilation technique – initial experience. Radiology. 1999;212(2):588–93.
78. Oppenheim C. Bronchopulmonary dysplasia: value of CT in identifying pulmonary sequelae. Am J Roentgenol. 1994;163(1):4.
79. Aukland SM, Rosendahl K, Owens CM, Fosse KR, Eide GE, Halvorsen T. Neonatal bronchopulmonary dysplasia predicts abnormal pulmonary HRCT scans in long-term survivors of extreme preterm birth. Thorax. 2009;64(5):405–10.
80. Kubota J. Ultrafast CT scoring system for assessing bronchopulmonary dysplasia: reproducibility and clinical correlation. Radiat Med. 1998;16(3):8.
81. Sarria E. Computed tomography score and pulmonary function in infants with chronic lung disease of infancy. Eur Respir J. 2011;38(4):6.
82. Shin S. Bronchopulmonary dysplasia: new high resolution computed tomography scoring system and correlation between the high resolution computed tomography score and clinical severity. Korean J Radiol. 2013;14(2):10.

83. Tonson la Tour AMD, Spadola LMD, Sayegh YMD, et al. Chest CT in bronchopulmonary dysplasia: Clinical and radiological correlations. Pediatr Pulmonol. 2013;48(7):693–8.

84. Ochiai MM, Hikino SMP, Yabuuchi HMP, et al. A new scoring system for computed tomography of the chest for assessing the clinical status of bronchopulmonary dysplasia. J Pediatr. 2008;152(1):90–5. 95e91-95e93

85. Mahut B, De Blic J, Emond S, et al. Chest computed tomography findings in bronchopulmonary dysplasia and correlation with lung function. Arch Dis Child Fetal Neonatal Ed. 2007;92(6):F459–64.

86. Aukland SM, Halvorsen T, Fosse KR, Daltveit AK, Rosendahl K. High-resolution CT of the chest in children and young adults who were born prematurely: findings in a population-based study. AJR Am J Roentgenol. 2006;187(4):1012–8.

87. Boechat MCB, Mello RR, Silva KS, et al. A computed tomography scoring system to assess pulmonary disease among premature infants. Sao Paulo Med J. 2010;128(6):328–35.

88. Howling SJ, Northway Jr WH, Hansell DM, Moss RB, Ward S, Muller NL. Pulmonary sequelae of bronchopulmonary dysplasia survivors: high-resolution CT findings. AJR Am J Roentgenol. 2000;174(5):1323–6.

89. de Mello RR, Dutra MVP, Ramos JR, Daltro P, Boechat M, de Andrade Lopes JM. Lung mechanics and high-resolution computed tomography of the chest in very low birth weight premature infants. Sao Paulo Med J. 2003;121(4):167–72.

90. Wong PM, Lees AN, Louw J, et al. Emphysema in young adult survivors of moderate-to-severe bronchopulmonary dysplasia. Eur Respir J. 2008;32(2):321–8.

91. van Mastrigt EMD, Logie KP, Ciet PMD, et al. Lung CT imaging in patients with bronchopulmonary dysplasia: a systematic review. Pediatr Pulmonol. 2016;51(9):975–86.

92. Walkup LL, Roach DJ, Fleck RJ, Brody AS, Woods JC, Stein J. Quantitative CT Of bronchopulmonary dysplasia in the pediatric lung. C27 Neonat Pediatr Crit Care Am Thoracic Soc. 2015;A4090:A4090.

93. Muller NL. Computed tomography and magnetic resonance imaging: past, present and future. Eur Respir J Suppl. 2002;35:3s–12s.

94. Wielputz M, Kauczor H-U. MRI of the lung: state of the art. Diagn Interv Radiol. 2012;18(4):344–53.

95. Hatabu H, Alsop DC, Listerud J, Bonnet M, Gefter WB. T2* and proton density measurement of normal human lung parenchyma using submillisecond echo time gradient echo magnetic resonance imaging. Eur J Radiol. 1999;29(3):245–52.

96. Stock KW, Chen Q, Hatabu H, Edelman RR. Magnetic resonance T2* measurements of the normal human lung in vivo with ultra-short echo times. Magn Reson Imaging. 1999;17(7):997–1000.

97. Mulkern R, Haker S, Mamata H, et al. Lung parenchymal signal intensity in MRI: a technical review with educational aspirations regarding reversible versus irreversible transverse relaxation effects in common pulse sequences. Concep Magn Reson A. 2014;43(2):29–53.

98. Adams EW, Harrison MC, Counsell SJ, et al. Increased lung water and tissue damage in bronchopulmonary dysplasia. J Pediatr. 2004;145(4):503–7.

99. Adams EW, Counsell SJ, Hajnal JV, et al. Magnetic resonance imaging of lung water content and distribution in term and preterm infants. Am J Respir Crit Care Med. 2002;166(3):397–402.

100. Strang LB. Lung development: biological and clinical perspectives. Edited by Philip M. Farrell. Vol. I, Biochemistry and physiology. Pp. 407. £31.40, $47.50. Vol. II, Neonatal respiratory distress. Pp. 307. £24.80, $37.50. (Academic Press, 1982.). Q J Exp Physiol. 1984;69(1):212.

101. O'Brodovich HM. Immature epithelial Na+ channel expression is one of the pathogenetic mechanisms leading to human neonatal respiratory distress syndrome. Proc Assoc Am Physicians. 1996;108(5):345–55.

102. Walkup LL, Tkach JA, Higano NS, et al. Quantitative magnetic resonance imaging of bron-chopulmonary dysplasia in the neonatal intensive care unit environment. Am J Respir Crit Care Med. 2015;192(10):1215–22.
103. Altes TA, Mata J, de Lange EE, Brookeman JR, Mugler III JP. Assessment of lung develop-ment using hyperpolarized helium-3 diffusion MR imaging. J Magn Reson Imaging. 2006;24(6):1277–83.
104. Narayanan M, Beardsmore CS, Owers-Bradley J, et al. Catch-up alveolarization in ex-preterm children: evidence from (3)He magnetic resonance. Am J Respir Crit Care Med. 2013;187(10):1104–9.

Longer Term Sequelae of Prematurity: The Adolescent and Young Adult

Andrew Bush and Charlotte E. Bolton

Introduction

Preterm birth is an important public health problem, accounting for around 8 % of all deliveries [1], and the prevalence may be increasing (below). Worldwide, it is estimated that 15 million babies a year are born preterm [2], with more than one million babies dying as a consequence of prematurity. There are various different definitions of bronchopulmonary dysplasia (BPD, also used interchangeably with chronic lung disease of prematurity) which are current [3], for example, oxygen dependency at 36 weeks postconceptional age or 28 days after birth (which are not interchangeable), and the definition probably needs revisiting in the modern era. When comparing studies, it is important to be clear how BPD is defined. Allowing for this, estimates of BPD prevalence are 25 % if birth weight is less than 1.5 kg, and 68 % if gestational age is less than 26 weeks [4, 5].

AB was supported by the NIHR Respiratory Disease Biomedical Research Unit at the Royal Brompton and Harefield NHS Foundation Trust and Imperial College London.

A. Bush, MD, FRCP, FRCPCH, FERS (✉)
Paediatrics, Imperial College, London, UK

Paediatric Respirology, National Heart and Lung Institute, Royal Brompton Harefield NHS Foundation Trust, London, UK

Department of Paediatric Respiratory Medicine, Royal Brompton Hospital, Sydney Street, London SW3 6NP, UK
e-mail: a.bush@imperial.ac.uk

C. E. Bolton, BM BS, MD, FRCP
Respiratory Medicine, University of Nottingham, Clinical Sciences, City Hospital Campus, Hucknall road, Nottingham NG5 1PB, UK

Nottingham University Hospitals Trust, Clinical Sciences, City Hospital Campus, Hucknall road, Nottingham NG5 1PB, UK
charlotte.bolton@nottingham.ac.uk

© Springer International Publishing AG 2017
A.M. Hibbs, M. S. Muhlebach (eds.), *Respiratory Outcomes in Preterm Infants*,
Respiratory Medicine, DOI 10.1007/978-3-319-48835-6_7

Adult respiratory physicians will encounter preterm survivors in one of three contexts:

1. A known preterm survivor who has been followed up through childhood. This will usually mean that there have been substantial neurodevelopmental or other comorbidities which have driven follow-up, or really significant respiratory issues; those with subclinical respiratory issues will usually have been lost to follow-up in early childhood.
2. De novo presentation with, usually, airway disease in an adult who has not connected their present problems with previous preterm birth. We and others have shown that, unfortunately, adult physicians rarely even attempt to try to take a neonatal history [6, 7]. As we will show, this puts the patient at risk of wrong treatment (below).
3. Detection of abnormal spirometry in an asymptomatic adult as a result of pre-employment or other screening check; again, the adult patient and physician may have failed to appreciate the significance of their early life events.

The baby born preterm may have long-term sequelae for a number of interlocking reasons:

- The effects of prematurity itself.
- The effects of treatment of prematurity (especially supplemental oxygen, barotrauma, and systemic corticosteroids, but also delivery by caesarian section, which has long-term effects on the microbiome [8]). It should be noted that treatment of premature babies is a fast-moving area (below), and modern ventilatory strategies, for example, may lead to very different sequelae compared to older, now discontinued practices.
- The effects of the underlying cause of premature delivery (e.g., maternal smoking or hypertension [9, 10])
- The effects of low birth weight independent of prematurity (including small vs. appropriate for gestational age, SGA and AGA, respectively); these effects may be direct or indirect, via increase in susceptibility to respiratory infections which impacts adult lung function [11], a risk factor for later asthma [12].
- Genetic effects: a recent study, which will not be discussed further identified 258 genes associated with BPD [13].
- Conceivably, the effect of programming by events at a critical time period; there is some evidence for this in animal studies in particular (below).
- The indirect effect of premature delivery on the baby, operating through the mother. There is an extensive literature on the effects of maternal stress on fetal outcomes [14–16]; whether and to what extent this is operative in children born prematurely is unknown.

The sequelae of prematurity are thus both heterogeneous (multiple components, which are not all present in the same subject) and complex (components are not linearly related). The effects of all the above are impossible to untangle in a given individual; so, the reader is cautioned against attributing any particular long-term disease to prematurity per se. Furthermore, comparisons between populations and manuscripts mandate extreme caution. Much of the most striking temporal change is in approaches to treatment [17]. Neonatal ventilation has evolved from slow rate, high pressures (leading to the so-called "old BPD," predominantly but not exclusively an airway disease) to fast rate with low airway pressures and tidal volumes; antenatal steroids, and in particular the therapeutic use of surfactants, have also been transformative. Continuous positive airway pressure (CPAP) is being used increasingly to avoid intubation. These survivors have "new BPD" characterized more by impaired alveolar development. Neonatal resuscitation has also recently changed from a very aggressive approach of intubation and ensuring high oxygen saturation very rapidly, to allowing a much slower rise in oxygenation, which may further impact outcomes [18]. These changes in neonatal practice mean there is a time component to studies – it cannot be assumed that today's survivors will have the same respiratory issues when they reach their 20s as do today's adults, nor that the pioneering papers which first delineated long-term sequelae are relevant to today's survivors.

Nonetheless, preterm birth delineates a group at risk for respiratory disease in adolescence and adult life. Such consequences include increased respiratory morbidity; airflow obstruction (distal and large airway); parenchymal disease; impaired exercise performance; abnormal control of breathing; and pulmonary circulatory disease, all of which will be considered in this chapter, which updates recent reviews and meta-analyses [2, 19–22].

It is also important to be clear at what level prematurity is of clinical significance. There is ample evidence that even very late premature delivery has important long-term consequences. The Avon Longitudinal Study of Parents and Children (ALSPAC) showed that at age 8–9 years, reduction in spirometry in the 33–34 week gestation babies was the same as the 25–32 week gestation babies; and at 14–17 years, first second forced expired volume (FEV_1), forced expiratory flows between 25 and 75 % of vital capacity (FEF_{25-75}), and the ratio of FEV_1 and forced vital capacity (FVC) were all still reduced [23]. Studies relating asthma prevalence (usually defined rather simplistically as reimbursement for asthma medication or doctor-diagnosed asthma) to gestational age at delivery have shown an increased risk even in those born at 37–38 weeks' gestation [24–26]. The conclusion from these and other studies is that even those born just short of term, who require no neonatal intervention, are at risk for respiratory sequelae. Worryingly, preterm birth may be increasing [27], despite the improvements made by increasingly stringent tobacco legislation [28]. The consequences of this conclusion are (a) that despite the fact that we are doing better, and decrements in spirometry in BPD are less now than before [29], we will not abolish the long-term consequences of prematurity, no matter how treatment improves (and indeed prevalence may be increasing [2]; and (b) there is a larger population at risk than might be thought. The respiratory consequences of late premature birth have recently been reviewed [30].

The Big Picture: 2012 and 2015 Meta-analyses

Although there have been more reports since the publication of these meta-analyses [2, 19], the general conclusions remain the same. The 2012 report [19] found 14 studies (only eight being of high quality); all BPD survivors had more symptoms and impairment of lung function than their peers; five radiological studies reported persistent radiological changes; and three small studies suggested exercise impairment. The meta-analysis was updated in 2015 [2]. The conclusions of both meta-analyses have remained broadly unchallenged over time. Newer manuscripts and additional details from some older ones are discussed below.

Respiratory Symptoms and Morbidity

A number of studies report increased symptoms, in particular cough and wheeze, and respiratory morbidity in adult life. In the longest follow-up cohort in the modern era, BPD survivors' mean SD 24.1± 4 years, mean gestational age 27.1 + 2.1 weeks, birth weight 955 + 256 gm were twice as likely to report symptoms and three times as likely to use asthma medications compared with the term controls, and also had impaired quality of life and obstructive spirometry [31]. These patients were largely not treated with surfactant neonatally and did not have the benefits of antenatal steroids. Another study reported equivalent quality of life, but increased utilization of healthcare resources, in preterm survivors compared with controls; a diagnosis of asthma and pneumonia was more likely in the BPD group [32]. Overall, reports suggest that health-related quality of life is good in preterm survivors [33]. The use of asthma medications, confirming the findings of others [34], is particularly concerning, given the likely nature of the airway disease (below); the type of prescription short-acting β-2 agonists, which might be justified versus inhaled corticosteroids (which probably are not), was not discussed. Other studies have also reported increased respiratory symptoms [35, 36] and the purchase of asthma medications, in even early-term survivors, although prevalence usually declined with age [24–26]. There is an increased risk of hospitalization for respiratory disease in early adult life (age 18–27 years); the odds ratios for low birth weight (LBW, here defined as 1.5–2.5kg) were 1.34 (1.17–1.53), and for very low birth weight (VLBW, <1.5 kg) 1.83 (1.28–2.62) compared with term controls [37]. Worryingly, a Swedish study showed a strong inverse association between gestational age at birth and mortality in early (1–5 years) childhood, which disappeared until young adult life when it reappeared, even in those born 34–36 weeks (late preterm). Deaths were due to congenital anomalies and respiratory, endocrine, and cardiovascular disorders. The adjusted hazard ratio for adult mortality from respiratory disease was 0.85 (0.76–0.94 95 % CI) [38]. To summarize, there is a substantial burden of respiratory symptoms, morbidity, airway disease, and even early death, even in those with relatively modest degrees of prematurity and decrements in birth weight.

Airway Disease After Premature Delivery

Airway disease is typically most severe in "old" BPD. The assessment of airway disease in adult preterm survivors is best performed using the recently proposed framework, focusing on treatable clinical traits [39], and expected benefit of treatments, using the three domains of pulmonary, extrapulmonary, and behavioral and lifestyle issues. These are summarized in Table 1.

Normal Airway Development This topic is reviewed in detail in chapter "Structural and Functional Changes in the Preterm Lung" of this book and elsewhere [40, 41]. For normal lifelong lung health, airway caliber must be normal at birth; spirometry improves to a plateau at age 20–25 years, and thereafter declines with age. These changes are best described by Global Lung Initiative (GLI) equations [42]. The threshold for respiratory disability will be crossed prematurely if there is

Table 1 Deconstructing the respiratory sequelae of prematurity in adult life. Treatable traits are underlined

	Clinical traits	Treatment	Expected benefits of treatment
Pulmonary	– Fixed airflow obstruction – Variable airflow obstruction – Airway inflammation – Alveolar hypoplasia – Focal parenchymal defects	Bronchodilators Stop inappropriate ICS	Better lung function Reduce side effects
	– Reduced exercise performance	Exercise prescription or pulmonary rehabilitation	Well-being improved Prevent progression
	– Pulmonary hypertension – Sleep-disordered breathing – Abnormal control of breathing	Ensure normoxia CPAP if needed (rare) Ensure normoxia	Improved symptoms Prevent progression
Extrapulmonary (comorbidities)	– Neurological – reflux and aspiration – Abnormal swallow – Retinopathy – Bone disease – Renal disease	Rehabilitation services Reflux medication Thicken liquids or PEG	Better QoL Airway-protected Prevent pneumonia
Lifestyle	– Smoking – Pollution – Susceptibility to infection	Smoking cessation Avoidance Immunizations	Preservation of lung function (all traits)

Abbreviations: *CPAP* continuous positive airway pressure, *ICS* inhaled corticosteroids, *PEG* percutaneous endoscopic gastrostomy, *QoL* quality of life impairment at birth, suboptimal growth in childhood, or accelerated decline in adult life. The developmental track of airway disease of prematurity is not clear. There are no large prospective cohort studies of preterm survivors extending from birth into middle age. Although a series of overlapping large birth cohort studies (term babies) have shown that spirometry tracks from the preschool years into the sixth decade [43–45], with no evidence of catch-up growth, this may not be the case in preterm airways disease [46, 47]. Indeed, in one cohort, there was evidence of airflow obstruction at age 7–9 years, which was no longer present at age 20–22 years [36]. However, these were relatively large babies by modern standards, and these data are not totally reassuring.

Pulmonary As with any airway disease, deconstructing the components allows logical treatment; this is to be preferred to asking meaningless questions like "do BPD survivors have asthma?" – which is only interpretable if all concerned have a common definition of asthma. Survivors of prematurity generally have fixed and variable airflow obstruction, the latter of which is responsive to short-acting β-2 agonists [31, 46, 48, 49]. The severity of airflow obstruction varies between studies, with some, but by no means all, reporting significant airflow obstruction in adult BPD survivors [50]. The differences between studies likely reflect that different types of populations were studied. Generally, a greater extent and duration of neonatal intensive care predicts worse lung function long term, although there is considerable overlap between groups, and the relationship is not close. Although acute bronchodilator response to short-acting β-agonists, more peak flow variability and bronchial responsiveness to methacholine have all been reported, the pathophysiology of the variable airflow is unclear; despite fixed and variable airflow obstruction, the evidence is that these patients do not have airway inflammation; the underlying cause may be airway wall thickening and increased airway smooth muscle [51]. Alternatively, genetic factors predisposing to airway hyperresponsiveness may also contribute with other insults to the development of BPD. What is clear is that there is little evidence for ongoing airway inflammation in adult preterm survivors. Hence neither exhaled breath temperature nor exhaled nitric oxide (both indirect surrogates for airway inflammation) are elevated [52, 53], implying in this largely inhaled steroid naïve population that there is no eosinophilic, Type 2 inflammation. The logical corollary is that, unless there is a superposed component of atopic airways disease, inhaled corticosteroids should not be prescribed; and indeed, there was no benefit in one admittedly small trial [54]. One study using exhaled breath condensate showed increased oxidative stress(elevated exhaled breath condensate 8-isoprostane) in adolescent survivors, which, although the clinical significance is unclear, given there was no correlation with symptoms or spirometry [55]. A metabolomics approach also showed differences between BPD survivors and normals, also suggesting there may be ongoing airway abnormalities [56]. There are no studies on the airway microbiome or the cough reflex, and mucus hypersecretion is not generally a component of this airway disease. Finally, proximal airway disease should be considered, including tracheobronchomalacia, subglottic stenosis, and left vocal cord palsy secondary to surgery for patent arterial duct; this last is considered in more detail below.

Among the determinants of adult life lung function is birth weight [57]. In the wider population, low birth weight and low weight gain in the first 3 years of life were correlated with reductions in adulthood FEV_1, lung volumes and transfer factor (DLCO), but not the presence of airflow obstruction [58]. Other studies have suggested an inverse relationship between weight gain in the first year of life and accrual of lung function [59–61]. Excessive weight gain after age 5 years may by contrast have later adverse effects [61]. However, there may be an increased risk of developing asthma if early weight gain is excessive [62]. In one cohort, birth weight in the SGA, but not AGA babies was an important determinant of spirometry age 20–22 years [36].This is important, because frequently this information is not reported. The study also did not demonstrate a greater prevalence of bronchial hyper-responsiveness to methacholine in adult survivors, which was reassuring; however this was not confirmed in a more recent study of a more severely affected population [63]. Another group [64] reported airflow obstruction in VLBW survivors (here defined as birth weight <1.5 kg) irrespective of any neonatal complications, worse those with BPD. There was an adverse an effect of maternal smoking in pregnancy, most marked in BPD survivors, but no effect of growth patterns at any developmental stage. In the longest follow up population based cohort [65] the effects of birth weight gradually declined with age, likely because environmental factors became increasingly important determinants.

It has been suggested that the survivors of premature birth will represent a new cohort of COPD patients. There are only very limited data on the very long-term outcome of BPD. Such data as exist do not suggest an accelerated rate of decline [63], at least in the early 20s, although factors such as the presence of bronchial hyper-responsiveness suggest this is a high-risk population for accelerated decline. A cohort of more than 6000 adults born between 1925 and 1949, reported in 2013, showed that women but not men born before 32 weeks gestation had a hazard ratio for any obstructive airway disease of 2.77 (95 % CI 1.39–1.54), with both low birth weight and prematurity being significant risk factors [66]. In a healthy population, lower birth weight was associated with a more rapid decline in FEV_1/FVC ratio, but not in FEV_1 or FVC; no gender effect was reported [67]. Whether bronchial hyper-responsiveness has the same adverse association with the attainment of poorer spirometry and greater decline in lung function in BPD survivors as in the general population is unclear [68–70]. Indeed, the basis of the hyper-responsiveness may well be different in the two groups (above). Low birth weight was associated with an increased risk of death from COPD [71]. The data would support the hypothesis that survivors are at risk from premature airflow obstruction, both by virtue of failing to reach the expected lung function plateau and also from having an accelerated rate of decline. In a population-based study, 26 % of those with an abnormal FEV_1 at age 40 years went on to develop premature airflow obstruction [72]; whether this also applies to preterm survivors is not known, but the data do suggest a high risk in those born preterm if they fail to attain a normal lung function plateau. However, as with airways disease in childhood (above), it is important to deconstruct airways disease in the elderly; it should not be assumed that these patients have the same airway problems as lifelong smokers, nor should it be assumed that management is the same [73]. This is a fruitful area for future research, but until adult physicians are in the habit of taking a history of early life events [6, 7], research will likely be stalled.

Extrapulmonary The range and treatment of comorbidities is beyond the scope of this chapter. There may be direct impact on the lung, for example, neurodevelopmental handicap leading to incoordinated swallow and aspiration, and impaired cough; and other organ manifestations, including visual impairment from retinopathy of prematurity, and renal and bone disease. Neurodevelopmental handicap may impact on the ability to use inhalers, and special attention needs to be paid to technique if these are prescribed. In one study, twice as many BPD patients reported difficulty with mobility and self-care compared with controls [31], although this did not reach statistical significance. Another group [32] reported that attention-deficit hyperactivity disorder (ADHD) was commoner in preterm survivors; however, another group suggested this was only the case for SGA survivors [74]. Cerebral palsy was commoner in adult BPD survivors, and they were less likely to access higher education or be in full-time employment; whether this relates to BPD itself, or associated low socioeconomic status, could not be determined. BPD survivors were more likely to use antipsychotic, sedative, and anxiolytic medication, although this is not a uniform finding [75]. Although it is difficult to unpick the pathways leading to these comorbidities, nevertheless, these data underscore that this is a needy group of young adults. Some of these young adults need access to holistic care; unfortunately, in most parts of even the developed world, this is not forthcoming, and transition from pediatric care, where there is a strong network of school and community-based services, is a nonevent because of total lack of services to which to transition.

Behavioral and Lifestyle Issues Maternal smoking is an important risk factor for prematurity, and anecdotally, in our study [36], survivors of prematurity are more likely to smoke, although whether prematurity conveys an extra risk of taking up smoking, as against the risks if the parents smoke, was unclear. Whether these young adults are more likely to abuse other substances is not known. By contrast, in another study [75], survivors were no more likely to abuse alcohol than their peers, and the only criminal behavior that was more common in preterm survivors was fare-dodging. If possible, other forms of environmental pollution, in addition to tobacco smoke, should be avoided. Immunization especially against influenza is also important.

Parenchymal Disease

Alveolar Hypoplasia "New BPD" in particular appears to be characterized by arrest of alveolar development. In animal models, hyperoxic gas mixtures, positive pressure ventilation, and systemic corticosteroids, all lead to alveolar simplification and failure of secondary septation. Previously, it was thought that the phase of maximal alveolar growth was within the first 2 years of life, the time of maximal exposure to iatrogenic toxicity. However, this may in fact not be the case (below). Hyperpolarized Helium (He^3) data [76, 77], confirming animal work [78], suggest that in fact alveolar numbers continue to increase throughout the period of somatic growth. This is rather a double-edged finding; on the one hand, this gives more opportunity for catch-up growth, and on the other hand, the period of vulnerability is much greater.

Diffusing capacity of the lungs for carbon monoxide (DL_{CO}) has been used as a surrogate for pulmonary capillary blood volume and can be measured reproducibly in preterm survivors [79]. Both the membrane and blood volume components of DL_{CO} are reduced in preschool children born prematurely, suggestive of early alveolar hypoplasia [80]. Two studies suggest that there may be alveolar catch-up growth. He^3 work in preterm survivors aged 10–14 years showed normal alveolar size [77]. An exercise study in 20–22-year-old survivors that used DL_{CO} measured using CO^{18} rebreathing and respiratory mass spectrometry as a surrogate for alveolar capillary blood volume showed normal results at maximal exercise, implying the alveolar–capillary bed size was normal and normally distensible [81]. This study also highlights the difficulties in interpreting DL_{CO} in the absence of a simultaneous measurement of pulmonary blood flow, since higher blood flows (as in exercise) lead to recruitment and distension of the pulmonary capillary bed and elevation of DL_{CO}. Effective pulmonary blood flow (Qp.eff, which in this context is virtually equivalent to pulmonary blood flow) was also measured using C_2H_2. The results showed that there were differences in SGA and AGA survivors; the SGA survivors had reduced DL_{CO} and Qp.eff at rest, normalizing on maximal exercise, which implies that the low resting DL_{CO} was not due to lung or heart disease, but because cardiac output at rest had been set to a lower level, presumably as a result of intrauterine adverse circumstances. The AGA survivors were normal both at rest and on maximal exercise. These studies are reassuring, but in neither study were measurements made in early childhood, and neither studied the very small, extremely preterm babies; so, it would be wrong to be too reassured by these data. Others have reported lower DL_{CO} at rest in preterm survivors [79, 82, 83], but without measurements of cardiac output, the significance of these findings is difficult to assess.

More recently, He^3 data [84], backed up by animal work [85], suggests that maternal nicotine exposure reduces secondary septation, thus increasing alveolar size and reducing numbers. Taken together, it is likely that there is early onset of an emphysema-like disease as a result of prematurity and not merely premature airflow obstruction.

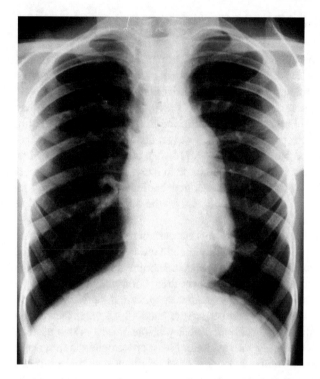

Fig. 1 Chest radiograph of an ex 24-week gestation baby with bronchopulmonary dysplasia, now aged 10 years. There are low flat diaphragms and very featureless lung fields, reminiscent of adult emphysema

Focal Parenchymal Abnormalities Imaging abnormalities usually reflect the consequences of prematurity and its treatment, but just occasionally, an interstitial lung disease may present in a preterm baby, and will not be suspected unless appropriate imaging is carried out. The chest radiograph may be obviously abnormal (Fig. 1). High-resolution computerized tomography (HRCT) may reveal extensive abnormalities that were not immediately obvious on the chest radiograph. However, there is no current indication for routine HRCT in preterm survivors [86]. The classical HRCT appearances of "old BPD" are well-defined linear densities, hypoattenuated areas, and subpleural triangular densities, suggestive of patchy atelectasis and hyperinflation [87] (Fig. 2). The largest imaging series [88] showed confirmed these findings, but perhaps surprisingly, BPD was not associated with worst change over and above prematurity itself, underscoring that there is only a loose association between neonatal events and long-term outcomes. There was a relationship however with duration of oxygen therapy [89]. Subsequent studies have frequently shown often quite extensive areas of focal lung destruction in BPD survivors, even if lung function is not particularly abnormal [89–91]. Studies in "new BPD" are more limited [92, 93].

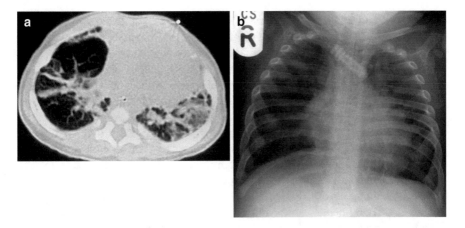

Fig. 2 (**a**) Chest radiograph of a 3-month old, ex-preterm baby with "old" BPD, still oxygen-dependent. There appears to be only relatively mild areas of hyperinflation with some opacification. (**b**) The CT scan of the same child shows very severe changes, classical of "old BPD" with coarse fibrotic strands and atelectasis, alternating with severe hyperinflation. The child subsequently dies

Perhaps surprisingly, the changes are quite similar to "old BPD," at least in the relatively younger populations studied. Thus, although the relatively mild lung function abnormalities are reassuring to some degree, there may still be quite marked structural changes. It is likely that advances in MRI will allow this modality to be used more, elucidating both structure and function [94].

Impaired Exercise Performance

In general, exercise performance in daily life in preterm survivors is good in adolescence and adult life, and the results of exercise testing, although not normal, often only reveal subtle abnormalities [81, 82, 95, 96], with no difference in longitudinal changes when these have been reported. Generally, exercise hypoxemia is not reported in these survivors [83]. Overall, neonatal events do not predict exercise performance [97]. Adults born preterm may exercise less than term born controls [98], and leisure time exercise rather than airflow obstruction or degree of prematurity correlates with formal exercise performance, and perhaps this is an area in which some form of pulmonary rehabilitation may be helpful. There is a differential hemodynamic response to exercise in SGA and AGA children, as discussed above, underscoring the need to try to separate out these two groups in future studies.

Notwithstanding, exercise testing does unmask physiological differences between preterm survivors and controls. Narang et al. [81] found that a minor elevation in FRC at end-exercise was the only difference between survivors of prematurity and controls, suggestive that there may have been some dynamic hyperinflation, despite no differences in resting spirometry. In a much more premature group of survivors than that studied by Narang et al., Lovering et al. [99] reported that, compared with normal controls, inspiratory reserve volume reduced at lower workloads in preterm survivors, who also developed severe dyspnea and leg pain on exercise, this despite having only relatively minor airflow obstruction at rest. The BPD survivors had more expiratory flow limitation at an early stage of exercise than the other groups. They suggested that there was a mechanical constraint to raising Vt during exercise (by contrast with Narang et al. [81]). There were no measurements of muscle blood flow or muscle oxygen extraction, which might have shed light on the mechanism of leg pain. It is surely conceivable that if auto-PEEP increases on exercise as pleural pressures rise, then venous return and hence cardiac output might drop, although again this was not found by Narang et al. [81]. The dyspnea was attributed to loss of inspiratory reserve capacity [100].

Exercise performance may also be reduced by upper airway obstruction. The left recurrent laryngeal nerve closely abuts the arterial duct on its course into and out of the thorax to innervate the left vocal cord. In one study, adults who were born preterm (defined as birth weight $\leq$1000 gm or gestational age $\leq$28/40) were studied using transnasal flexible laryngoscopy (at rest and on exercise) [101]. Thirteen had undergone cardiac surgery for a patent arterial duct, a common complication of prematurity, of whom seven had a left vocal cord palsy. Exercise-induced noisy breathing had previously been put down to prematurity or asthma, but unsurprisingly there had been no response to treatment. Increasing exercise symptoms correlated with increasing aryepiglottic collapse at endoscopy.

In summary, levels of activity are reduced in preterm survivors, and this is associated with what are usually mild impairments of exercise performance. The data suggest these subjects may benefit from fitness training, although this needs to be tested in future studies.

Abnormal Control of Breathing

There are extensive studies on the multiple mechanisms whereby control of breathing is disordered in infancy after premature birth [102]. There is very little information relating to adolescents and adulthood. Sleep-disordered breathing is more common in mid-childhood after prematurity [103], but whether BPD confers an extra risk is unclear [104, 105]. A very small study documented abnormal responses to hypoxia and hyperoxia in adult preterm survivors [106]. This is an area for future research, and certainly there should be a low threshold for performing polysomnography in adult preterm survivors. Whether there is any deficit in control of breathing during exercise is unclear [102].

Pulmonary Circulatory Disease

Pulmonary hypertension, which is multifactorial, and increased pulmonary vasoreactivity are well described in preterm infants. It is said that the elevation in pulmonary vascular resistance disappears by childhood [107]. However, pulmonary vascular reactivity to hypoxemia and inhaled nitric oxide may persist into adolescence [108]. There are only scanty data on pulmonary circulation in adult survivors. The most intriguing data are from a comparison of 10 survivors of persistence of the fetal circulation (PFC) compared with 10 matched controls at age 21 years [109]. The investigators performed echocardiographic estimates of pulmonary arterial pressure at sea level and altitude. There was no difference in change in mean arterial oxygen saturation, but the PFC survivors had a much greater pulmonary hypertensive response (mean 62.3 vs.49.7 mm Hg). Another group showed a greater pulmonary hypertensive response to hypoxemia in preterm survivors [110]; this has implications for air travel, given that flying in a commercial jet is equivalent to breathing 15 % oxygen [111]. The systemic cardiovascular consequences of prematurity are out of the scope of this chapter, but have been reviewed elsewhere [112].

In summary, the possibility that an adult survivor of prematurity may have reduced pulmonary vascular reserve, and have or develop frank pulmonary arterial hypertension during aging, should be borne in mind. It is clearly important to ensure that such patients do not develop significant hypoxemia due, for example, to sleep-disordered breathing (above).

Developmental Origins of Health and Disease Hypothesis (DOHAD)

This hypothesis states that in utero events at critical times can reprogram an individual to respond better to current adverse circumstances, but at a cost of later maladaptive responses. Speculatively, this may account for the pulmonary hypertensive responses in preterm survivors described earlier. Unsurprisingly, the best data come from murine models; tobacco smoke exposure of pregnant dams leads to enhanced allergic responses postnatally in the offspring [113], and neonatal hyperoxia alters pulmonary immune responses and oxidative stress [114, 115]. It is possible, but speculative, that the increased oxidative stress in human preterm survivors (above) may be a DOHAD manifestation. Clearly, more research is needed, but the clinician should be alert to the possibility that these survivors may react differently to adverse later life insults.

Management of the Adult Survivor of Prematurity

The first essential is, if at all possible, to establish the birth history; this should in fact be routine in all adults with airway disease because of the differences in the nature of the disease documented above. If this is to happen, there needs to be a change in emphasis during the years of medical training. There are currently no specific remedies for the airway disease of prematurity. Obviously, general respiratory health measures should be implemented, including annual influenza immunization and the avoidance of active or passive tobacco exposure, and where possible, environmental pollution. This group should actively be targeted for smoking cessation programs. The nature of any airway disease should be carefully characterized, because some will have atopic asthma and type 2 inflammation as well as being born preterm, and any inappropriately prescribed anti-inflammatory medication weaned. Ideally induced sputum for eosinophilia should be performed, or at the very least a measurement of exhaled nitric oxide or blood eosinophil count obtained. If there is any suggestion of sleep-disordered breathing, then polysomnography should be performed. If there is significant impairment of spirometry, then pulmonary hypertension must be excluded, and, if present, overnight saturations monitored to exclude nocturnal hypoxemia as an exacerbating factor. The burden of comorbidity should be assessed and appropriate referrals made. It would seem sensible to review even relatively well adult survivors with spirometry as a minimum at least every 1–2 years to understand the trajectory of the airway problem; but, this is clearly an area where a better understanding and more research are needed. There are no guidelines for imaging either at presentation or follow-up, but, as with ordering any investigation, it would seem sensible only to repeat imaging if it is likely to change clinical management.

The management of those presenting with nonrespiratory problems, or those who are found to have abnormal spirometry at a screening test, is even less clear. Any adult born preterm who has abnormal spirometry must be considered at least as at risk for premature airflow obstruction, and it would seem sensible to repeat spirometry every 1–2 years to track any progression, as well as give general lung health advice on exercise, avoidance of tobacco and pollution, and the need for immunizations. If despite the lack of symptoms, airway obstruction is severe, then management should be more aggressive, along the lines suggested above.

Summary and Conclusions

Respiratory sequelae of preterm birth are diverse, and much remains to be learned about them. There has been a tendency to lump together all those with low birth weight or prematurity, and this has likely masked differences between SGA and AGA survivors, for example. Their health care needs may be very different from those of the adult with asthma or COPD; they are a needy group, both in terms of clinical care, in particular, those with complex comorbidities, and research. It seems likely that a large number of these survivors are receiving inappropriate prescriptions of inhaled corticosteroids, putting them at risk of side effects and also wasting resources. This group throws down a challenge to young clinicians and researchers respectively to improve clinical care and the evidence base for management!

References

1. Office for National Statistics. Preterm births, preterm births data, press release based on 2005 data.2005.Available from:http://www.ons.gov.uk/ons/publications/re-reference-tables.html? edition=tcm%3A77-50818.
2. Islam JY, Keller RJ, Aschner JL, Hartert TV, Moore PE. Understanding the short- and long-term respiratory outcomes of prematurity and bronchopulmonary dysplasia. Am J Respir Crit Care Med. 2015;192:134–56.
3. Poindexter BB, Feng R, Schmidt B, Aschner JL, Ballard RA, Hamvas A, Reynolds AM, Shaw PA, Jobe AH. Prematurity and Respiratory Outcomes Program. Comparisons and limitations of current definitions of bronchopulmonary dysplasia for the prematurity and respiratory outcomes program. Ann Am Thorac Soc. 2015;12:1822–30.
4. Stocks J, Hislop A, Sonnappa S. Early lung development: lifelong effect on respiratory health and disease. Lancet Respir Med. 2013;1:728–42.
5. McGrath-Morrow SA, Ryan T, Rickert K, Lefton-Greif MA, Eakin M, Collaco JM. The impact of bronchopulmonary dysplasiaon caregiver health-related quality of life during the first 2 years of life. Pediatr Pulmonol. 2013;48:579–86.
6. Crump C. Medical history taking in adults should include questions about preterm birth. Br Med J. 2014;349:g4860.
7. Bolton CE, Bush A, Hurst JR, Kotecha S, McGarvey L, Stocks J, Walshaw MJ. Are early life factors considered when managing respiratory disease?A British Thoracic Society survey of current practice. Thorax. 2012;67:1110.
8. van Nimwegen FA, Penders J, Stobberingh EE, Postma DS, Koppelman GH, Kerkhof M, Reijmerink NE, Dompeling E, van den Brandt PA, Ferreira I, Mommers M, Thijs C. Mode and place of delivery, gastrointestinal microbiota, and their influence on asthma and atopy. J Allergy Clin Immunol. 2011;128:948–55.
9. Stick SM, Burton PR, Gurrin L, Sly PD, LeSouëf PN. Effects of maternal smoking during pregnancy and a family history of asthma on respiratory function in newborn infants. Lancet. 1996;348:1060–4.
10. Rusconi F, Galassi C, Forastiere F, Bellasio M, De Sario M, Ciccone G, Brunetti L, Chellini E, Corbo G, La Grutta S, Lombardi E, Piffer S, Talassi F, Biggeri A, Pearce N. Maternal complications and procedures in pregnancy and at birth and wheezing phenotypes in children. Am J Respir Crit Care Med. 2007;175:16–21.
11. Shaheen SO, Sterne JAS, Tucker JS, Florey CD. Birth weight, childhood lower respiratory tract infection, and adult lung function. Thorax. 1998;53:549–53.
12. Svanes C, Sunyer J, Plana E, Dharmage S, Heinrich J, Jarvis D, de Marco R, Norbäck D, Raherison C, Villani S, Wjst M, Svanes K, Antó JM. Early life origins ofchronic obstructive pulmonary disease. Thorax. 2010;65:14–20.
13. Li J, Yu KH, Oehlert J, Jeliffe-Pawlowski LL, Gould JB, Stevenson DK, Snyder M, Shaw GM, O'Brodovich HM. Exome sequencing of neonatal blood spots and the identification of genes implicated in bronchopulmonary dysplasia. Am J Respir Crit Care Med. 2015;192:589–96.

14. Cookson H, Granell R, Joinson C, Ben-Shlomo Y, Henderson JA. Mothers' anxiety during pregnancy is associated with asthma in their children. J Allergy Clin Immunol. 2009;123:847–53.
15. Wright RJ. Epidemiology of stress and asthma: from constricting communities and fragile families to epigenetics. Immunol Allergy Clin North Am. 2011;31:19–39.
16. Mathilda Chiu YH, Coull BA, Cohen S, Wooley A, Wright RJ. Prenatal and postnatal maternal stress and wheeze in urban children: effect of maternal sensitization. Am J Respir Crit Care Med. 2012;186:147–54.
17. Stoll BJ, Hansen NI, Walsh MC, Carlo WA, Shankaran S, Lapook AR, et al. Eunice Kennedy Shriver National Institute of Child Health and Human Development Neonatal Research Network. Trends in care practices, morbidity and mortality of extremely preterm neonates, 1993-2012. JAMA. 2015;314:1039–51.
18. Diaz-Rosello JL, Gisore P, Niermeyer S, Paul VK, Quiroga A, Saugstad OL, Silvestre MA, Singhal N, Sugiura T, Uxa F. Guidelines on basic newborn resuscitation 2012. Geneva: World Health Organization; 2012.
19. Gough A, Spence D, Linden M, Hallikday HL, McGarvey LPA. General and respiratory health outcomes in adult survivors of bronchopulmonary dysplasia. Chest. 2012;141:1554–67.
20. Mazloum DEI, Moschino L, Bozzetto S, Baraldi E. Chronic lung disease of prematurity: long-term respiratory outcomes. Neonatology. 2014;105:352–6.
21. Gibson A-M, Doyle LW. Respiratory outcomes for the tiniest or most immature infants. Semin Fetal Neonatal Med. 2014;39:105–11.
22. Bolton CE, Bush A, Hurst JR, Kotecha S, McGarvey L. Lung consequences in adults born prematurely. Thorax. 2015;70:574–80.
23. Kotecha SJ, Watkins WJ, Paranjothy S, Dunstan FD, Henderson AJ, Kotecha S. Effect of late preterm birth on longitudinal lung spirometry in school age children and adolescents. Thorax. 2012;67:54–61.
24. Harju M, Keski-Nisula L, Georgiadis L, Raisanen S, Gissler M, Heinionen S. The burden of childhood asthma and late preterm and early term births. J Pediatr. 2014;164:295–9.
25. Vogt H, Lindstrom K, Brabak L, Hjern A. Preterm birth and inhaled corticosteroid use in 6-70 19-year-olds: a Swedish national cohort study. Pediatrics. 2011;127:1052–9.
26. Damgaard AL, Hansen BM, Mathiasen R, Buchvald F, Lange T, Greisen G. PLoS One. 2015;10:e0117253.
27. Langhoff-Roos J, Kesmodel U, Jacobsson B, Rasmussen S, Vogel I. Spontaneous preterm delivery in primiparous women at low risk in Denmark: population based study. Br Med J. 2006;332:937–9.
28. Cox B, Martens E, Nemery B, Vangronsveld J, Nawrot TS. Impact of a stepwise introduction of smoke-free legislation on the rate of preterm births: analysis of routinely collectedbirthdata. BMJ. 2013;346:f441.
29. Kotecha SJ, Edwards MO, Watkins WJ, Henderson AJ, Paranjothy S, Dunstan FD, Kotecha S. Effect of preterm birth on later FEV1: a systematic review and meta-analysis. Thorax. 2013;68:760–6.
30. Pike KC, Lucas JS. Respiratory consequences oflate preterm birth. Paediatr Respir Rev. 2015;16:182–8.
31. Gough A, Linden M, Spence D, Patterson CC, Halliday HL, McGarvey LPA. Impaired lung function and health status in adult survivors of bronchopulmonary dysplasia. Eur Respir J. 2014;43:808–16.
32. Beaudoin S, Tremblay GM, Croitoru D, Benedetti A, Landry JS. Healthcare utilization and health-related quality of life of adult survivors of preterm birth complicated by bronchopulmonary dysplasia. Acta Paediatr. 2013;102:607–12.
33. Landry JS, Tremblay GM, Li PZ, Wong C, Benedetti A, Taivassalo T. Lung function and bronchial hyperresponsiveness in adults born prematurely: acohort study. Ann Am Thorac Soc2015. [Epub ahead of print]

34. Crump C, Winkleby MA, Sundquist J, et al. Risk of asthma in young adults who were born preterm: a Swedish national cohort study. Pediatrics. 2011;127:e913–20.
35. Doyle LW, Faber B, Callanan C, et al. Bronchopulmonary dysplasia in very low birth weight subjects and lung function in late adolescence. Pediatrics. 2006;118:108–13.
36. Narang I, Rosenthal M, Cremonesini D, Silverman M, Bush A. Longitudinal evaluation of airway function 21 years after preterm birth. Am J Respir Crit Care Med. 2008;178:74–80.
37. Walter EC, Ehlenbach WJ, Hotchkin DL, Chien JW, Koepsell TD. Low birth weight and respiratory disease in adulthood: a population-based case-control study. Am J Respir Crit Care Med. 2009;180:176–80.
38. Crump C, Sundquist K, Sundquist J, Winkleby MA. Gestational age at birth and mortality in young adulthood. JAMA. 2011;306:1233–40.
39. Agusti A, Bel E, Thomas M, Vogelmeier C, Brusselle G, Holgate S, Humbert M, Jones P, Gibson PG, Vestbo J, Beasley R, Pavord ID. Treatable traits: toward precision medicine of chronic airway diseases. Eur Respir J. 2016;47(2):410–9.
40. Roth-Kleiner M, Post M. Similarities and dissimilarities of branching and septation during lungdevelopment. Pediatr Pulmonol. 2005;40:113–34.
41. Kho AT, Bhattacharya S, Tantisira KG, Carey VJ, Gaedigk R, Leeder JS, Kohane IS, Weiss ST, Mariani TJ. Transcriptomic analysis of humanlung development. Am J Respir Crit Care Med. 2010;181:54–63.
42. Quanjer PH, Stanojevic S, Cole TJ, Baur X, Hall GL, Bruce H, et al., the ERS Global Lung Function Initiative. Multi-ethnic reference values for spirometry for the 3–95-yr age range: the global lung function 2012 equations. Eur Respir J. 2012;40:1324–43.
43. Morgan WJ, Stern DA, Sherrill DL, Guerra S, Holberg CJ, Guilbert TW, Taussig LM, Wright AL, Martinez FD. Outcome of asthma and wheezing in the first 6 years of life: follow-up through adolescence. Am J Respir Crit Care Med. 2005;172:1253–8.
44. Sears MR, Greene JM, Willan AR, Wiecek EM, Taylor DR, Flannery EM, Cowan JO, Herbison GP, Silva PA, Poulton R. A longitudinal, population-based, cohort study of childhood asthma followed to adulthood. N Engl J Med. 2003;349:1414–22.
45. Tai A, Tran H, Roberts M, Clarke N, Wilson J, Robertson CF. The association between childhood asthma and adult chronic obstructive pulmonary disease. Thorax. 2014;69:805–10.
46. Vollsaeter M, Roksund OD, Eide GE, Markestad T, Halvorsen T. Lung function after preterm birth: development from mid-childhood to adulthood. Thorax. 2013;68:767–76.
47. Bolton CE, Bush A. Coming now to a chest clinic near you. Thorax. 2013;68:707–8.
48. Brundage KL, Mohsini KG, Froese AB, Fisher JT. Bronchodilatorresponse to ipratropium bromide in infants with bronchopulmonary dysplasia. Am Rev Respir Dis. 1990;142:1137–42.
49. Fawke J, Lum S, Kirkby J, Hennessy E, Marlow N, Rowell V, Thomas S, Stocks J. Lung function and respiratory symptoms at 11 years in children born extremely preterm: the EPICure study. Am J Respir Crit Care Med. 2010;182:237–45. Gough A, Linden M, Spence D et al. Impaired lung function and health status in adult survivors of bronchopulmonary dysplasia. Eur Respir J.2014;43:808–16.
50. Tiddens HA, Hofhuis W, Casotti V, Hop WC, Hulsmann AR, de Jongste JC. Airway dimensions in bronchopulmonary dysplasia: implications for airflow obstruction. Pediatr Pulmonol. 2008;43:1206–13.
51. Baraldi E, Bonetto G, Zachello F, Filippone M. Low exhaled nitric oxide in school-age children with bronchopulmonary dysplasia and airflow limitation. Am J Respir Crit Care Med. 2005;171:68–72.
52. Carraro S, Piacentini G, Lusiani M, Uyan ZS, Filippone M, Schiavon M, Boner AL, Baraldi E. Exhaled air temperature in bronchopulmonary dysplasia. Pediatrics. 2010;45:1240–5.
53. Chan N, Silverman M. Increased airway responsiveness in children of low birth weight at school age: effect of topical corticosteroids. Arch Dis Child. 1993;69:120–4.
54. Filippone M, Bonetto G, Corradi M, Frigo AC, Baraldi E. Evidence of unexpected oxidative stress in airways of adolescents born very preterm. Eur Respir J. 2012;40:1253–9.

55. Carraro S, Giordano G, Pirillo P, Maretti M, Reniero F, Cogo PE, Perilongo G, Stocchero M, Baraldi E. Airway metabolic anomalies in adolescents with bronchopulmonary dysplasia: new insights from the metabolomic approach. J Pediatr. 2015;166:234–9.

56. Lawlor DA, Ebrahim S, Davey SG. Association of birth weight with adult lung function: findings from the British Women's Heart and Health Study and a meta-analysis. Thorax. 2005;60:851–8.

57. Hancox RJ, Poulton R, Greene JM, McLachlan CR, Pearce MS, Sears MR. Associations between birth weight, early childhood weight gain and adult lung function. Thorax. 2009;64:228–32.

58. Lucas JS, Inskip HM, Godfrey KM, Foreman CT, Warner JO, Gregson RK, Clough JB. Small size at birth and greater postnatal weight gain: relationships to diminished infant lung function. Am J Respir Crit Care Med. 2004;170:534–40.

59. Turner S, Zhang G, Young S, Cox M, Goldblatt J, Landau L, Le Souëf P. Associations between postnatal weight gain, change in postnatal pulmonary function, formula feeding and early asthma. Thorax. 2008;63:234–9.

60. Suresh S, O'Callaghan M, Sly PD, Mamun AA. Impact of childhood anthropometry trends on adult lung function. Chest. 2015;147:1118–26.

61. Lin MH, Hsieh CJ, Caffrey JL, et al. Fetal growth, obesity, and atopic disorders in adolescence: a retrospective birth cohort study. Paediatr Perinat Epidemiol. 2015;29:472–9.

62. der Voort AM S-v, Arends LR, de Jongste JC, et al. Preterm birth, infantweight gain, and childhoodasthmarisk: ameta-analysisof 147,000 European children. J Allergy Clin Immunol. 2014;133:1317–29.

63. Halvorsen T, Skadberg BT, Eide GE, Røksund OD, Carlsen KH, Bakke P. Pulmonary outcome in adolescents of extreme preterm birth: a regional cohort study. Acta Paediatr. 2004;93:1294–300.

64. Saarenpaa H-K, Tikanmaki M, Sipola-Leppanen M, et al. Lung function in very low birth weight adults. Pediatrics. 2015;136:642–50.

65. Cai Y, Shaheen SO, Hardy R, Kuh D, Hansell AL. Birth weight, early childhood growth and lung function in middle to early old age: 1946 British birth cohort. Thorax. 2016;71:916–22.

66. Brostrom EB, Akre O, Katz-Salamon M, Jaraj D, Kaijser M. Obstructive pulmonary disease in old age among individuals born preterm. Eur J Epidemiol. 2013;28:79–85.

67. Baumann S, Godtfredsen NS, Lange P, Pisinger C. The impact of birth weight on the level of lung function and lung function decline in the general adult population. The Inter99 study. Respir Med. 2015;109:1293–9.

68. Grol MH, Gerritsen J, Vonk JM, Schouten JP, Koëter GH, Rijcken B, Postma DS. Risk factors for growth and decline of lung function in asthmatic individuals up to age 42 years. A 30-year follow-up study. Am J Respir Crit Care Med. 1999;160:1830–7.

69. Grol MH, Postma DS, Vonk JM, Schouten JP, Rijcken B, Koëter GH, Gerritsen J. Risk factors from childhood to adulthood forbronchialresponsiveness at age 32-42 yr. Am J Respir Crit Care Med. 1999;160:150–6.

70. Bisgaard H, Jensen SM, Bønnelykke K. Interaction between asthma and lung function growth in early life. Am J Respir Crit Care Med. 2012;185:1183–9.

71. Barker DJP, Godfrey KM, Fall C, Osmond C, Winter PD, Shaheen SO. Relation of birth weight and childhood respiratory infection to adult lung function and death from chronic obstructive pulmonary disease. BMJ. 1991;303:671–5.

72. Lange P, Celli B, Agustí A, Boje Jensen G, Divo M, Faner R, Guerra S, Marott JL, Martinez FD, Martinez-Camblor P, Meek P, Owen CA, Petersen H, Pinto-Plata V, Schnohr P, Sood A, Soriano JB, Tesfaigzi Y, Vestbo J. Lung-function trajectories leading to chronic obstructive pulmonary disease. N Engl J Med. 2015;373:111–22.

73. Postma DS, Brusselle G, Bush A, Holloway JW. I have taken my umbrella, so of course it does not rain. Thorax. 2012;67:88–9.

74. Strang-Karlsson S, Raikkonen K, Pesonen A-K, et al. Very low birth weightand behavioural symptoms of attention deficit hyperactivity disorder in young adulthood: the Helsinki study of very-low-birth-weight adults. Am J Psychiatry. 2008;165:1345–53.

75. Hille ETM, Dorrepaal C, Pirenboom R, Gravenhorst JB, Brand R, Virloove-Vanhorick SP. Social lifestyle, risk-taking behaviour, and psychopathology in young adults born very preterm or with a very low birthweight. J Pediatr. 2008;152:793–800.

76. Narayanan M, Beardsmore CS, Owers-Bradley J, Dogaru CM, Mada M, Ball I, Garipov RR, Kuehni CE, Spycher BD, Silverman M. Catch-up alveolarization in ex-preterm children: evidence from (3)He magnetic resonance. Am J Respir Crit Care Med. 2013;187:1104–9.

77. Waters B, Owers-Bradley J, Silverman M. Acinar structure in symptom-free adults by Helium-3 magnetic resonance. Am J Respir Crit Care Med. 2006;173:847–51.

78. Hyde DM, Blozis SA, Avdalovic MV, et al. Alveoli increase in number but not size from birth to adulthood in rhesus monkeys. Am J Physiol Lung Cell Mol Physiol. 2007;293:L570–9.

79. Satrell E, Roksund O, Thorsen E, Halvorsen T. Pulmonary gas transfer in children and adults born extremely preterm. Eur Respir J. 2013;42:1536–44.

80. Chang DV, Assaf SJ, Tiller CJ, Kisling JA, Tepper RS. Membrane and capillary components of lung diffusion in infants with bronchopulmonary dysplasia. Am J Respir Crit Care Med. 2016;193(7):767–71.

81. Narang I, Bush A, Rosenthal M. Gas transfer and pulmonary blood flow at rest and during exercise in adults, 21 years after preterm birth. Am J Respir Crit Care Med. 2009;180:339–45.

82. Mitchell SH, Teague WH. Reduced gas transfer at rest and during exercise in school-age survivors of bronchopulmonary dysplasia. Am J Respir Crit Care Med. 1998;157:1406–12.

83. Lovering AT, Laurie SS, Elliott JE, et al. Normal pulmonary gas exchange efficiency and absence of exercise-induced arterial hypoxemia in adults with bronchopulmonary dysplasia. J Appl Physiol. 2013;115:1050–6.

84. Narayanan M. PhD thesis, University of Leicester; 2014.

85. Maritz GS, Thomas RA. The influence of maternal nicotine exposure on the interalveolar septal status of neonatal rat lung. Cell Biol Int. 1994;18:747–57.

86. Wilson AC. What does imaging the chest tell us about bronchopulmonary dysplasia? Paediatr Respir Rev. 2010;11:158–61.

87. Oppenheim C et al. Bronchopulmonary dysplasia: value of CT in identifying pulmonary sequelae. AJR Am J Roentgenol. 1994;163:169–72.

88. Auckland SM et al. High-resolution CT of the chest in children and young adults who were born prematurely: findings in a population based study. AJR Am J Roentgenol. 2006;187:1012–8.

89. Auckland SM, Rosendahl K, Owens CM, Fosse KR, Eide GE, Halvorsen T. Neonatal bronchopulmonary dysplasia predicts abnormal pulmonary HRCT scans in long-term survivors of extreme preterm birth. Thorax. 2009;64:505–10.

90. Wong PM, Lees AN, Louw J, Lee FY, French N, Gain K, Murray CP, Wilson A, Chambers DC. Emphysema in young adult survivors of moderate-to-severebronchopulmonary dysplasia. Eur Respir J. 2008;32:321–8.

91. Aquino SL, Schechter MS, Chiles C, Ablin DS, Chipps B, Webb WR. High-resolution inspiratory and expiratory CT in older children and adults with bronchopulmonary dysplasia. AJR Am J Roentgenol. 1999;173:963–7.

92. Mahut B et al. Chest computed tomography findings in bronchopulmonary dysplasia and correlation with lung function. Arch Dis Child Fetal Neonatal Ed. 2007;92:F459–64.

93. Ochiai M et al. A new scoring system for computed tomography of the chest for assessing the clinical status of bronchopulmonary dysplasia. J Pediatr. 2008;152:90–5.

94. Walkup LL, Tkach JA, Higano NS, Thomen RP, Fain SB, Merhar SL, Fleck RJ, Amin RS, Woods JC. Quantitative magnetic resonance imaging of bronchopulmonary dysplasia in the neonatal intensive care unit environment. Am J Respir Crit Care Med. 2015;192:1215–22.

95. Clemm HH, Vollsaeter M, Roksund OD, Eide GE, Markestad T, Halvorsen T. Exercise capacity after extremely preterm birth. Development from adolescence to adulthood. Ann Am Thorac Soc. 2014;11:537–45.
96. Clemm H, Roksund O, Thorsen E, Eide GE, Markestad I, Halvorsen T. Aerobic capacity and exercise performance in young people born extremely preterm. Pediatrics. 2012;129:e97–e105.
97. O'Donnell DE. Adult survivors of preterm birth. What spirometry conceals, exercise tests reveal. Ann Am Thorac Soc. 2014;10:1606–7.
98. Kjantie E, Strang-Karlsson S, Hovi P, et al. Adults born at very low birth weight exercise less than their peers born at term. J Pediatr. 2010;157:610–6.
99. Lovering AT, Elliott JE, Laurie SS, et al. Ventilatory and sensory responses in adult survivors of preterm birth and bronchopulmonary dysplasia with reduced exercise capacity. Ann Am Thorac Soc. 2014;11:1528–37.
100. Guenette JA, Webb KA, O'Donnell DE. Does dynamic hyperinflation contribute to dyspnoea during exercise in patients with COPD? Eur Respir J. 2012;40:322–9.
101. Røksund OD, Clemm H, Heimdal JH, Aukland SM, Sandvik L, Markestad T, Halvorsen T. Left vocal cord paralysis after extreme preterm birth, a new clinical scenario in adults. Pediatrics. 2010;126:e1569–77.
102. Bates ML, Pillers D-AM, Palta M, Farrell ET, Eldridge MW. Ventilatory control in infants, children and adults with bronchopulmonary dysplasia. Respir Physiol Neurobiol. 2013;189:329–37.
103. Rosen CL, Larkin EK, et al. Prevalence and risk factors for sleep-disordered breathing in 8- to 11-year-old children: association with race and prematurity. J Pediatr. 2003;142:383–9.
104. Sharma PB, Barody F, et al. Obstructive sleep apnea in the formerly preterm infant: an overlooked diagnosis. Front Neurol. 2011;2:73.
105. Hibbs AM, Johnson NL, et al. Prenatal and neonatal risk factors for sleep disordered breathing in school-aged children born preterm. J Pediatr. 2008;153:176–82.
106. Bates ML, Farrell ET, Eldridge MW. Abnormal ventilatory responses in adults born prematurely. N Engl J Med. 2014;370:584–5.
107. Vrijlnadt EJLE, Boezen HM, Gerritsen J, Stremmelaar EF, Duiverman EJ. Respiratory health in prematurely born preschool children with and without bronchopulmonary dysplasia. J Pediatr. 2007;150:256–61.
108. Mourami PM, Ivy DD, Gao D, Abman SH. Pulmonary vascular effects of inhaled nitric oxide nd oxygen tension in bronchopulmonary dysplasia. Am J Respir Crit Care Med. 2004;170:1006–13.
109. Sartori C, Allemann Y, Trueb L, Delabays A, Nicod P, Scherrer U. Augmented vasoreactivity in adult life associated with perinatal vascular insult. Lancet. 1999;353:2205–7.
110. Poon CY, Watkins WJ, Evans CJ, Tsai-Goodman B, Bolton CE, Cockcroft JR, Wise RG, Kotecha S. Pulmonary arterial response to hypoxia in survivors of chronic lung disease of prematurity. Arch Dis Child Fetal Neonatal Ed. 2016;101(4):F309–13.
111. Harding RM, Mills FJ. Aviation medicine. 2nded ed. Plymouth: BMA Publications; 1988.
112. Poon MGS, Edwards MO, Kotecha S. Long term cardiovascular consequences of chronic lung disease of prematurity. Paediatr Respir Rev. 2013;14:242–9.
113. Penn AL, Rouse RL, Horohov DW, Kearney MT, Paulsen DB, Lomax L. In utero exposure to environmental tobacco smoke potentiates adult responses to allergen in BALB/c mice. Environ Health Perspect. 2007;115:548–55.
114. Buczynski BW, Yee M, Martin KC, Lawrence BP, O'Reilly MA. Neonatal hyperoxia alters the host response to influenza A virus infection in adult mice through multiple pathways. Am J Physiol Lung Cell Mol Physiol. 2013;305:L282–90.
115. Bouch S, O'Reilly M, Harding R, Sozo F. Neonatalexposure to mildhyperoxiacauses persistent increases inoxidative stressand immune cells in the lungs of mice without altering lung structure. Am J Physiol Lung Cell Mol Physiol. 2015;309:L488–96.

Adverse Outcomes Do Not Stop at Discharge: Post-NICU Health Care Use by Prematurely Born Infants

Scott A. Lorch and Shawna Calhoun

The health care needs of prematurely born infants do not stop upon discharge from the neonatal intensive care unit (NICU). Costs and resource utilization by preterm, low birth weight infants (those at the highest risk of readmission) are substantially higher than infants born at term [1, 2], with an estimated 35 % of all health care costs in the first year of life stemming from the care of the infants born at a birth weight <1500 g. However, there are limited data to help counsel families about the health care use of their prematurely born infant after the child is discharged from the NICU, and how these expectations may change based on the child's medical conditions and the family's social and economic factors. This chapter will present a summary of the postdischarge health care use of prematurely born infants, including future hospitalizations, emergency department visits, and outpatient health care use including medications and nonwell visits. Each section will present information on the prevalence of each outcome and risk factors for differences in rates based on specific medical risk factors. Finally, we

S.A. Lorch, MD, MSCE (✉)
Center for Outcomes Research, The Children's Hospital of Philadelphia,
Philadelphia, PA, USA

Division of Neonatology, Department of Pediatrics, The Children's Hospital of Philadelphia,
Philadelphia, PA, USA

Center for Clinical Epidemiology and Biostatistics, University of Pennsylvania School of
Medicine, Philadelphia, PA, USA

Leonard Davis Institute for Health Economics, University of Pennsylvania,
Philadelphia, PA, USA
e-mail: lorch@email.chop.edu

S. Calhoun, MPH
Center for Outcomes Research, The Children's Hospital of Philadelphia,
Philadelphia, PA, USA

© Springer International Publishing AG 2017
A.M. Hibbs, M.S. Muhlebach (eds.), *Respiratory Outcomes in Preterm Infants*,
Respiratory Medicine, DOI 10.1007/978-3-319-48835-6_8

will end with a conceptual framework for increased health care use in these infants and directions for future research in the field.

Hospital Readmissions

The most commonly examined postdischarge outcome for preterm infants is hospital admission. One reason for this emphasis is the high costs, both financial and psychosocial, associated with them, and the potential role of variations in care quality to explain these hospitalizations. The so-called "preventable" readmissions, described because ostensibly some change in practice at either the inpatient or outpatient level could have prevented the readmission, may provide insight into care practices that could limit hospitalizations. Preventing hospital readmissions is an area of emphasis by insurers and public health professionals, because hospital readmissions may represent either poor quality of care during the hospitalization or poor discharge planning and transition of care from inpatient to outpatient providers [3–8]. Readmissions can be used to define or measure the effectiveness of infant discharge criteria [9, 10] or the effect of performance-based quality metrics [11]. Analysis of readmissions on longer time intervals can also be used to assess quality of outpatient care or the dyad of inpatient and outpatient care providers [3]. These methods may also provide insight into the overall structure of the health care system for managing the care of the prematurely born infant.

The second major reason for evaluating hospital readmissions is the increased financial and social costs to families associated with a return admission to the hospital. Several studies have found elevated levels of hostility, anxiety, and/or depression among parents of NICU infants [12, 13]. These alterations in parental attitudes and family well-being can produce long-term effects on the development of the child and family. Caring for a premature infant also requires more maternal/family education, failure of which can further increase risk of readmission [11, 14].

For this section, we will present descriptive data from the United States and internationally, outlining the increased risk of hospital admission after NICU discharge in prematurely born infants. Then, we will discuss how specific risk factors, such as extreme prematurity or bronchopulmonary dysplasia (BPD) influence these rates. We will finish with a brief discussion about hospital admissions secondary to respiratory syncytial virus (RSV), given the large number of studies on this topic.

Epidemiology of Readmissions in the Prematurely Born Infants

There is extensive literature describing the elevated risk of hospitalizations in the preterm population. A representative sample of the literature across the past 20 years in both the United States and internationally is shown in Table 1. We see a wide

Table 1 Unadjusted total readmission rates

Author	Pub year	Organization	Group studied	Years studied	Time frame after discharge	N	Readmission rate (%)	Term admission rate if presented (%)
United States studies								
Lorch [49]	2014	California	23–34	1995–2009	7 days	343,625	2.2	
Goyal [68]	2013	California	34–36, vaginal births	1993–2005	7 days	231,831	3.3	
Lorch [49]	2014	California	23–34	1995–2009	14 days	343,625	3.3	
Ray [20]	2013	California	24–36	1993–2005	14 days	702,468	3.6	
Escobar [22]	1999	Kaiser Permanente, Northern California	24–33	1992–1995	14 days	2328	3.4	2.2
McLaurin [19]	2009	US, Commercially insured	33–36	2004	15 days	1683	3.8	1.3
Lorch [49]	2014	California	23–34	1995–2009	30 days	343,625	5.5	
Ray [20]	2013	California	24–36	1993–2005	30 days	702,468	5.3	
Kuzniewicz [18]	2013	Kaiser Permanente, Northern California	31–37	2003–2012	30 days	23,190	6.8	3.3
Moyer [69]	2014	Cincinnati	34–36	2009	28 days	1861	3.6	
Young [25]	2013	Intermountain Health Care (Utah)	34–36	2000–2010	28 days	19,081	3.5	1.5
Lorch [49]	2014	California	23–34	1995–2009	90 days	343,625	9.9	

(continued)

Table 1 Unadjusted total readmission rates (continued)

Author	Pub year	Organization	Group studied	Years studied	Time frame after discharge	N	Readmission rate (%)	Term admission rate if presented (%)
Ray [20]	2013	California	24–36	1993–2005	90 days	702,468	8.8	
Lorch [3]	2010	Kaiser Permanente, Northern California	24–33	1998–2001	1 year	892	37	
Smith [70]	2004	Kaiser Permanente, Northern California	24–33, BPD	1995–1999	1 year	238	26.7	
Ray [42]	2010	Kaiser Permanente, Northern California	24–34	1998–2001	1 year	663	19	
Lorch [49]	2014	California	23–34	1995–2009	1 year	343,625	19	
Ray [20]	2013	California	24–36	1993–2005	1 year	702,468	13.4	
Furman [17]	1996	Rainbow Babies, Cleveland	VLBW, BPD	1988–1990	1 year	98	50	
McLaurin [19]	2009	US, Commercially insured	33–37	2005	1 year	1683	15.2	7.9
Morris [21]	2005	NICHD NRN	ELBW	1998–2000	18–22 months	1405	49	
Ambalavanan [24]	2011	NICHD NRN	ELBW	2002–2005	18–22 months	3787	45	
International studies								
Stephens [27]	2016	New South Wales, Australia	24–33	2001–2011	30 days	19,901	16.2	3.4
Slimings [71]	2014	Western Australia	24–37	1980–2010	30 days	44,650	6.2	

Author	Pub year	Organization	Group studied	Years studied	Time frame after discharge	N	Readmission rate (%)	Term admission rate if presented (%)
Tseng [72]	2010	Taiwan	24–37	2000–2002	31 days	18,421	13.5	
Martens [23]	2004	Manitoba	24–37	1997–2001	6 weeks	4492	7.7	3.7
Lamarche-Vadel [73]	2004	EPIPAGE	24–28	1997	9 months	376	47.4	
Stephens [27]	2016	New South Wales, Australia	24–33	2001–2011	1 year	19,901	43.6	16.8
Gray [47]	2006	Christchurch Women's hospital	24–32	1998–2000	1 year	100	40	12
Elder [26]	1999	Western Australia	24–33	1990–1991	1 year	538	42	
Chien [16]	2002	National Taiwan Hospital	ELBW	1993–1998	2 years	60	72	
Doyle [15]	2003	Royal Women's Hospital, Melbourne, Australia	ELBW	1997	2 years	72	66	23
Ralser [74]	2012	Northern Tyrol, Austria	24–32	2003–2008	2 years	377	40.1	

range of rates that vary by the length of follow-up after NICU discharge, the location studied, and the years studied. Overall, for the very low birth weight infant (VLBW) with a birth weight < 1500 g and for the extremely low birth weight infant (ELBW) with a birth weight < 1000 g, rates typically range from 2 to 3 % within 2 weeks of NICU discharge to widely variable rates by 1 year after discharge between 20 and 50 %, although some smaller studies from Australia and Taiwan during the 1980s–1990s found rates as high as 72 % [15, 16]. Data are similar between studies of infants born in the United States and studies from other countries, even though the baseline readmission rates in infants born at term may differ somewhat. Finally, in general, these rates do not substantively change by the years of birth, although much of the work includes information from the 1990s.

Some of these studies report on the primary diagnoses for readmissions in prematurely born infants [15–26]. The majority of early readmissions within 7–14 days of NICU discharge are for jaundice and feeding difficulties, especially in infants born at a gestational age (GA) between 34 and 36 weeks. In the first year after discharge, respiratory diagnoses and infections make up the majority of admissions, regardless of country or years of birth.

Impact of Gestational Age and Infant Complications

As expected, younger GA and the presence of common complications of preterm birth are associated with a higher risk of readmission at all time periods after discharge (Tables 2 and 3). In general, rates of readmission in infants born at a gestational age between 24 and 28 weeks have a threefold to fourfold increase in readmissions compared with moderately preterm infants born at a GA between 32 and 34 weeks, and a fivefold to tenfold increase rate compared with infants born at term [18, 27]. Readmissions within 7–14 days of discharge in infants born between 32 and 36 weeks GA are elevated in several studies compared to infants born at an earlier GA, likely secondary to discharge of these moderate to late preterm infants at a chronological age that places them at risk for readmission secondary to jaundice or feeding disorders. The best example of this changing risk of readmission at various time periods is shown in the study of Ray et al. [20]. Using data from over 7 million births in California over a 13-year period, Fig. 1 shows the declining trend in hospital readmissions with older gestational ages, except for a hump in readmission risk within 14 days of discharge in the infants born at a GA between 34 and 36 weeks. These odds ratios remain increased compared to term infants for all GA below 38 weeks.

The primary infant complication examined for its association with postdischarge health care use is BPD. BPD places a prematurely born infant at higher risk for severe RSV disease and hospitalization, pulmonary insufficient associated with respiratory infections overall, and the development of reactive airways disease in future years. Numerous investigators shown in Table 3 show elevated risk of future hospital admission in infants with BPD compared to those of similar gestational

Table 2 Impact of gestational age on readmission rates

Author	Years studied	Readmission time period	Gestational age group	Rate (%)
Lorch [49]	1995–2009	7 days	< 28	2.6
			29–32	2.1
			33–34	2.2
Lorch [49]	1995–2009	14 days	< 28	4.1
			29–32	3.2
			33–34	3.1
Ray [20]	1993–2005	14 days	< 28	3.7
			28–32	3.6
Lorch [49]	1995–2009	30 days	< 28	6.7
			29–32	5.2
			33–34	4.9
Ray [20]	1993–2005	30 days	< 28	6
			28–32	5
Kuzniewicz [18]	2003–2012	30 days	31–33	2.9
			34–36	8
Lorch [49]	1995–2009	90 days	< 28	12.2
			29–32	9.9
			33–34	9.3
Ray [20]	1993–2005	90 days	< 28	10.6
			28–32	8.2
Ray [42]	1998–2001	1 year	< 28	[a]
Lorch [49]	1995–2009	1 year	< 28	20.3
			29–32	19.2
			33–34	18.7
Ray [20]	1993–2005	1 year	< 28	16
			28–32	12.5
Stephens [27]	2001–2011	30 days	24–27	30.7
			28–31	19.9
			32–33	10.1
Slimings [71]	1980–2010	30 days	< 28	2.3
			28–31	4
			32–33	8.9
			34–36	8.9
Tseng [72]	2000–2002	31 days	< 28	22.9
			28–36	12.9
Lamarche-Vadel [73]	1997	9 months	24–25	53.2
			26	46.7
			27	46.1
			28	46.8
Stephens [27]	2001–2011	1 year	24–27	62.1
			28–31	47.7
			32–33	36.2

[a]RR 4.4

Table 3 Impact of complications of preterm birth on readmission rates

Author	Years studied	Readmission time period	BPD odds ratio	Other factor odds ratio
Lorch [3]	1998–2001	1 year	2.2	
Smith [70]	1995–1999	1 year	1.8	
Morris [21]	1998–2000	18–22 months	2.6	NEC 2.5, VP Shunt 5.0
Tseng [72]	2000–2002	31 days	1.2[b]	
Lamarche-Vadel [73]	1997	9 months	1.7	
Elder [26]	1990–1991	1 year	1.4	
Doyle [15]	1997	2 years	[a]	
Ralser [74]	2003–2008	2 years	2.2	

[a]Readmission in BPD 82 %, versus 53 % in infants without BPD
[b]Hazard ratio

ages without BPD, with odds ratios ranging from 1.4 to 2.6. For other complications, Morris [21] used data on infants born at a birth weight < 1000 g at a NICHD Neonatal Research Network center to report an elevated risk of hospital admission associated with a history of necrotizing enterocolitis and placement of a ventriculo-peritoneal shunt (Table 3).

RSV Hospitalizations

As mentioned above, RSV is a primary etiology for the elevated readmission risk in prematurely born infants. RSV has been studied both for its prevalence of disease, its impact on hospitalizations of infants in the first year of life regardless of their gestational age at birth, and the severity of bronchiolitis symptoms in preterm infants who contract the illness. RSV typically results in hospitalization for an estimated 17/1000 infants' ages 0–6 months, and 5/1000 infants' ages 6–12 months in US studies [28, 29], with rates as high as 20/1000 infants in European studies [30, 31]. Overall, prematurely born infants have a twofold to fourfold higher rate of hospitalization, depending on season, location, and the use of palivizumab or monoclonal anti-RSV IgG in the community. As with data from general hospitalizations, younger GA and the presence of BPD are associated with a marked increase in risk of RSV hospitalization [32]. For example, in the pre-palivizumab time period, the estimated number of hospitalizations per 1000 children enrolled in Medicaid was 388 for infants with BPD; 70 for infants born at a GA ≤ 28 weeks; 66 for infants born at a GA between 29 and 32 weeks; 57 for infants born at a GA 33–35 weeks; and 30 for infants born at a GA ≥ 36 weeks [33]. Another study confirmed the higher risk of RSV hospitalization seen in infants

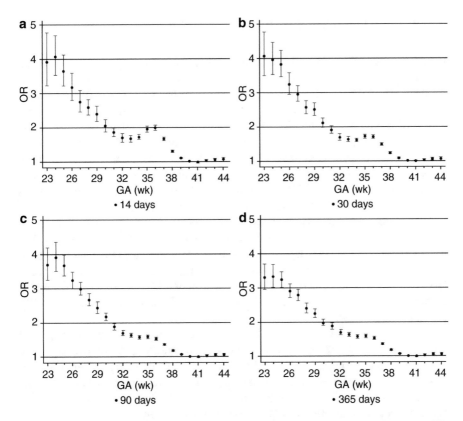

Fig. 1 Impact of gestational age on risk of future hospitalization (Taken from Ray et al. [20], Figure 1)

born between 33 and 35 weeks GA with an adjusted risk of disease being as high as 2.45 compared with infants born at term in the US military health care system [34].Other studies demonstrate longer length of hospital stay, higher use of intensive care services, and higher rates of intubation in these infants [35–37]. Reasons for this risk are not clear.

The impact of RSV in the prematurely born infant is not limited to the acute illness, especially for the highest risk infants. A study from the United Kingdom found that infants with BPD who required hospitalization for RSV had longer length of initial hospital stay, higher use of respiratory medications and inhalers over the first 5 years of age, and 80 % higher health care costs compared to infants with BPD who did not have a hospitalization for RSV [38]. As a result, many countries have protocols in place to encourage the use of palivizumab, a monoclonal IgG against an epitope in the A antigenic site of the F protein of RSV, although the eligibility requirements for receipt of this treatment continue to change frequently.

Emergency Department Visits

Unlike hospital admissions, there are few studies on the use of emergency department by prematurely born infants after NICU discharge. The limited epidemiological data, primarily from single center studies or within staff model HMOs such as Kaiser Permanente, suggest that the rate of emergency department use ranges from 4–5 % of infants within the first 30 days after discharge to 30–40 % of infants by 1 year of age [18, 39–41]. Rates do appear to be increased in the moderate to late preterm infant compared to infants born at term. For example, moderately preterm infants have a 1.4-fold increase in the odds of an emergency department visit, and late preterm infants have a 1.2-fold increase in the odds compared to term infants within the Northern California Kaiser Permanente system [18].

Risk factors for increased use have focused more on social factors compared to medical factors. Preterm infants born to teenaged mothers were found to have a 3.6-fold increase in emergency department use [42], while day care attendance has been associated with a 3.7-fold increase in emergency department use in infants born at a $GA \leq 32$ weeks with BPD [43]. The visits are likely related to the increased report by parents of respiratory symptoms at least weekly in day care attendees (52.2 % compared to 28.5 %).

Even with these data, there have been few studies on the mechanisms to reduce this increased use of the emergency department. In Ohio, weekly to biweekly home visits in the late preterm infant failed to change the use of emergency rooms, with 35–40 % of infants having at least one visit in the first year of life regardless of the frequency of home visits [41]. Intensive pulmonary follow-up at a single medical center for infants with BPD was not associated with difference in ED visits, with a mean of 0.73 visits in the first year for participants compared to 0.53 visits per year for nonparticipants. As participants had a greater respiratory illness severity, with a four times higher rate of BPD, it is possible that the intensive follow-up program may have normalized the emergency department use in a group of infants at risk for elevated use of the emergency department [44]. Little other data are known about the risk factors and mechanisms to ameliorate the influence of these factors on emergency department use.

Outpatient Health Care Use

As with emergency department use, there is almost no data on the outpatient health care use of infants born prematurely. The primary work comes from the Kaiser Permanente system in 892 infants born between 1998 and 2001 [45]. Here, these infants had over 18,346 visits, 91 % of which were to the primary care physician or a pediatric subspecialist. Fifty-eight percent of visits were nonwell visits to the

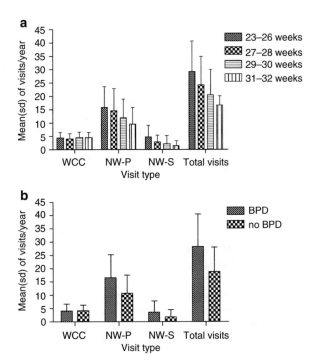

Fig. 2 Total number of outpatient visits, by gestational age (panel **a**) or BPD status (panel **b**) (Taken from Wade et al. [45], Figure 1)

physician, while 22 % of the visits were for well-child checks. This study found increased numbers of visits with decreasing GA and the presence of BPD (Fig. 2), although infants born between 30 and 32 weeks GA had almost 50 % greater number of visits compared to the expected number of visits for an infant born at term. Visits peaked within 3 months of hospital discharge (Fig. 3), with the smallest infants having four to five visits monthly over the first 3 months after NICU discharge. Risk factors for having over 30 visits in the first year after discharge (15.2 % of the cohort) included BPD (OR 1.87), grade 3–4 IVH (OR 3.21), NEC (OR 4.16), and earlier GA at birth (GA 23–26 weeks: OR 8.04; 27–28 weeks: OR 4.42; 29–30 weeks: OR 2.91, compared to 31–32 week GA infants).

Prematurely born infants were high users of prescription medications during the first year after discharge, with 43 % of the cohort filling at least one prescription during this time period. Similar factors predicted the 13.1 % of the cohort that filled over five medications in the first year after discharge, including BPD (OR 2.27) and earlier GA at birth (23–26 weeks: GA OR 2.62; 27–28 weeks: GA OR 2.43; 29–30 weeks: GA OR 2.07).

Similar results have been shown in other countries. BPD and IVH are associated with increased use of therapies such as speech therapy, physical therapy, and occupational therapy in Quebec [46]. In this study, the single most predictive risk factor for therapy use was single parenthood, emphasizing the potential influence of social

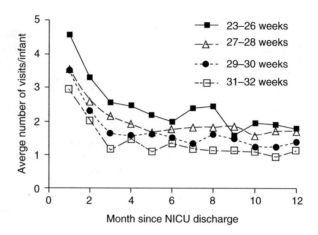

Fig. 3 Average number of outpatient visits per child by month, stratified by gestational age (Taken from Wade et al. [45], Figure 2)

factors on postdischarge health care use in these infants. Higher overall outpatient health care use was seen in preterm infants born in New Zealand [47]. However, in general, the data are sparse for outpatient health care use in preterm infants, with no data on moderate or late preterm infants.

Discussion and Future Directions

As these studies show, there is extensive evidence describing the increased health care use in premature infants after discharge from the NICU. While most of the literature focuses on the highest risk infants – the ELBW infant or the infant discharged home with a diagnosis of BPD – there are studies that suggest that moderate to late preterm infants have an increased risk of future health care use after discharge, especially readmissions for jaundice, feeding difficulties, and RSV.

This overview also demonstrates the limited scope of research and policy concerning this increased use of health care services. To truly reduce the risk of HC use in these infants, one must understand the drivers of this use in prematurely born infants, as these drivers offer opportunities for future quality improvement studies. To this end, we present a conceptual framework for the increased risk of postdischarge health care use, exemplified by readmissions in Fig. 4, although one could substitute other outpatient use or emergency department visits in the center of this figure. This model is based off of other work in pediatric readmissions [48], and attempts to incorporate not only the medical drivers of increased health care use, but also hospital and outpatient quality, transitions of care, and the social and economic factors that may drive health care use. The roles of these factors are discussed in future research directions below.

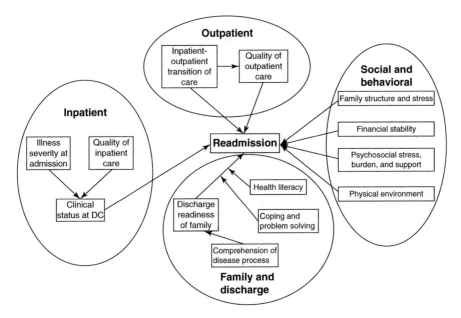

Fig. 4 Conceptual framework for postdischarge health use

Role of Hospital and Outpatient Care

Readmissions can be used to define or measure the effectiveness of infant discharge criteria [9, 10] or the effect of performance-based quality metrics [11]. Analysis of readmissions on longer time intervals can also be used to assess quality of outpatient care or the dyad of inpatient and outpatient care providers [3]. These methods may also provide insight into the overall structure of the health care system for managing the care of the prematurely born infant. Of note, rates of readmissions of prematurely born infants vary substantially between hospitals, both statewide [49] and within a health care system [3] .This variation can be substantial: variation in the unadjusted readmission rates among all California delivery hospitals regardless of time period, as assessed using standardized differences in readmission rates, ranged from 578 to 683 %. The large variation between hospitals persisted after adjusting for gestational age and sociodemographic factors [49].

Readmissions may also result from differences in outpatient providers and practices after discharge. For example, recent data from our group found increased rates of hospital readmission for preterm infants receiving care at outpatient providers with a higher use of unnecessary antibiotics or other medications [3]. Coller, in a systematic review of pediatric hospitals published in 2014, found that the primary method of preventing readmissions in children with complex health issues was improved continuity and care coordination [50]. When studies account for all aspects of the health care system, both inpatient and outpatient, it may inform observed interhospital differences in readmission rates shown by our data and others using Medicare [51] or individual hospital data [52].

Unfortunately, much less is known about the underlying processes of care, reflected by the "Family and Discharge" bubble in the conceptual framework, which may alter this trajectory in health care use potentially driven by the health care system. Readmission rates in NICUs do not correlate with complication rates, although, as we and others have argued [53, 54] this lack of association with some measures of hospital quality may reflect the theory that readmission measures a different aspect of care – the discharge/transition to home process, including education of the family – that fails to affect other quality measures such as complication or mortality rates [50]. There is no evidence that the timing of discharge alters future health care use once the infant achieves the necessary feeding, breathing, and temperature regulation skills needed for discharge [55]. Thus, future research into the specific drivers for these observed variations in readmission rates across health care providers is needed to effect substantial change.

Social Determinants of Health

Social determinants of health, or those personal and community factors represented by the bubble on the far right of our conceptual framework, have increased in their public health importance over time, especially the role of socioeconomic status and financial hardship. Data from numerous adult studies show that infants of lower socioeconomic status have higher rates of hospital readmissions [56], leading to higher rates of readmissions at safety-net hospitals for surgical procedures [57] and congestive heart failure [58]. Other studies show associations between readmission rates within ZIP codes and rates of poverty and other measures of social deprivation [59–61]. Family socioeconomic status, as measured by insurance status [60, 62–65] and financial hardship [66], is associated with readmission risk. Children with publicly financed insurance have higher rates of readmission, with prematurely born infants in some states having rates as high as 30 % [49].

The specific role of these factors in the prematurely born infant is less understood. Since preterm birth is associated with socioeconomic status, these data could reflect the contribution from childhood poverty, resulting in increased use of day care, less health physical environment, chronic and acute toxic stress, and reduced access to high-quality outpatient care. Other potential factors include community factors such as social segregation and social deprivation [67]. While there is a growing interest in the role of social determinants of health on pediatric care, much less is known about the role of these determinants on the short-term and long-term health of preterm infants and the contribution of these factors on the future health care use of high risk infants.

Moderate and Late Preterm Infants

Work presented in this chapter suggests that born at 32–37 weeks GA are not "small-term infants," but rather have an elevated risk of future health care use compared to infants born at term. Data suggest that some acute health care use may be related to physiological immaturity of these infants at the time of discharge from the NICU, especially bilirubin metabolism and feeding coordination. However, the impact of moderate–late preterm birth on long-term health care use is not clear, nor the use of services in the outpatient setting. Given the large number of infants born within this gestational age range, even small increases to health care use may have a large impact on health care costs.

Preterm Infants in a Population's Health

In the United States, there has been substantial change in policy since 2010, with Medicaid expansion in some states, the passage and implementation of the Affordable Care Act, and the growing implementation of Accountable Care Organizations. How these programs will impact preterm infants, particularly as part of Accountable Care Organizations, is unclear given that few programs have targeted perinatal care or newborn care in their mandates. Thus, there are no data on program structure or implementation to optimize health and health care use of preterm infants.

Summary

In short, these results suggest an increased use of health care in prematurely born infants after discharge from the NICU. Much of the available data identifies patient-level risk, particularly for high-cost outcomes such as hospital admission. More work is needed on the more prevalent infants born at later gestations and the overall use of outpatient services and emergency departments. The role of nonmedical factors, such as social factors, suggested in some of the work in emergency departments, and provider quality remains unknown. Further understanding of the global drivers for increased health care use in these high-risk infants will allow for the development of optimal models of care to minimize postdischarge health care use and minimize stress in families and caregivers.

References

1. Gilbert WM, Nesbitt TS, Danielsen B. The cost of prematurity: quantification by gestational age and birth weight. Obstet Gynecol. 2003;102(3):488–92.

2. Russell RB, Green NS, Steiner CA, et al. Cost of hospitalization for preterm and low birth weight infants in the United States. Pediatrics. 2007;120(1):e1–9.
3. Lorch SA, Baiocchi M, Silber JH, et al. The role of outpatient facilities in explaining variations in risk-adjusted readmission rates between hospitals. Health Serv Res. 2010;45(1):24–41.
4. Tsai TC, Joynt KE, Orav EJ, et al. Variation in surgical-readmission rates and quality of hospital care. N Engl J Med. 2013;369(12):1134–42.
5. Berry JG, Toomey SL, Zaslavsky AM, et al. Pediatric readmission prevalence and variability across hospitals. JAMA. 2013;309(4):372–80.
6. Morse RB, Hall M, Fieldston ES, et al. Hospital-level compliance with asthma care quality measures at children's hospitals and subsequent asthma-related outcomes. JAMA. 2011;306(13):1454–60.
7. Escobar GJ, Greene JD, Hulac P, et al. Rehospitalisation after birth hospitalisation: Patterns among infants of all gestations. Arch Dis Child. 2005;90(2):125–31.
8. Profit J, McCormick MC, Escobar GJ, et al. Neonatal intensive care unit census influences discharge of moderately preterm infants. Pediatrics. 2007;119(2):314–9.
9. Seki K, Iwasaki S, An H, et al. Early discharge from a neonatal intensive care unit and rates of readmission. Pediatr Int. 2011;53(1):7–12.
10. Kotagal UR, Perlstein PH, Gamblian V, et al. Description and evaluation of a program for the early discharge of infants from a neonatal intensive care unit. J Pediatr. 1995;127(2):285–90.
11. Paul IM, Lehman EB, Hollenbeak CS, et al. Preventable newborn readmissions since passage of the Newborns' and Mothers' Health Protection Act. Pediatrics. 2006;118(6):2349–58.
12. Doering LV, Moser DK, Dracup K. Correlates of anxiety, hostility, depression, and psychosocial adjustment in parents of NICU infants. Neonatal Netw. 2000;19(5):15–23.
13. Carter JD, Mulder RT, Bartram AF, et al. Infants in a neonatal intensive care unit: parental response. Arch Dis Child Fetal Neonatal Ed. 2005;90(2):F109–13.
14. Bakewell-Sachs S, Gennaro S. Parenting the post-NICU premature infant. MCN Am J Matern Child Nurs. 2004;29(6):398–403.
15. Doyle LW, Ford G, Davis N. Health and hospitalistions after discharge in extremely low birth weight infants. Semin Neonatol. 2003;8(2):137–45.
16. Chien YH, Tsao PN, Chou HC, et al. Rehospitalization of extremely-low-birth-weight infants in first 2 years of life. Early Hum Dev. 2002;66(1):33–40.
17. Furman L, Baley J, Borawski-Clark E, et al. Hospitalization as a measure of morbidity among very low birth weight infants with chronic lung disease. J Pediatr. 1996;128(4):447–52.
18. Kuzniewicz MW, Parker SJ, Schnake-Mahl A, et al. Hospital readmissions and emergency department visits in moderate preterm, late preterm, and early term infants. Clin Perinatol. 2013;40(4):753–75.
19. McLaurin KK, Hall CB, Jackson EA, et al. Persistence of morbidity and cost differences between late-preterm and term infants during the first year of life. Pediatrics. 2009;123(2):653–9.
20. Ray KN, SA L. Hospitalization of early preterm, late preterm, and term infants during the first year of life by gestational age. Hospital Pediatrics. 2013;3(3):194–203.
21. Morris BH, Gard CC, Kennedy K. Rehospitalization of extremely low birth weight (ELBW) infants: are there racial/ethnic disparities? J Perinatol. 2005;25(10):656–63.
22. Escobar GJ, Joffe S, Gardner MN, et al. Rehospitalization in the first two weeks after discharge from the neonatal intensive care unit. Pediatrics. 1999;104(1):e2.
23. Martens PJ, Derksen S, Gupta S. Predictors of hospital readmission of Manitoba newborns within six weeks postbirth discharge: a population-based study. Pediatrics. 2004;114(3):708–13.
24. Ambalavanan N, Carlo WA, McDonald SA, et al. Identification of extremely premature infants at high risk of rehospitalization. Pediatrics. 2011;128(5):e1216–25.
25. Young PC, Korgenski K, Buchi KF. Early readmission of newborns in a large health care system. Pediatrics. 2013;131(5):e1538–44.

26. Elder DE, Hagan R, Evans SF, et al. Hospital admissions in the first year of life in very preterm infants. J Paediatr Child Health. 1999;35(2):145–50.
27. Stephens AS, Lain SJ, Roberts CL, et al. Survival, hospitalization, and acute-care costs of very and moderate preterm infants in the first 6 years of life: a population-based study. J Pediatr. 2016;169:61–8. e63
28. Hall CB, Weinberg GA, Iwane MK, et al. The burden of respiratory syncytial virus infection in young children. N Engl J Med. 2009;360(6):588–98.
29. Hall CB, Weinberg GA, Blumkin AK, et al. Respiratory syncytial virus-associated hospitalizations among children less than 24 months of age. Pediatrics. 2013;132(2):e341–8.
30. Munoz-Quiles C, Lopez-Lacort M, Ubeda-Sansano I, et al. Population-based analysis of bronchiolitis epidemiology in Valencia, Spain. Pediatr Infect Dis J. 2016;35(3):275–80.
31. Fjaerli HO, Farstad T, Bratlid D. Hospitalisations for respiratory syncytial virus bronchiolitis in Akershus, Norway, 1993-2000: a population-based retrospective study. BMC Pediatr. 2004;4(1):25.
32. Figueras-Aloy J, Carbonell-Estrany X, Quero-Jimenez J, et al. FLIP-2 Study: risk factors linked to respiratory syncytial virus infection requiring hospitalization in premature infants born in Spain at a gestational age of 32 to 35 weeks. Pediatr Infect Dis J. 2008;27(9):788–93.
33. Boyce TG, Mellen BG, Mitchel Jr EF, et al. Rates of hospitalization for respiratory syncytial virus infection among children in medicaid. J Pediatr. 2000;137(6):865–70.
34. Helfrich AM, Nylund CM, Eberly MD, et al. Healthy late-preterm infants born 33-36+6 weeks gestational age have higher risk for respiratory syncytial virus hospitalization. Early Hum Dev. 2015;91(9):541–6.
35. Forbes ML, Hall CB, Jackson A, et al. Comparative costs of hospitalisation among infants at high risk for respiratory syncytial virus lower respiratory tract infection during the first year of life. J Med Econ. 2010;13(1):136–41.
36. Horn SD, Smout RJ. Effect of prematurity on respiratory syncytial virus hospital resource use and outcomes. J Pediatr. 2003;143(5 Suppl):S133–41.
37. Greenberg D, Dagan R, Shany E, et al. Increased risk for respiratory syncytial virus-associated, community-acquired alveolar pneumonia in infants born at 31-36 weeks of gestation. Pediatr Infect Dis J. 2014;33(4):381–6.
38. Greenough A, Alexander J, Burgess S, et al. Health care utilisation of prematurely born, preschool children related to hospitalisation for RSV infection. Arch Dis Child. 2004;89(7):673–8.
39. Lee JH, Chang YS, Committee on Data C, et al. Use of medical resources by preterm infants born at less than 33 weeks' gestation following discharge from the Neonatal Intensive Care Unit in Korea. J Korean Med Sci. 2015;30(Suppl 1):S95–S103.
40. Jain S, Cheng J. Emergency department visits and rehospitalizations in late preterm infants. Clin Perinatol. 2006;33(4):935–45. abstract xi.
41. Goyal NK, Folger AT, Hall ES, et al. Effects of home visiting and maternal mental health on use of the emergency department among late preterm infants. J Obstet Gynecol Neonatal Nurs. 2015;44(1):135–44.
42. Ray K, Escobar GJ, Lorch SA. Premature infants born to adolescent mothers: Health care utilization after initial discharge academic pediatrics. Acad Pediatr. 2010;10(5):302–8.
43. McGrath-Morrow SA, Lee G, Stewart BH, et al. Day care increases the risk of respiratory morbidity in chronic lung disease of prematurity. Pediatrics. 2010;126(4):632–7.
44. Rhein LM, Konnikova L, McGeachey A, et al. The role of pulmonary follow-up in reducing health care utilization in infants with bronchopulmonary dysplasia. Clin Pediatr (Phila). 2012;51(7):645–50.
45. Wade KC, Lorch SA, Bakewell-Sachs S, et al. Pediatric care for preterm infants after NICU discharge: High number of office visits and prescription medications. J Perinatol. 2008;28(10):696–701.
46. Luu TM, Lefebvre F, Riley P, et al. Continuing utilisation of specialised health services in extremely preterm infants. Arch Dis Child Fetal Neonatal Ed. 2010;95(5):F320–5.

47. Gray D, Woodward LJ, Spencer C, et al. Health service utilisation of a regional cohort of very preterm infants over the first 2 years of life. J Paediatr Child Health. 2006;42(6):377–83.
48. Nakamura MM, Toomey SL, Zaslavsky AM, et al. Measuring pediatric hospital readmission rates to drive quality improvement. Acad Pediatr. 2014;14(5 Suppl):S39–46.
49. Lorch SA, Passarella M, Zeigler A. Challenges to measuring variation in readmission rates of neonatal intensive care patients. Acad Pediatr. 2014;14(5 Suppl):S47–53.
50. Coller RJ, Nelson BB, Sklansky DJ, et al. Preventing hospitalizations in children with medical complexity: a systematic review. Pediatrics. 2014;134(6):e1628–47.
51. Herrin J, St Andre J, Kenward K, et al. Community factors and hospital readmission rates. Health Serv Res. 2015;50(1):20–39.
52. McMillan JE, Meier ER, Winer JC, et al. Clinical and geographic characterization of 30-day readmissions in pediatric Sickle Cell crisis patients. Hosp Pediatr. 2015;5(8):423–31.
53. Lorch SA. Quality measurements in pediatrics: What do they assess? JAMA Pediatr. 2013;167(1):89–90.
54. Krumholz HM, Lin Z, Keenan PS, et al. Relationship between hospital readmission and mortality rates for patients hospitalized with acute myocardial infarction, heart failure, or pneumonia. JAMA. 2013;309(6):587–93.
55. Silber JH, Lorch SA, Rosenbaum PR, et al. Time to send the preemie home? Additional maturity at discharge and subsequent healthcare costs and outcomes. Health Serv Res. 2009;44(2, Part I):444–463.
56. Srivastava R, Keren R. Pediatric readmissions as a hospital quality measure. JAMA. 2013;309(4):396–8.
57. Hoehn RS, Wima K, Vestal MA, et al. Effect of hospital safety-net burden on cost and outcomes after surgery. JAMA Surg. 2016;151(2):120–8.
58. Joynt K, Jha AK. Which hospitals have higher readmission rates for patients with heart failure? J Am Coll Cardiol. 2010;55(10s1):A143.E1348.
59. Beck AF, Simmons JM, Huang B, et al. Geomedicine: Area-based socioeconomic measures for assessing risk of hospital reutilization among children admitted for asthma. Am J Public Health. 2012;102(12):2308–14.
60. Liu SY, Pearlman DN. Hospital readmissions for childhood asthma: The role of individual and neighborhood factors. Public Health Rep. 2009;124(1):65–78.
61. Ray KN, Lorch SA. Hospitalization of rural and urban infants during the first year of life. Pediatrics. 2012;130(6):1084–93.
62. Rice-Townsend S, Hall M, Barnes JN, et al. Variation in risk-adjusted hospital readmission after treatment of appendicitis at 38 children's hospitals: An opportunity for collaborative quality improvement. Ann Surg. 2013;257(4):758–65.
63. Auger KA, Kahn RS, Davis MM, et al. Medical home quality and readmission risk for children hospitalized with asthma exacerbations. Pediatrics. 2013;131(1):64–70.
64. Bloomberg GR, Trinkaus KM, Fisher Jr EB, et al. Hospital readmissions for childhood asthma: A 10-year metropolitan study. Am J Respir Crit Care Med. 2003;167(8):1068–76.
65. Coller RJ, Klitzner TS, Lerner CF, et al. Predictors of 30-day readmission and association with primary care follow-up plans. J Pediatr. 2013;163(4):1027–33.
66. McGregor MJ, Reid RJ, Schulzer M, et al. Socioeconomic status and hospital utilization among younger adult pneumonia admissions at a Canadian hospital. BMC Health Serv Res. 2006;6:152.
67. Lorch SA, Enlow E. The role of social determinants in explaining racial/ethnic disparities in perinatal outcomes. Pediatr Res. 2016;79(1–2):141–7. doi:10.1038/pr.2015.199. Epub 2015 Oct 14.
68. Goyal N, Zubizarreta JR, Small DS, et al. Length of stay and readmissions among late preterm infants: an instrumental variable approach. Hosp Pediatr. 2013;3(1):7–15.
69. Moyer LB, Goyal NK, Meinzen-Derr J, et al. Factors associated with readmission in late-preterm infants: a matched case-control study. Hosp Pediatr. 2014;4(5):298–304.

70. Smith VC, Zupancic JA, McCormick MC, et al. Rehospitalization in the first year of life among infants with bronchopulmonary dysplasia. J Pediatr. 2004;144(6):799–803.
71. Slimings C, Einarsdottir K, Srinivasjois R, et al. Hospital admissions and gestational age at birth: 18 years of follow up in Western Australia. Paediatr Perinat Epidemiol. 2014;28(6):536–44.
72. Tseng YH, Chen CW, Huang HL, et al. Incidence of and predictors for short-term readmission among preterm low-birthweight infants. Pediatr Int. 2010;52(5):711–7.
73. Lamarche-Vadel A, Blondel B, Truffer P, et al. Re-hospitalization in infants younger than 29 weeks' gestation in the EPIPAGE cohort. Acta Paediatr. 2004;93(10):1340–5.
74. Ralser E, Mueller W, Haberland C, et al. Rehospitalization in the first 2 years of life in children born preterm. Acta Paediatr. 2012;101(1):e1–5.

Opportunities to Promote Primary Prevention of Post Neonatal Intensive Care Unit Respiratory Morbidity in the Premature Infant

Cindy T. McEvoy

Introduction

The Importance of Lung Trajectories in the Prevention of Post-NICU Respiratory Morbidity in the Premature Infant

There is increasing evidence that lung function tracks from infancy to early adulthood along percentiles established very early in life [1]. Therefore, it is critical to develop early perinatal prevention strategies and life strategies to maximize the lung growth and development which begin very early in gestation and follow very precisely orchestrated steps. Any premature birth at <37 weeks of gestation can impair normal lung growth and development since fetal lung development is interrupted during a critical time-sensitive period. This can occur without the clinical manifestation of respiratory disease postnatally [2]. Infants born with low lung function due to premature birth coupled with other potential in utero and early life insults to the developing lung are likely to remain at a decreased percentile of lung function and are more likely, during the normal aging process, to develop chronic obstructive pulmonary disease (COPD), as discussed in chapter "Sequelae of Prematurity: The Adolescent and Young Adult Patient". COPD is increasing worldwide and is predicted to be the third largest cause of mortality by 2030 [1]. Prevention of post neonatal intensive care unit (NICU) respiratory morbidity should focus on maximizing the

C.T. McEvoy, MD, MCR
Department of Pediatrics, Oregon Health & Science University, Portland, OR, USA
e-mail: mcevoyc@ohsu.edu

© Springer International Publishing AG 2017
A.M. Hibbs, M. S. Muhlebach (eds.), *Respiratory Outcomes in Preterm Infants*,
Respiratory Medicine, DOI 10.1007/978-3-319-48835-6_9

preterm infant's lung potential to attain maximum potential respiratory health into adulthood. Primary efforts should be twofold: decrease preterm deliveries whenever feasible, and decrease or avoid postnatal insults. Considering the "normal premature" lung as a critical reference point for the concept of lung function trajectories may enhance prevention of post NICU respiratory morbidity.

A variety of positive and negative environmental exposures can promote lung health or disease throughout life, but fetal and infant lung health is particularly important as it correlates with adult lung function and establishes the lifelong lung function trajectory. Lung development is directly related to fetal growth and the duration of gestation, and prematurity/low birth weight is a marker of impaired fetal growth that is associated with lower lifetime lung function. About 15–20 % of adult asthma is attributable to low birth weight [3] which is likely a combination of the direct effect of impaired lung function from prematurity and/or the effect of other insults such as environmental exposures on the premature lung. With regard to the prevention of post NICU respiratory morbidities, this chapter will focus on the modifiable insults that, if decreased, could assist in preventing subsequent life-long lung disease, focusing particularly on in utero smoke, its physiological basis, and the potential for in utero intervention. Preterm deliveries are the most common cause of abnormal lung development [1], but subsequent lung function in this scenario can also be affected by a number of additional adverse in utero and early postnatal insults.

Preterm Birth Epidemiology and Complications

Despite intense research, the occurrence of preterm birth remains a global health problem with 14.9 million babies born before 37 weeks gestation in year 2010 [4]. Preterm birth is associated with increased mortality and morbidity including increased respiratory complications. Preterm birth is the most common cause of altered lung development and one with potential lifelong ramifications [5]. As discussed in other chapters in this book, at one end of this spectrum are the extremely premature infants who commonly have acute neonatal respiratory morbidity and are at risk for the development of bronchopulmonary dysplasia (BPD). However, lung development is a continuum, and compared to term infants, late preterm infants also manifest increased neonatal respiratory morbidity including altered pulmonary function [6], respiratory distress syndrome, transient tachypnea, pneumonia [2, 7], and increased wheezing, asthma, and respiratory morbidity as they age [8, 9]. Any approaches that decrease preterm birth will likely decrease the respiratory morbidity associated with the spectrum of prematurity.

Preconception Interventions Before Pregnancy to Prevent Post NICU Respiratory Morbidities

Maternal Nutrition and Weight Preconception

The Barker hypothesis classically highlights the importance of maternal nutrition to offspring lung development. Barker et al. demonstrated that fetal undernutrition in middle to late gestation leads to disproportionate fetal growth and permanent changes in body structure [10]. Perinatal vitamin deficiencies including those in vitamin A [11], vitamin D [12], and vitamin E [13] have been linked to deficiencies in offspring pulmonary function, but few of these nutritional deficiencies have been studied in the scenario of preterm deliveries and their subsequent respiratory health. One might speculate that the effects would likely be more pronounced in extremely preterm, very preterm (<30–32 weeks gestation), and late preterm infants.

There is evidence from multiple large epidemiological trials [14–21] that maternal preconception obesity increases the risk of preterm birth [14], and is also significantly associated with subsequent wheezing, bronchodilator prescriptions, and asthma development in the offspring [14, 15, 19, 21]. Reichman et al. [19] and Kumar et al. [15] independently found preconception obesity (body mass index [BMI] > 30 kg/m^2) was associated with increased risk for asthma diagnosis or recurrent wheezing. Several of these studies conducted in the United States were done in minority, urban, and disadvantaged populations. However, MacDonald et al. [21] demonstrated a significant association in the electronic medical record documented bronchodilator dispensings and preconception maternal obesity in an insured, nonurban largely White population in the United States, demonstrating the generalizability of this association. Haberg and colleagues [14] analyzed data from 33,192 pregnancies and found that preterm birth and maternal obesity increased the risk of wheezing by 4.3 % and 3.3 %, respectively. These increased risks of wheezing were in addition to the baseline risk of 39.2 % found in the term infants of uncomplicated pregnancies and born to moms with a normal BMI [14]. Thus, the risk of wheezing in preterm infants born to mothers with an obese BMI is estimated to be 46.8 % [14]. The mechanism of this association is postulated to be inflammatory, but still unproven. There are few studies targeting preconception weight management [22], but decreased obesity would likely prevent increased post NICU respiratory morbidities in premature infants.

Preconception and Intergenerational Smoking Cessation

As outlined below, maternal smoking during pregnancy is associated with adverse perinatal outcomes including increased prematurity and adverse childhood respiratory outcomes [23, 24]. Although intuitively preconception smoking cessation would be ideal, a recent systematic review [22] identified only three studies that focused on decreasing preconception smoking, and pregnancy outcomes were not reported. In addition, studies [25] have shown that a grandmother's smoking can affect the grandchild's lung development even if the mother did not smoke, likely via effects on methylation pathways. This emphasizes the importance of inter-generational smoking cessation, although the impact of this benefit will be delayed.

Prenatal Interventions to Decrease Post NICU Respiratory Morbidities

Decreasing In Utero (and Second Hand) Smoke Exposure During Pregnancy

Clinical Benefits

There is strong evidence that smoking cessation or decreased in utero smoke/tobacco/nicotine exposure is effective on multiple levels to promote lung health in the offspring. Importantly, maternal smoking during pregnancy is the largest preventable cause of low birth weight (LBW), prematurity and perinatal mortality [23, 24]. About one-third of preterm births occur secondary to maternal indications or fetal concerns and two-thirds are due to spontaneous rupture of membranes and/or onset of labor [26]. Maternal smoking during pregnancy is associated with many of the obstetrical complications that precipitate indicated preterm birth such as pla-centa previa, placental abruption, or fetal growth restriction [4]. One of the common risk factors for premature labor includes maternal smoking during pregnancy. Smoking predisposes to intrauterine infection, cervical insufficiency, and preterm prelabor rupture of membranes, all key causes of spontaneous preterm delivery [27]. There are several confounding factors in the relationship between maternal smoking during pregnancy and preterm birth, but the evidence supports the likely causality [4]. A meta-analysis of 20 prospective studies of over 100,000 women [28] found that smoking in pregnancy increased preterm births by about 25 %. The asso-ciation between second hand smoke exposure during pregnancy and preterm birth is less clear [29].

In addition to its association with increased preterm deliveries, maternal smok-ing during pregnancy is also the largest preventable cause of childhood respiratory illness, and children whose mothers smoked during pregnancy show lifetime decreases in pulmonary function and increased respiratory illnesses and asthma [30, 31]. A population-based Canadian cohort of over 29,000 infants <33 weeks gesta-tion demonstrated that maternal smoking during pregnancy was also associated with the development of BPD with an adjusted odds ratio of 1.21, 95 % confidence interval of 1.04–1.41 [32]. Despite being the focus of the Surgeon General for at least 40 years, at least 12 % of American women continue to smoke during pregnancy, and in low and middle income countries, the incidence is increasing. A recent large study from the ENRIECO Consortium reported the incidence of smoking in pregnancy in Europe was 20–40 % [33].

Pulmonary Function Tests and Lung Development After Maternal Smoking in Pregnancy

The decreases in offspring pulmonary function caused by maternal smoking during pregnancy occur in both preterm and term infants, are present prior to any significant exposure to postnatal smoke, and are lifelong. One of the initial reports indicating a connection between maternal smoking and children's respiratory function was from Tager et al. [34] who reported decreases of 7–10 % in the forced expiratory volume in 1 s (FEV_1) in children 1–5 years of age with smoking mothers. Hanrahan et al. [35] examined pulmonary function of infants shortly after birth (~4.2 weeks) as a function of maternal smoking during pregnancy and found a significant decrease in maximal expiratory flow at functional residual capacity (VmaxFRC). Important to this focus on premature infants, Hoo et al. [36] performed pulmonary function tests at 36.5 weeks of postmenstrual age in 108 infants who delivered preterm at <36 weeks gestation (mean gestational age of 33.5 weeks). These infants manifested no clinical respiratory disease, but those who had been exposed to in utero smoke had a significantly decreased time to peak tidal expiratory flow to expiratory time ratio (TPTEF:TE) and a decreased VmaxFRC compared to the preterm infants not exposed to in utero smoke. TPTEF:TE remained significant after allowing for sex, ethnic group, body size, postnatal age, and socioeconomic status. Since TPTEF:TE is a parameter that has been shown to precede and predict wheezing [37], this study of pulmonary function in late preterm infants emphasizes the impact of in utero smoke exposure in this population. This study also demonstrates that the changes seen in pulmonary function tests after in utero tobacco smoke exposure are not caused just by exposures at the end of the gestation.

The decreases in pulmonary function after in utero smoke appear long-lasting. Cunningham et al. [38] performed tests on 8800 school children aged 8–12 years of age who were nonsmokers and found reduced forced expiratory flows in children whose mothers smoked during pregnancy, which was not explained by postnatal smoke exposure. A recent prospective study with a 21-year follow-up has now extended the decreases in FEV_1 and FEF_{25-75} (forced expiratory flows between 25 % and 75 % of forced vital capacity [FVC]) to 21 years of age in males [31]. Birth cohorts demonstrate that the changes in pulmonary function after in utero smoke exposure persist, which support the structural changes that have been demonstrated, as outlined below. This strongly suggests that the incidence and severity of subsequent respiratory illnesses in preterm infants would be decreased [32] by programs to reduce maternal smoking in pregnancy or block the effects of in utero smoke on lung development as a modifiable factor in the face of prematurity.

The critical importance of decreasing exposure to in utero smoke is highlighted by studies demonstrating structural changes in lung development by postmortem exams as well as in animal models after in utero smoke exposure. Elliot et al. [39] demonstrated that children who died of sudden infant death syndrome (SIDS) whose mothers had smoked prenatally and postnatally had increased airway wall thickness compared to infants who died of SIDS whose mothers had not smoked. Spindel et al. [40] in a nonhuman primate model, have demonstrated extensive expression of nicotinic acetylcholine receptors (nAChR) in fetal monkey lung [40] and demonstrated that nicotine crossed the placenta of the pregnant monkey and upregulated the α7nAChR in the airway epithelial cells and fibroblasts in the fetal monkey lung (Fig. 1), which translated into increases in collagen in a similar distribution [41]. These nicotine-induced changes in lung structure translated into alterations in pulmonary function in the newborn rhesus monkeys similar to those changes measured in children born to smoking mothers [42]. The increased collagen and decreased elastin caused by prenatal nicotine exposure likely underly the changes in pulmonary function with decreased respiratory compliance and forced expiratory flows caused by maternal smoking in pregnancy.

Studies in mice have suggested the potential mechanism by which prenatal nicotine exposure leads to decreases in expiratory flows is by affecting airway growth. Nicotine stimulated lung branching and dysnaptic/disproportionate lung growth in a dose-dependent fashion in embryonic murine lung explants [43]. This was further studied in vivo in a murine model of in utero nicotine exposure in which pregnant mice were treated with nicotine from gestation day 7 to postnatal day 14. Similar to changes seen in humans and nonhuman primates, this combination of prenatal and postnatal nicotine exposure caused significant decreases in forced expiratory flows in the offspring [44]. A primary mediator of this effect appeared to be the α7 nAChR, as the effect of nicotine was lost in α7 nAChR knockout mice [44]. Further studies in this model demonstrated that the critical period for perinatal nicotine exposure to alter forced expiratory flows was exposure that corresponded to the end of the pseudoglandular period through the canalicular and saccular periods, but before most of the alveolarization [44] and suggests a primary effect of nicotine on airway growth. This was confirmed by stereological analysis of airway size and diameter which showed an increased number of airways of small diameter with nicotine treatment. These data suggest that prenatal nicotine exposure leads to decreased forced expiratory flows by stimulating epithelial cell growth and potentially lung branching to result in longer and more tortuous airways.

Smoking Cessation/Decreasing Maternal Smoking Reduces Preterm Birth

A recent Cochrane review [45] concluded that smoking cessation programs reduce the proportion of women who smoke and reduce the rate of preterm birth. This review concluded that the effect was larger when counseling was combined with other strategies such as providing feedback with biochemical measures. It also found incentive-based interventions to be effective, but these randomized controlled

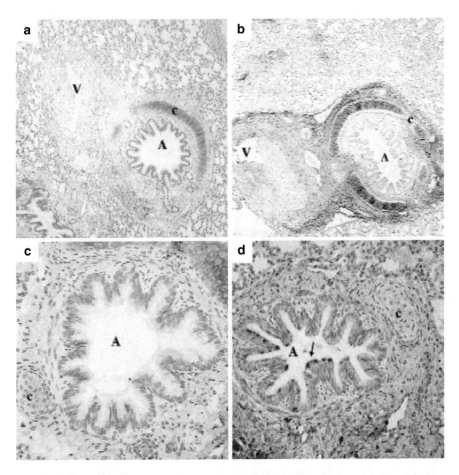

Fig. 1 Prenatal nicotine exposure increases α7 nAChR expression in fetal monkey lung (134 days gestation). Immunohistochemical localization of nicotinic receptor subtypes in 134- day fetal monkey lung. *a* and *c* from control fetus; *b* and *d* from nicotine-exposed fetus. (*a*) Anti-α7 (MAB 319) showing brownish-red staining in fibroblast cell layer in cartilaginous airways and vessel walls. ×100. (*b*) In nicotine-exposed fetus, greatly enhanced α7 staining is seen in cartilaginous airway and vessel walls. ×100. No immunostaining was seen with nonimmune serum (not shown). (*c* and *d*) High-power view of smaller cartilaginous airways showing relatively little α7 in airway wall and epithelial cell lining in control lung, but intense staining in airway wall and epithelial cells (*arrows*) from nicotine-exposed lung. ×400. AEC was used as immunoperoxidase substrate, and hematoxylin was used as counterstain. *A* airway lumen, *V* blood vessel lumen, *C* cartilage, *AEC3*-amino-9-ethylcarbazole, *MAB* monoclonal antibody (Reprinted with permission obtained from the American Society for Clinical Investigation publications Sekhon et al. [40])

trials (RCTs) were underpowered to assess the effect on preterm births. A recent meta-analysis [46] involving 1.3 million women demonstrated that the introduction of antismoking legislation reduced preterm birth rates by 10 %. This was likely due to cessation in the smoking mother but also in those around her with subsequent decreased exposure to passive smoke. Cnattingius et al. [47] studied 250,000 women who delivered consecutive singletons examining women who either began smoking or stopped smoking in between the two deliveries. The risk of preterm birth was either increased or decreased respectively in a dose-dependent fashion, indicating that effective smoking cessation efforts should reduce preterm birth and by translation decrease post NICU respiratory morbidities.

Nicotine Replacement Therapies (NRT)

Nicotine replacement therapies have also been studied as a means of smoking cessation; however, based on the studies discussed above, nicotine itself will continue to have significant adverse effects on lung development. Also, randomized clinical trials have not demonstrated that nicotine replacement is effective or safe in promoting smoking cessation during pregnancy. A recent Cochrane review [48] examined the safety and efficacy of six trials of NRT in 1745 pregnant smokers, and no significant differences for smoking cessation or other important birth-related outcomes were demonstrated between randomized groups. The U.S. Food and Drug Administration recently announced that it is extending its regulatory authority over all the electronic nicotine delivery systems which are being increasingly used, especially by middle and high school students [49].

Vitamin Supplementation to Decrease the Effects of In Utero Nicotine on Offspring Pulmonary Function

Evidence from animal studies [50] and from a recent randomized clinical trial [37] of vitamin C supplementation (500 mg/day) to pregnant smokers unable to quit smoking indicates that vitamin C may help mediate some of the effects of in utero smoke exposure on offspring respiratory health. The newborns whose mothers had been randomized to vitamin C had significantly improved newborn pulmonary function tests and a decreased incidence of wheeze at 1 year of age compared to those whose mothers had been randomized to placebo. The effect of maternal smoking on newborn lung function was also associated with the maternal genotype for the $\alpha5$ nAChR (rs16969968) ($p < 0.001$ for interaction), which is the $\alpha5$ nAChR structural polymorphism that has the strongest link to lung disease [51] (Fig. 2). This study was not powered to examine preterm births between the randomized groups, but a large RCT [52] of vitamin C (1000 mg) and vitamin E (400 IU) supplementation during pregnancy found a reduction in preterm birth (RR 0.76; 95 % CI 0.58–0.99) and placenta abruption in the treated versus untreated smokers. Although the results of the initial trial of vitamin C supplementation to pregnant smokers were encouraging, a second randomized trial of a more diverse population with measurements of offspring forced expiratory flows as a sensitive measure of the peripheral airways is currently underway.

The independent and joint effects of prenatal smoking and LBW on subsequent childhood asthma were studied in 3389 prospectively followed children at

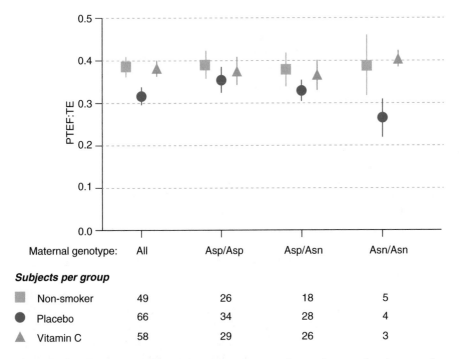

Fig. 2 Effect of maternal smoking during pregnancy on newborn pulmonary function as modulated by maternal α5 genotype (rs16969968). Newborns whose mothers were homozygous for the risk allele in which amino acid 398 of the α5 nAChR is changed from Asp to Asn showed the largest decrease in TPTEF:TE comparing placebo to vitamin C treatment. Values presented are means and 95 % confidence intervals. Asp/Asp indicates mothers homozygous for nonrisk allele, Asp/Asn indicates heterozygous mothers, Asn/Asn indicates mothers homozygous for risk allele. *P* values comparing TPTEF:TE values from newborns of mothers randomized to vitamin C versus placebo are 0.02, 0.32, 0.07, and <0.0001 for mothers of all genotypes, Asp/Asp, Asp/Asn, and Asn/Asn, respectively. *P* values are from linear mixed models (used to allow for unequal variance) adjusting for gestational age at randomization (≤16 versus >16 weeks), birth weight, and gestational age <37 weeks, and allowing for different SDs within each genotype (Reprinted with permission from the American Medical Association publications McEvoy et al. [37])

11–12 years of age [53]. This study demonstrated a strong interaction of LBW and prenatal smoking on the risk of physician-diagnosed asthma. The association of prenatal smoking with physician-diagnosed asthma in LBW infants had a risk ratio of 8.8 versus a risk ratio of 1.3 in normal birth weight children [53].

Decrease in Air Pollution to Decrease Preterm Birth

A recent meta-analysis of 62 studies examining the association of LBW and preterm birth with outdoor air pollution demonstrated that third trimester exposure to carbon monoxide (CO) and particulate matter with aerodynamic diameter of <10 μm

(PM_{10}) was significantly associated with a higher preterm birth risk [54]. Particulate matter with aerodynamic diameter of <2.5 μm ($PM_{2.5}$) and sulfur dioxide (SO_2) have also been associated with higher risks of preterm delivery as have polycyclic aromatic hydrocarbons [55]. A study of 223,502 electronic medical records in the United Stated found that mothers with asthma may experience a higher risk for preterm birth after exposure to traffic-related pollutants such as CO and nitrogen dioxide (NO_2), especially for exposures 3 months preconception and in the early weeks of pregnancy [55]. In the last 6 weeks of pregnancy, preterm birth risk associated with particulate matter with aerodynamic diameter of <10 μm was higher among women with asthma [55].

The association between prenatal exposure to fine particulate matter $PM_{2.5}$ (inhalable material <2.5 μm diameter) and early childhood lung function was investigated by Jedrychowski et al. [56]. Pregnant women had measurements of $PM_{2.5}$ performed over a 48-h period during the second trimester of pregnancy, and the offspring were followed through 5 years of age. Pulmonary function tests were done in 176 children of nonsmokers at 5 years of age and showed a significant decrease in FVC at the highest quartile of $PM_{2.5}$ exposure [56]. The increased exposure to $PM_{2.5}$ was in turn associated with increased wheezing at 2 years, though this effect was no longer significant by 4 years of age [57]. Mortimer et al. similarly saw negative associations with prenatal and early exposures to PM_{10} (inhalable material <10 μm in diameter), NO_2, and CO in asthmatic children, though associations were for specific subgroups of children [58]. Conversely, exposure to increased levels of CO during pregnancy increased allergic sensitization in children with asthma [59]. In a retrospective study of 37,401 children born in British Columbia [60], the incidence of asthma in 3–4 year olds was correlated with estimated levels of in utero and first year of life exposures to air pollution, and an increase in asthma risk was seen with increased exposure to NO_2, CO, and PM_{10}. Animal models have been developed to examine effects of both particulate and gaseous pollution, but the exact mechanisms by which exposure to air pollution alters lung development and leads to increased respiratory disease are still not completely clear.

Normalizing or Maximizing Prenatal Growth

Although it is difficult to distinguish the effects of prematurity and intrauterine growth restriction (IUGR) due to frequent difficulties in establishing gestational age, epidemiological data [61] suggest that IUGR is associated with persistently impaired respiratory development. In sheep, it was demonstrated that fetal growth restriction affected lung structure at 8 weeks, and 2 years after birth with thicker intra-alveolar septa and thicker alveolar blood–air barrier [62]. Fetal lambs with induced IUGR have decreased alveolar and vascular growth [63]. Therefore, decreasing any modifiable underlying etiology for IUGR such as in utero smoke or optimizing prenatal growth in the face of IUGR would likely improve lung development and decrease postnatal NICU respiratory morbidities.

Perinatal Interventions

Avoiding Iatrogenic Preterm Deliveries and Cesarean Sections

Decreasing preterm delivery is the holy grail in the protection of lung development, since premature delivery is the most common cause of altered lung development [1]. Recent studies have shown that progesterone administration in high-risk women with a prior spontaneous preterm birth and those with ultrasound confirmed shortened cervix can decrease preterm deliveries including births at <37 weeks [64]. Preterm delivery can be spontaneous or indicated in response to adverse maternal or fetal conditions. The risks and benefits of iatrogenic pregnancy interruption need to be carefully considered and reviewed. In the United States, the preterm birth rate increased by 31 % from 1981 to 2003, largely because of increased deliveries of late preterm infants ($34^{0/7}$ to $36^{6/7}$ weeks gestation) [65]. In 2003, 12.3 % of births in the United States were preterm [65]. This increased rate of preterm deliveries was highlighted by a number of organizations, and since 2005, there has been consistent decrease with 9.6 % of deliveries being preterm in 2014 [66]. A recent study noted that this decline was due to a decrease of equal magnitude in both spontaneous and indicated preterm deliveries [67]. This should enhance the optimization of lung development of those infants who avoided a preterm delivery and therefore their post NICU respiratory morbidities. Delivery by cesarean section can also influence the relationship between the gut microbiota, immune regulation, and offspring lung health [68], but further study is required.

Postnatal Interventions

Growth and Nutrition

Optimizing postnatal growth in preterm infants is critical to respiratory outcomes and therefore decreasing post NICU morbidities. In extremely preterm infants, BPD occurs more frequently in those with poor somatic growth [69], and nutritional intake in these infants at 7 days is associated with their growth velocity over the first month of life [70], and important factor for lung development. Vitamin A administration has also been shown to decrease BPD in at-risk patients [71], but translation to the bedside has been variable. With reference to late preterm infants, the importance of early postnatal nutrition is extrapolated from data in term infants who develop growth restriction during the final weeks of the pregnancy [72]. In these infants, the lower rates of fetal growth are associated with impaired lung development [72]. Late preterm infants are at increased risk of decreased nutritional intake due to their immature suck and swallow, but there have been no studies evaluating nutrition and growth velocities in late preterm infants and subsequent respiratory outcomes.

Breast-Feeding

Early and comprehensive lactation and breast-feeding support may present a unique opportunity to improve the respiratory health of all preterm and especially late-preterm infants. The global benefits of breast milk are such that the American Academy of Pediatrics (AAP) recommends all preterm infants receive human milk, either mother's own milk or pasteurized donor milk [73]. Breast-feeding or the administration of human milk has been associated with decreased occurrence of factors associated with long-term respiratory health of preterm infants including infections, necrotizing enterocolitis, and rehospitalization for respiratory illness [74]. The anti-infective and anti-inflammatory action of human milk is thought to be related to its unique composition, which includes high concentrations of Lactoferrin [75], antibodies including targeted IgA, glycoproteins, interleukin-2 receptor antagonist, and other anti-infectious agents [76].

Difficulty with breast-feeding also effects postnatal growth in preterm infants, which as previously been discussed is another component driving respiratory outcomes [77]. For the mother and her late preterm infant, breast-feeding or mechanical/manual expression of human milk may be altered by maternal factors (delayed lactogenesis) [78], offspring factors (immature feeding behaviors, comorbidities, and increased nutrition requirements) [78], and/or facility factors (maternal–infant separation, inaccessible mechanical expression equipment, lack of provider knowledge) [78]. As late preterm infants may remain on nonspecialized obstetrical units, it is important that clinicians and their interdisciplinary colleagues who care for these mother–infant dyads strive to follow the World Health Organization's "Ten Steps to Successful Breastfeeding" endorsed by the AAP [73].

Several studies suggest that breast-feeding may be protective against respiratory disease in infancy. The Italian FLIP study [79] (Factors Leading to Respiratory Syncytial Virus-related Infection and Hospitalization among Premature infants) reported breast-feeding as one of the seven variables predicting RSV-related hospitalization in infants born at 33–35 weeks' gestation [79]. A follow-up study of 39 infants with birth weights <2000 g demonstrated those who received human milk had significantly fewer days of upper respiratory symptoms at 1 month and at 7 months corrected age ($p < 0.025$) [80]. A birth cohort in the study by Copenhagen [81] was followed through 2 years of age and demonstrated that breast-feeding reduced the risk of wheezy episodes and severe wheezy exacerbations, but preterm infants were not specifically broken out in the analysis.

Avoidance of Second Hand Smoke

Second hand tobacco smoke remains a significant burden to young children who spend the majority of their time in their home environment where second hand smoke (SHS) is present. This continues despite the implementation of laws requiring smoke-free public and working places. Former preterm infants are particularly vulnerable to the effects of SHS, which is an additional predictor of increased respiratory morbidity, asthma, and worsened asthma morbidity throughout childhood [82]. Smoke-free legislation in England was immediately followed by a decrease in admissions for respiratory tract infections (RTI) in children <15 years old, primarily lower RTI with upper RTI being more incremental, and 11,000 fewer hospital admissions for RTI per year [83]. A randomized trial of brief asthma education plus motivational interviewing counseling versus asthma education alone to families with infants ≤ 32 weeks gestation demonstrated more home smoking bans, but these differences did not persist [82]. At 8 months post NICU discharge, the treatment group had lower salivary cotinine levels, but there was no difference in respiratory clinical outcomes of the children in the groups.

Avoiding Early Postnatal Pollution Exposure

Multiple studies have associated increased environmental air pollution with increased risk of childhood asthma, respiratory infections, and indices of reduced lung function [84, 85], although the specific impact on people born preterm is unknown. Types of air pollution that have been associated with altered lung development include particulate matter, ozone, NO_2, SO_2, and CO. Studies exposing infant monkeys to ozone demonstrated decreased lung branching, hyperplastic airway epithelium, alterations in alveolar development, and smooth muscle remodeling [86]. The combination of ozone and allergen also leads to hyperinnervation of airway epithelium [87] and increased CD25+ cells in airway epithelium, which could provide a link between ozone and asthma. Thus, there is likely a considerable interaction between multiple pollutants and prenatal and postnatal exposures.

Importance of Avoidance of Viral Infections and Prophylaxis When Available

As discussed in other chapters in this book, the preterm infant is vulnerable to viral infections due to underlying structural weaknesses in lung development and issues with innate immunity. Olicker et al. [88] compared the incidence of respiratory morbidity in preterm infants born between 32 $^0/_7$ and 34 $^6/_7$ weeks gestation (without BPD) before and after the American Academy of Pediatric (AAP) change in the administration guidelines of palivizumab, and found a significant increase in the incidence of recurrent wheeze through 12 months of age (46.2 % vs 28.8 %; $p = 0.03$) after the administration policy change. The Dutch RSV Neonatal Network [89] randomized 429 healthy preterm infants born at 33–35 weeks of gestational age to monthly palivizumab or placebo during the RSV season. The palivizumab-treated infants had a relative reduction of 61 % in the total number of wheezing days during the first year of life and significantly less demonstrated recurrent wheeze (11 % vs 21 %; $p = 0.01$). This double-blinded RCT further implicates RSV infection as an important mechanism of recurrent wheeze in healthy preterm infants born at 32–35 weeks of gestation and revisits the importance of prophylaxis to decrease both short-term and long-term respiratory morbidity.

The Barry Caerphilly Growth Study [90] collected information on childhood upper and lower RTI from birth to 5 years on 14 occasions and followed subjects prospectively with lung function measured at 25 years. They found that the lower RTI were associated with an obstructive lung function deficit, and the first year of life appeared to be a sensitive period for these infections. Drysdale et al. [91] prospectively studied the impact of lower RTI in 70 infants born at 24–35 weeks gestation with pulmonary function tests measured at 36 weeks postmenstrual age and at 1 year corrected age. There were no significant differences in lung function at 36 weeks, but at 1 year, the infants who had suffered a viral RTI had a significantly higher mean airway resistance (23 vs 17 cm $H2O/L/s$; $p = 0.0068$), which remained after adjustments for significant covariates [91]. One hundred and fifty-three infants born at 23–35 weeks were followed to 12 months of age, and in this cohort, human rhinovirus C infection was associated with increased wheeze, use of respiratory medication, and use of inhaler [92].

Avoidance of Personal Smoking in Former Premature Infants

Doyle et al. [93] reported follow-up of a cohort of 60 consecutive extremely low birth weight survivors with pulmonary function testing at 8 and 20.2 years of age. Respiratory function was compared between the smokers ($n = 14$) and the nonsmokers ($n = 30$). There was a significantly larger decrease in the FEV1/FVC ratio between the ages of 8 and 20 in the smokers versus nonsmokers demonstrating that active smoking by young adult survivors of extremely low birth weight is associated with reduced respiratory function. Upton et al. [94] studied the effects of former and current personal smoking on FEV1/FVC across the range of exposure to maternal (and paternal) smoking in adult offspring of couples who also had participated in a population study conducted from 1972 to 1976. They documented that maternal smoking-impaired lung volume, regardless of personal smoking, was associated with greater smoking intensity and less quitting in the offspring who took up smoking, and synergized with the offspring's smoking to increase airflow limitation in adults. Although this study did not focus specifically on preterm infants, the implication for preterm infants is likely even more significant.

Treatment of Post-NICU Respiratory Morbidity

As outlined in other chapters, prematurity including late preterm birth increases the risk of a number of respiratory morbidities including childhood wheeze, asthma, and viral and bacterial pneumonias [1]. As outlined in chapter "The Bronchopulmonary Dysplasia Diagnosis: Definitions, Utility, Limitations", there also continues to be discussion with regards to the limitations of the current definition of BPD. In addition, investigation continues into the likely multifactorial etiology of wheeze in former preterm infants [95]. Interestingly, there is relatively little evidence available on the pathophysiology and treatment of wheezing in preschool children (whether born term or preterm) in general [96, 97]. Currently, the treatment of the respiratory symptoms in former preterm infants, both late preterm and survivors with the diagnosis of BPD, is primarily symptomatic with their symptoms decreasing over time as they age, similar to that of the general history of preschool wheeze [5]. There are few randomized trials of therapy in the general population of children with preschool wheeze (and even fewer/none done specifically in populations of preterm infants), but increasing publications of the incidence of clinical symptoms and treatment approaches.

Vrijlandt et al. [8] reported follow-up at 12 months of age in 77 preterm infants delivered at a mean gestational age of 28–29 weeks with and without BPD. Of those with BPD, 39 % used a beta-agonist bronchodilator and 37 % used an inhaled corticosteroid versus 50 % and 31 %, respectively of those without BPD [8]. A number of large trials in extremely preterm infants have recently reported the respiratory follow-up of the children through 1–2 years of age [98, 99]. Follow-up of the Support Trial by Stevens et al. [98] reported follow-up on 918 infants born between $24^{0/7}$ to $27^{6/7}$ weeks for the first 18–22 months of life. Overall, 47.9 % of patients reported wheezing more than twice per week during the worst 2-week period, 31 % reported a cough lasting more than 3 days without a cold, 26.3 % used inhaled steroids, and/or 9.4 % used systemic steroids [98]. Hibbs et al. [99] reported follow-up at 12 months of age on 456 infants with birth weights of 500–1250 g who had been ventilated and randomized to inhaled nitric oxide versus placebo. Overall, the incidence of wheeze was 52.3 %, with the use of bronchodilators at 47 % and inhaled steroids at 25.9 %.

Vrijlandt et al. [9] also reported that at 4 years of age, moderate preterm infants born at 32–36 weeks gestation were receiving the following therapies: 13 % were receiving treatment with a beta-agonist, 9 % an inhaled corticosteroid, and 2 % a combination of a beta-agonist and an inhaled corticosteroid. For the most part, these therapies were used less in moderate preterm infants than early preterm infants, but more in the moderate preterm infants than in the term infants.

Research Priorities for the Primary Prevention of Post NICU Respiratory Morbidities in Premature Infants

The key to treatment of post NICU respiratory morbidity is the optimization of lung development in the face of prematurity, particularly since lung function tracks from infancy through early adulthood along percentiles established very early in life [1]. There are multiple opportunities to address specific research priorities in the prenatal and early perinatal focus to promote lifelong lung health in the premature infant as outlined in Table 1. Foremost is the prevention and cessation of smoking which promotes lung health at multiple levels.

Table 1 Research opportunities to prevent/decrease post NICU respiratory morbidities grouped by the timing of the factors on lung development

Preconception
Study the effectiveness of smoking cessation strategies on incidence of preterm birth and offspring respiratory outcomes
Evaluate the impact of preconception weight loss in obese patients on subsequent preterm birth and respiratory outcomes
Investigate the role of epigenetic modification in mediating effects of nicotine and air pollution
Prenatal
Increased study into effective approaches to increase smoking cessation in all populations
Evaluate the effect of Electronic Nicotine Delivery Systems on the developing lung
Determine the combination of vitamin supplementation to pregnant women to improve offspring respiratory outcomes
Increased evaluation of critical exposure windows and pathophysiological mechanisms of air pollution on birth outcomes
Studies of interventions to optimize prenatal fetal growth
Establishment of prebirth cohorts to characterize the effects of specific obstetrical scenarios on preterm birth and offspring pulmonary outcomes
Perinatal (at delivery)
Continued focus on decreasing preterm deliveries, particularly iatrogenic ones
Detailed evaluation of the variety of scenarios currently ending in indicated preterm deliveries
Evaluation of the effectiveness of antenatal steroids in subgroups of late preterm infants
Early postnatal/childhood
Increased study into effective approaches to decrease second hand smoke exposure in former preterm infants
Evaluation of interventions to maximize and protect lung growth including physiological assessments and longitudinal studies
Increased study into decreasing the initiation of personal smoking in former preterm infants
Longitudinal studies of growth in late preterm infants including the impact of breast-feeding and relation to wheeze
Further study into the potential long-term benefits of RSV prophylaxis

References

1. Stocks J, Hislop A, Sonnappa S. Early lung development: lifelong effect on respiratory health and disease. Lancet Respir Med. 2013;1:728–42.
2. Colin AA, McEvoy C, Castile RG. Respiratory morbidity and lung function in preterm infants of 32 to 36 weeks' gestational age. Pediatrics. 2010;126:115–28.
3. Jaakkola JJ, Ahmed P, Leromnimon A, et al. Preterm delivery and asthma: a systematic review and meta-analysis. J Allergy Clin Immunol. 2006;118:823–30.
4. Wagijo MA, Sheikh A, Duijts L, Been JV. Reducing tobacco smoking and smoke exposure to prevent preterm birth and its complications. Paediatr Respir Rev. 2015. http://dx.doi.org/10.1016/j.prrv.2015.09.002.
5. McEvoy CT, Jain L, Schmidt B, Abman S, Bancalari E, Aschner JL. Bronchopulmonary dysplasia: NHLBI Workshop on the Primary Prevention of Chronic Lung Diseases. Ann Am Thorac Soc. 2014;11(Suppl 3):S146–53.
6. McEvoy C, Venigalla S, Schilling D, Clay N, Spitale P, Nguyen T. Respiratory function in healthy late preterm infants delivered at 33-36 weeks of gestation. J Pediatr. 2013;162:464–9.
7. Hibbard JU, Wilkins I, Sun L, et al. Respiratory morbidity in late preterm births. JAMA. 2010;304:419–25.
8. Vrijlandt EJ, Boezen HM, Gerritsen J, Stremmelaar EF, Duiverman EJ. Respiratory health in prematurely born preschool children with and without bronchopulmonary dysplasia. J Pediatr. 2007;150:256–61.
9. Vrijlandt EJ, Kerstjens JM, Duiverman EJ, Bos AF, Reijneveld SA. Moderately preterm children have more respiratory problems during their first 5 years of life than children born full term. Am J Respir Crit Care Med. 2013;187:1234–40.
10. Barker DJ. In utero programming of chronic disease. Clin Sci (Lond). 1998;95:115–28.
11. Checkley W, West Jr KP, Wise RA, et al. Maternal vitamin A supplementation and lung function in offspring. N Engl J Med. 2010;362:1784–94.
12. Zosky GR, Hart PH, Whitehouse AJ, et al. Vitamin D deficiency at 16 to 20 weeks' gestation is associated with impaired lung function and asthma at 6 years of age. Ann Am Thorac Soc. 2014;11:571–7.
13. Turner S, Prabhu N, Danielan P, et al. First- and second-trimester fetal size and asthma outcomes at age 10 years. Am J Respir Crit Care Med. 2011;184:407–13.
14. Haberg SE, Stigum H, London SJ, Nystad W, Nafstad P. Maternal obesity in pregnancy and respiratory health in early childhood. Paediatr Perinat Epidemiol. 2009;23:352–62.
15. Kumar R, Story RE, Pongracic JA, et al. Maternal pre-pregnancy obesity and recurrent wheezing in early childhood. Pediatr Allergy Immunol Pulmonol. 2010;23:183–90.
16. Leermakers ET, Sonnenschein-van der Voort AM, Gaillard R, et al. Maternal weight, gestational weight gain and preschool wheezing: the Generation R Study. Eur Respir J. 2013;42:1234–43.
17. Lowe A, Braback L, Ekeus C, Hjern A, Forsberg B. Maternal obesity during pregnancy as a risk for early-life asthma. J Allergy Clin Immunol. 2011;128:1107–9.
18. Pike KC, Inskip HM, Robinson SM, et al. The relationship between maternal adiposity and infant weight gain, and childhood wheeze and atopy. Thorax. 2013;68:372–9.
19. Reichman NE, Nepomnyaschy L. Maternal pre-pregnancy obesity and diagnosis of asthma in offspring at age 3 years. Matern Child Health J. 2008;12:725–33.
20. Scholtens S, Wijga AH, Brunekreef B, et al. Maternal overweight before pregnancy and asthma in offspring followed for 8 years. Int J Obes (Lond). 2010;34:606–13.
21. MacDonald KD, Vesco KK, Funk KL, et al. Maternal body mass index before pregnancy is associated with increased bronchodilator dispensing in early childhood: a cross-sectional study. Pediatr Pulmonol. 2016;51(8):803–11. doi:10.1002/ppul.23384.

22. Temel S, van Voorst SF, Jack BW, Denktas S, Steegers EA. Evidence-based preconceptional lifestyle interventions. Epidemiol Rev. 2014;36:19–30.
23. Dietz PM, England LJ, Shapiro-Mendoza CK, Tong VT, Farr SL, Callaghan WM. Infant morbidity and mortality attributable to prenatal smoking in the U.S. Am J Prev Med. 2010;39:45–52.
24. Salihu HM, Aliyu MH, Pierre-Louis BJ, Alexander GR. Levels of excess infant deaths attributable to maternal smoking during pregnancy in the United States. Matern Child Health J. 2003;7:219–27.
25. Li YF, Gilliland FD, Berhane K, et al. Effects of in utero and environmental tobacco smoke exposure on lung function in boys and girls with and without asthma. Am J Respir Crit Care Med. 2000;162:2097–104.
26. Ion R, Bernal AL. Smoking and preterm birth. Reprod Sci. 2015;22:918–26.
27. Hodyl NA, Grzeskowiak LE, Stark MJ, Scheil W, Clifton VL. The impact of aboriginal status, cigarette smoking and smoking cessation on perinatal outcomes in South Australia. Med J Aust. 2014;201:274–8.
28. Shah NR, Bracken MB. A systematic review and meta-analysis of prospective studies on the association between maternal cigarette smoking and preterm delivery. Am J Obstet Gynecol. 2000;182:465–72.
29. Been JV, Lugtenberg MJ, Smets E, et al. Preterm birth and childhood wheezing disorders: a systematic review and meta-analysis. PLoS Med. 2014;11:e1001596.
30. Best D. From the American Academy of Pediatrics: technical report – secondhand and prenatal tobacco smoke exposure. Pediatrics. 2009;124:e1017–44.
31. Hayatbakhsh MR, Sadasivam S, Mamun AA, Najman JM, O'callaghan MJ. Maternal smoking during and after pregnancy and lung function in early adulthood: a prospective study. Thorax. 2009;64:810–4.
32. Isayama T, Shah PS, Ye XY, et al. Adverse impact of maternal cigarette smoking on preterm infants: a population-based cohort study. Am J Perinatol. 2015;32:1105–11.
33. Neuman A, Hohmann C, Orsini N, et al. Maternal smoking in pregnancy and asthma in preschool children: a pooled analysis of eight birth cohorts. Am J Respir Crit Care Med. 2012;186:1037–43.
34. Tager IB, Weiss ST, Munoz A, Rosner B, Speizer FE. Longitudinal study of the effects of maternal smoking on pulmonary function in children. N Engl J Med. 1983;309:699–703.
35. Hanrahan JP, Tager IB, Segal MR, et al. The effect of maternal smoking during pregnancy on early infant lung function. Am Rev Respir Dis. 1992;145:1129–35.
36. Hoo AF, Henschen M, Dezateux C, Costeloe K, Stocks J. Respiratory function among preterm infants whose mothers smoked during pregnancy. Am J Respir Crit Care Med. 1998;158:700–5.
37. McEvoy CT, Schilling D, Clay N, et al. Vitamin C supplementation for pregnant smoking women and pulmonary function in their newborn infants: a randomized clinical trial. JAMA. 2014;311:2074–82.
38. Cunningham J, Dockery DW, Speizer FE. Maternal smoking during pregnancy as a predictor of lung function in children. Am J Epidemiol. 1994;139:1139–52.
39. Elliot J, Vullermin P, Robinson P. Maternal cigarette smoking is associated with increased inner airway wall thickness in children who die from sudden infant death syndrome. Am J Respir Crit Care Med. 1998;158:802–6.
40. Sekhon HS, Jia Y, Raab R, et al. Prenatal nicotine increases pulmonary alpha7 nicotinic receptor expression and alters fetal lung development in monkeys. J Clin Invest. 1999;103:637–47.
41. Sekhon HS, Keller JA, Proskocil BJ, Martin EL, Spindel ER. Maternal nicotine exposure upregulates collagen gene expression in fetal monkey lung. Association with alpha7 nicotinic acetylcholine receptors. Am J Respir Cell Mol Biol. 2002;26:31–41.
42. Sekhon HS, Keller JA, Benowitz NL, Spindel ER. Prenatal nicotine exposure alters pulmonary function in newborn rhesus monkeys. Am J Respir Crit Care Med. 2001;164:989–94.

43. Wongtrakool C, Roser-Page S, Rivera HN, Roman J. Nicotine alters lung branching morphogenesis through the alpha7 nicotinic acetylcholine receptor. Am J Physiol Lung Cell Mol Physiol. 2007;293:L611–8.
44. Wongtrakool C, Wang N, Hyde DM, Roman J, Spindel ER. Prenatal nicotine exposure alters lung function and airway geometry through alpha7 nicotinic receptors. Am J Respir Cell Mol Biol. 2012;46:695–702.
45. Chamberlain C, O'Mara-Eves A, Oliver S, et al. Psychosocial interventions for supporting women to stop smoking in pregnancy. Cochrane Database Syst Rev. 2013;10:CD001055.
46. Been JV, Nurmatov UB, Cox B, Nawrot TS, van Schayck CP, Sheikh A. Effect of smoke-free legislation on perinatal and child health: a systematic review and meta-analysis. Lancet. 2014;383:1549–60.
47. Cnattingius S, Granath F, Petersson G, Harlow BL. The influence of gestational age and smoking habits on the risk of subsequent preterm deliveries. N Engl J Med. 1999;341:943–8.
48. Coleman T, Chamberlain C, Davey MA, Cooper SE, Leonardi-Bee J. Pharmacological interventions for promoting smoking cessation during pregnancy. Cochrane Database Syst Rev. 2012;9:CD010078.
49. U.S. Food and Drug Administration. Vaporizers, e-cigarettes, and other electronic nicotine delivery systems (ENDS). Last edited: 2016-05-09.
50. Proskocil BJ, Sekhon HS, Clark JA, et al. Vitamin C prevents the effects of prenatal nicotine on pulmonary function in newborn monkeys. Am J Respir Crit Care Med. 2005;171:1032–9.
51. Bierut LJ. Convergence of genetic findings for nicotine dependence and smoking related diseases with chromosome 15q24-25. Trends Pharmacol Sci. 2010;31:46–51.
52. Abramovici A, Gandley RE, Clifton RG, et al. Prenatal vitamin C and E supplementation in smokers is associated with reduced placental abruption and preterm birth: a secondary analysis. BJOG. 2015;122:1740–7.
53. Bjerg A, Hedman L, Perzanowski M, Lundback B, Ronmark E. A strong synergism of low birth weight and prenatal smoking on asthma in schoolchildren. Pediatrics. 2011;127: e905–12.
54. Stieb DM, Chen L, Eshoul M, Judek S. Ambient air pollution, birth weight and preterm birth: a systematic review and meta-analysis. Environ Res. 2012;117:100–11.
55. Mendola P, Wallace M, Hwang BS, et al. Preterm birth and air pollution: critical windows of exposure for women with asthma. J Allergy Clin Immunol. 2016. pii: S0091-6749(16)00087-7. doi:10.1016/j.jaci.2015.12.1309.
56. Jedrychowski WA, Perera FP, Maugeri U, et al. Effect of prenatal exposure to fine particulate matter on ventilatory lung function of preschool children of non-smoking mothers. Paediatr Perinat Epidemiol. 2010;24:492–501.
57. Jedrychowski WA, Perera FP, Maugeri U, et al. Intrauterine exposure to polycyclic aromatic hydrocarbons, fine particulate matter and early wheeze. Prospective birth cohort study in 4-year olds. Pediatr Allergy Immunol. 2010;21:e723–32.
58. Mortimer K, Neugebauer R, Lurmann F, Alcorn S, Balmes J, Tager I. Air pollution and pulmonary function in asthmatic children: effects of prenatal and lifetime exposures. Epidemiology. 2008;19:550–7.
59. Mortimer K, Neugebauer R, Lurmann F, Alcorn S, Balmes J, Tager I. Early-lifetime exposure to air pollution and allergic sensitization in children with asthma. J Asthma. 2008;45:874–81.
60. Clark NA, Demers PA, Karr CJ, et al. Effect of early life exposure to air pollution on development of childhood asthma. Environ Health Perspect. 2010;118:284–90.
61. Edwards CA, Osman LM, Godden DJ, Campbell DM, Douglas JG. Relationship between birth weight and adult lung function: controlling for maternal factors. Thorax. 2003;58:1061–5.
62. Maritz GS, Cock ML, Louey S, Suzuki K, Harding R. Fetal growth restriction has long-term effects on postnatal lung structure in sheep. Pediatr Res. 2004;55:287–95.
63. Rozance PJ, Seedorf GJ, Brown A, et al. Intrauterine growth restriction decreases pulmonary alveolar and vessel growth and causes pulmonary artery endothelial cell dysfunction in vitro in fetal sheep. Am J Physiol Lung Cell Mol Physiol. 2011;301:L860–71.

64. Schmouder VM, Prescott GM, Franco A, Fan-Havard P. The rebirth of progesterone in the prevention of preterm labor. Ann Pharmacother. 2013;47:527–36.
65. Raju TN, Higgins RD, Stark AR, Leveno KJ. Optimizing care and outcome for late-preterm (near-term) infants: a summary of the workshop sponsored by the National Institute of Child Health and Human Development. Pediatrics. 2006;118:1207–14.
66. Hamilton BE, Martin JA, Osterman MJ, Curtin SC, Matthews TJ. Births: final data for 2014. Natl Vital Stat Rep. 2015;64:1–64.
67. Gyamfi-Bannerman C, Ananth CV. Trends in spontaneous and indicated preterm delivery among singleton gestations in the United States, 2005-2012. Obstet Gynecol. 2014;124:1069–74.
68. Manuck TA, Levy PT, Gyamfi-Bannerman C, Jobe AH, Blaisdell CJ. Prenatal and perinatal determinants of lung health and disease in early life: a National Heart, Lung, and Blood Institute Workshop Report. JAMA Pediatr. 2016;170:e154577.
69. Ehrenkranz RA, Dusick AM, Vohr BR, Wright LL, Wrage LA, Poole WK. Growth in the neonatal intensive care unit influences neurodevelopmental and growth outcomes of extremely low birth weight infants. Pediatrics. 2006;117:1253–61.
70. Martin CR, Brown YF, Ehrenkranz RA, et al. Nutritional practices and growth velocity in the first month of life in extremely premature infants. Pediatrics. 2009;124:649–57.
71. Tyson JE, Wright LL, Oh W, et al. Vitamin A supplementation for extremely-low-birth-weight infants. National Institute of Child Health and Human Development Neonatal Research Network. N Engl J Med. 1999;340:1962–8.
72. Lucas JS, Inskip HM, Godfrey KM, et al. Small size at birth and greater postnatal weight gain: relationships to diminished infant lung function. Am J Respir Crit Care Med. 2004;170:534–40.
73. Breastfeeding and the use of human milk. Pediatrics. 2012;129:e827–41.
74. Sisk PM, Lovelady CA, Dillard RG, Gruber KJ, O'Shea TM. Early human milk feeding is associated with a lower risk of necrotizing enterocolitis in very low birth weight infants. J Perinatol. 2007;27:428–33.
75. Sano H, Nagai K, Tsutsumi H, Kuroki Y. Lactoferrin and surfactant protein A exhibit distinct binding specificity to F protein and differently modulate respiratory syncytial virus infection. Eur J Immunol. 2003;33:2894–902.
76. Liu B, Newburg DS. Human milk glycoproteins protect infants against human pathogens. Breastfeed Med. 2013;8:354–62.
77. Meier PP, Engstrom JL, Patel AL, Jegier BJ, Bruns NE. Improving the use of human milk during and after the NICU stay. Clin Perinatol. 2010;37:217–45.
78. Meier PP, Furman LM, Degenhardt M. Increased lactation risk for late preterm infants and mothers: evidence and management strategies to protect breastfeeding. J Midwifery Womens Health. 2007;52:579–87.
79. Simoes EA, Carbonell-Estrany X, Fullarton JR, et al. A predictive model for respiratory syncytial virus (RSV) hospitalisation of premature infants born at 33-35 weeks of gestational age, based on data from the Spanish FLIP Study. Respir Res. 2008;9:78.
80. Blaymore Bier JA, Oliver T, Ferguson A, Vohr BR. Human milk reduces outpatient upper respiratory symptoms in premature infants during their first year of life. J Perinatol. 2002;22:354–9.
81. Giwercman C, Halkjaer LB, Jensen SM, Bonnelykke K, Lauritzen L, Bisgaard H. Increased risk of eczema but reduced risk of early wheezy disorder from exclusive breast-feeding in high-risk infants. J Allergy Clin Immunol. 2010;125:866–71.
82. Blaakman SW, Borrelli B, Wiesenthal EN, et al. Secondhand smoke exposure reduction after NICU discharge: results of a randomized trial. Acad Pediatr. 2015;15:605–12.
83. Been JV, Millett C, Lee JT, van Schayck CP, Sheikh A. Smoke-free legislation and childhood hospitalisations for respiratory tract infections. Eur Respir J. 2015;46:697–706.
84. Fedulov AV, Leme A, Yang Z, et al. Pulmonary exposure to particles during pregnancy causes increased neonatal asthma susceptibility. Am J Respir Cell Mol Biol. 2008;38:57–67.

85. Wang L, Pinkerton KE. Air pollutant effects on fetal and early postnatal development. Birth Defects Res C Embryo Today. 2007;81:144–54.
86. Fanucchi MV, Plopper CG, Evans MJ, et al. Cyclic exposure to ozone alters distal airway development in infant rhesus monkeys. Am J Physiol Lung Cell Mol Physiol. 2006;291:L644–50.
87. Kajekar R, Pieczarka EM, Smiley-Jewell SM, Schelegle ES, Fanucchi MV, Plopper CG. Early postnatal exposure to allergen and ozone leads to hyperinnervation of the pulmonary epithelium. Respir Physiol Neurobiol. 2007;155:55–63.
88. Olicker A, Li H, Tatsuoka C, Ross K, Trembath A, Hibbs AM. Have changing palivizumab administration policies led to more respiratory morbidity in infants born at 32–35 weeks? J Pediatr. 2015;171:31–37.
89. Blanken MO, Rovers MM, Molenaar JM, et al. Respiratory syncytial virus and recurrent wheeze in healthy preterm infants. N Engl J Med. 2013;368:1791–9.
90. Lopez Bernal JA, Upton MN, Henderson AJ, et al. Lower respiratory tract infection in the first year of life is associated with worse lung function in adult life: prospective results from the Barry Caerphilly Growth study. Ann Epidemiol. 2013;23:422–7.
91. Drysdale SB, Lo J, Prendergast M, et al. Lung function of preterm infants before and after viral infections. Eur J Pediatr. 2014;173:1497–504.
92. Drysdale SB, Alcazar M, Wilson T, et al. Respiratory outcome of prematurely born infants following human rhinovirus A and C infections. Eur J Pediatr. 2014;173:913–9.
93. Doyle LW, Olinsky A, Faber B, Callanan C. Adverse effects of smoking on respiratory function in young adults born weighing less than 1000 grams. Pediatrics. 2003;112:565–9.
94. Upton MN, Smith GD, McConnachie A, Hart CL, Watt GC. Maternal and personal cigarette smoking synergize to increase airflow limitation in adults. Am J Respir Crit Care Med. 2004;169:479–87.
95. Martin RJ, Prakash YS, Hibbs AM. Why do former preterm infants wheeze? J Pediatr. 2013;162:443–4.
96. Brand PL, Caudri D, Eber E, et al. Classification and pharmacological treatment of preschool wheezing: changes since 2008. Eur Respir J. 2014;43:1172–7.
97. Bush A, Grigg J, Saglani S. Managing wheeze in preschool children. BMJ. 2014;348:g15.
98. Stevens TP, Finer NN, Carlo WA, et al. Respiratory outcomes of the surfactant positive pressure and oximetry randomized trial (SUPPORT). J Pediatr. 2014;165:240–9.
99. Hibbs AM, Walsh MC, Martin RJ, et al. One-year respiratory outcomes of preterm infants enrolled in the Nitric Oxide (to prevent) Chronic Lung Disease trial. J Pediatr. 2008;153:525–9.

Sleep Outcomes in Children Born Prematurely

Kristie R. Ross and Susan Redline

Abbreviations

AHI	Apnea hypopnea index
AI	Apnea index
AS	Active sleep
BMI	Body mass index
BPD	Bronchopulmonary dysplasia
NREM	Nonrapid eye movement
OSAS	Obstructive sleep apnea syndrome
PSG	Polysomnogram
QS	Quiet sleep
RDI	Respiratory disturbance index
REM	Rapid eye movement
SDB	Sleep-disordered breathing
SIDS	Sudden infant death syndrome
UARS	Upper airway resistance syndrome
VLBW	Very low birth weight

Emergence and consolidation of sleep states and maturation of control of breathing during sleep and wake are critical developmental milestones in the first year of life. Additional maturation occurs throughout childhood, and early insults may impact sleep and breathing into childhood, adolescence, and adulthood. The developmental trajectories of sleep state maturation and control of breathing are impacted by premature birth across the spectrum from marked prematurity with infants born with

K.R. Ross, MD, MS (✉)
Case Western Reserve University School of Medicine, Rainbow Babies and Children's Hospital, Cleveland, OH, USA

S. Redline, MD, MPH
Harvard Medical School, Brigham and Women's Hospital and Beth Israel Deaconess Medical Center, Boston, MA, USA

© Springer International Publishing AG 2017   161
A.M. Hibbs, M.S. Muhlebach (eds.), *Respiratory Outcomes in Preterm Infants*,
Respiratory Medicine, DOI 10.1007/978-3-319-48835-6_10

very low birth weight (VLBW, <1500 g) to those born at 34–37 weeks gestation (late preterm and early term). In this chapter, we will review the association of premature birth with sleep outcomes once infants reach full term, through childhood, and into early adulthood. Our focus will be on the putative impact of premature birth on disordered breathing during sleep and sleep behaviors and circadian rhythm development, organized by age group. We will also highlight opportunities for further research to address important knowledge gaps.

Overview of Respiratory Control and Sleep State Maturation in Infancy

While a detailed review of normal maturation of breathing and sleep and the impact of prematurity on these processes during the period immediately after birth is outside the scope of this chapter and has been reviewed elsewhere [1–5], we will briefly review important concepts. The maturation of respiratory control, sleep state, and arousal is governed by complex interactions between the central and peripheral nervous systems during prenatal and immediate postnatal development, with voluntary and involuntary components. Maturation of neural control of breathing, including peripheral chemoreceptors, central chemoreceptors, and centers in the midbrain and forebrain, is a nonlinear developmental process that spans from prenatal to postnatal periods. In addition to central nervous system development, chest wall compliance, mechanoreceptors or stretch receptors, airway compliance, laryngeal reflexes, and responsiveness of chemoreceptors to hypoxia, hypercapnia, and changes in pH all undergo maturational changes in the postnatal period in healthy infants. In the immediate postnatal period, prematurity-related interruptions or delays in these developmental processes can lead to apnea of prematurity, periodic breathing, and difficulties coordinating sucking, swallowing, and breathing.

The maturation of control of breathing coincides with the emergence of mature sleep states. While ventilation generally decreases during sleep, there are significant variations in breathing patterns and respiratory chemosensitivity across sleep states, and these are evident throughout the life span. Sleep in children and adults can be divided into two primary states: nonrapid eye movement sleep (NREM) and rapid eye movement (REM) sleep. By about 32 weeks gestation, fetuses and neonates exhibit immature versions of these states, namely quiet sleep (QS) and active sleep (AS) [6]. QS and AS mature into NREM and REM sleep, respectively, during the first several months of life in term infants. The proportion of time humans spend in each sleep state changes dramatically during prenatal and postnatal development, with AS dominating in the prenatal period, with a transition to NREM dominance after birth. This maturational change is thought to be important for brain maturation and plasticity. Term infants spend approximately 50 % of sleep time in AS [7], and as AS matures into REM sleep, the proportion decreases to approximately 25 % as infants approach 1 year of age [8]. Maturation of sleep architecture during the first year of life does not appear to be significantly delayed in children who were born preterm [9, 10]. NREM sleep is characterized by a lack of behavioral controls, with more regular breathing and reduced tidal volume and respiratory rate compared with wakefulness. During REM sleep, respiratory rate and tidal volume become more irregular. REM sleep is also characterized by a reduction in muscle tone; short central respiratory pauses are common during REM sleep in healthy children. The loss of muscle tone and marked respiratory variability interact with the immature features of the infant respiratory and nervous systems to result in increased risk for apneas and periodic breathing in premature infants in the immediate postnatal period. Specifically, reduced neuromuscular input to respiratory muscles along with the increased chest wall compliance seen in infants leads to a reduction in ventilation during sleep. Increased laryngeal reflexes and increased sensitivity of central and peripheral reflexes may then precipitate apneas.

In summary, differences between adult and newborn respiratory systems that make infants more vulnerable to disordered breathing during sleep include central nervous system immaturity, exaggerated laryngeal reflexes, increased chest wall compliance, immaturity of chemoreceptors, and increased time in active sleep/REM sleep (summarized in Table 1). Premature birth, with interruption and delay of neurological and pulmonary maturation, along with increased susceptibility to pulmonary disease and exposure to adverse effects of treatment, exaggerates these influences.

Disordered Breathing During Sleep Across the Life Span (Fig. 1)

Preterm Infants at Term Postconceptual Age

While control of breathing and sleep state maturation becomes more normal as preterm infants approach term postconceptual ages, there is some evidence for residual effects of prematurity. Two early cross-sectional studies in late preterm

Table 1 Characteristics of the premature respiratory system that contribute to disordered breathing in infancy

Interrupted development of alveolar units, surfactant system, and pulmonary vasculature
Increased inflammation and oxidative stress (infection, treatment-related)
Immature chemoreceptors (enhanced peripheral sensitivity and reduced central sensitivity)
Increased laryngeal chemoreflexes with apnea, bradycardia, and vasoconstriction
Increased time in active sleep with loss of expiratory braking and stabilizing intercostal muscle tone
Increased chest wall compliance, lower specific lung compliance
Mechanical disadvantage due to barrel-shaped chest and more horizontal rib position

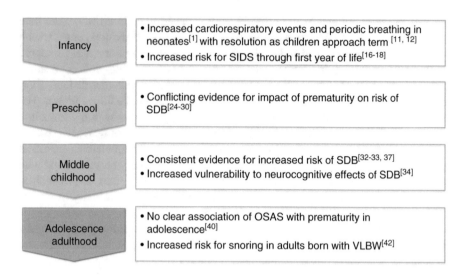

Infancy	• Increased cardiorespiratory events and periodic breathing in neonates[1] with resolution as children approach term [11, 12] • Increased risk for SIDS through first year of life[16-18]
Preschool	• Conflicting evidence for impact of prematurity on risk of SDB[24-30]
Middle childhood	• Consistent evidence for increased risk of SDB[32-33, 37] • Increased vulnerability to neurocognitive effects of SDB[34]
Adolescence adulthood	• No clear association of OSAS with prematurity in adolescence[40] • Increased risk for snoring in adults born with VLBW[42]

Fig. 1 Summary of associations between premature birth and sleep-disordered breathing during sleep throughout the life span

infants demonstrated minor increases in the number of short (2–15 s) central pauses in former late preterm infants [11], and shorter but similar numbers of pauses in preterm compared to term infants [12]. Neither study reported an increase in the number of prolonged apneas or apneas that resulted in significant cardiorespiratory consequences. Both of these studies assessed breathing during sleep only at a single time point.

Albani et al. prospectively studied a small group ($n = 12$, 50 % male) of late preterm (mean gestational age 35 weeks, range 32.2–36.6) infants and term ($n = 21$, 48 % male) infants with sequential polysomnograms (PSGs) at 40, 52, and 64 postconceptual weeks to characterize the number, duration, and character (obstructive, central, mixed) of apneas [13]. All infants in both groups were apparently healthy, and did not have evidence of apnea of prematurity requiring pharmacological treatment, bronchopulmomary dysplasia or other pulmonary disease, or intracranial hemorrhage. Apnea was defined as a pause of 3 s or greater, and classified as central if no respiratory effort was recorded, obstructive if respiratory effort was recorded, and mixed if both patterns were present in either order. Apnea density (number per unit time), duration, character, and the presence of periodic breathing were measured. Compared to term infants, preterm infants had significantly increased density of apneas at the 40-week recording (126 vs. 49 per 100 min recording, $p < 0.05$). Most of the observed differences were attributable to a higher density of obstructive/mixed apneas in NREM/quiet sleep among the preterm infants. At the 52-week postconceptual age recording, term infants had higher apnea density overall (50 vs. 20 per 100 min, $p < 0.05$), driven largely by findings in REM sleep, and there were no differences at 64 weeks postconceptual age in apnea density or type. Apneas in both groups were very rare during the final recording. The majority of preterm infants demonstrated periodic breathing at 40 weeks (75 % vs. 42 % term, $p < 0.05$), primarily during NREM sleep. Periodic breathing was rare in both groups during subsequent recordings. Somewhat surprisingly, two of the preterm infants died during the study; both deaths were attributed to sudden infant death syndrome (SIDS), one at 44 weeks after one PSG and one at 56 weeks after two PSGs. The infant who died at 44 weeks was described as having more frequent and longer apneas (obstructive and mixed) and more periodic breathing than the other preterm and term infants. The second infant was similar to preterm peers. This study, although small, suggests that variations in breathing during sleep in preterm infants in the immediate postnatal period largely resolve shortly after postconceptual term ages are reached in healthy late preterm infants. These findings cannot be extrapolated to children born extremely prematurely or with significant lung disease, and are limited by the very small sample size. Research studies also have shown that the presence and severity of bronchopulmonary dysplasia (BPD) may be associated with the severity of alterations in control of ventilation [14, 15]; therefore, BPD may influence propensity for persistent sleep-related breathing disturbances in preterm infants.

First Year of Life and Sudden Infant Death Syndrome

SIDS is defined as the unexplained death of a child during sleep before 1 year of age. While the precise pathophysiology and etiology of SIDS remain elusive, and is likely multifactorial, it is thought to be a disorder of respiratory control and arousal. Infants born prematurely are at increased risk for SIDS. Early descriptions of the relationship between preterm birth and SIDS suggested that rates rise substantially with increasing prematurity (1.06 deaths/1000 live births at term vs. 3.52 deaths/1000 live births at 24–28 weeks gestation) and that the peak age at death was 4–6 weeks earlier in preterm children [16]. Despite a decrease in overall rates of SIDS with the "Back to Sleep" campaign, preterm birth remains a risk factor for SIDS. In one population-based case-control study in five regions in England, preterm birth (<37 weeks gestation) was associated with a 3.44 (2.47–4.79) increased odds of SIDS, although this relationship was attenuated and no longer significant after multivariate adjustment [17]. Other studies, however, have found higher rates of SIDS in children born preterm in multivariate analyses that include adjustment for maternal smoking, markers of socioeconomic status, and race, including a study of linked US birth and death records from 1996 to 1998 [18]. In this study, adjusted odds ratios for SIDS in children born preterm compared with those born at 40–41 weeks gestation ranged from 1.52 (1.42–1.63) for children born at 36–37 weeks gestation to 2.88 (2.57–3.23) for children born at 28–32 weeks gestation. Halloran and colleagues also found that the postnatal age at death was slightly later in preterm infants than term infants (16 vs. 12 weeks), with a second peak at approximately 28 weeks in those born extremely prematurely (22–27 weeks gestation), although postconceptional age at death was earlier in preterm infants [18]. Similar to the findings by Malloy and Hoffman [16], when analyzed by postconceptional age, very preterm infants died, on average, more than 6 weeks earlier than term infants (46 vs. 54 weeks postconceptual age). The increased prevalence of SIDS in children who were born prematurely suggests that there are sustained abnormalities in respiratory control in some cases, although non respiratory (cardiac) differences may also play a role. Instability of central chemoreception, responses to carbon dioxide and hypoxia, and the impact of early chronic intermittent hypoxemia on the autonomic nervous system have all been implicated (reviewed in [4, 19]). Shared risk factors for prematurity and SIDS (maternal inflammation, nicotine exposure) have also been suggested to explain the association [19].

Sleep-Disordered Breathing: Preschool to Adolescence

SDB is a term that broadly describes abnormal breathing and/or gas exchange during sleep, and encompasses a spectrum of severity from primary snoring to upper airway resistance syndrome (UARS) to obstructive sleep apnea syndrome (OSAS). Untreated SDB is associated with behavioral and neurocognitive effects across its spectrum [20], and metabolic and cardiovascular effects in its more severe form [21]. The prevalence of snoring, as reported by caregivers, is highly variable depending on the definition used, but a meta-analysis of studies that included over 95,000 children (0–19 years of age) worldwide found the prevalence to be 7.45 % (95 % CI 5.75–9.61 %) [22]. Most studies suggest an OSAS prevalence of 4–11 % using questionnaires and 1–4 % using PSG in otherwise healthy children [22], with a peak prevalence occurring between ages 2 and 6 years. A second increase in prevalence is likely in adolescence, associated with obesity. Many studies have demonstrated prematurity to be a risk factor for obstructive sleep-disordered breathing during childhood [23–25]. However, these associations vary by age group. A longitudinal birth cohort showed that the association between SDB and prematurity was present in early childhood, but not during adolescence, when obesity emerged as a strong risk factor [26].

The pathophysiology of OSAS is complex, and reviewed in detail elsewhere [27]. While the defining feature is the partial or complete collapse of the upper airway during sleep, there are multiple factors that likely contribute to upper airway obstruction, including soft-tissue hypertrophy (adenoids, tonsils, airway fat deposition), skeletal craniofacial features, pharyngeal and laryngeal tone, lower respiratory tract neuromuscular tone, arousal threshold, and control of breathing [27, 28]. Gas exchange abnormalities due to lower respiratory tract disease, upper airway inflammation due to gastroesophageal reflux, or swallowing disorders may influence the development or presentation of OSAS. Premature birth may influence several of these factors, most notably ventilatory control, airway tone, craniofacial growth, lower airway disease, and increased risk for obesity in some premature populations. As these influences seem to change with age, we will discuss the relationship between prematurity and SDB by age category. When possible, differences in children with and without BPD will be discussed.

Sleep-Disordered Breathing in Preschool Children

While prematurity has been fairly consistently identified as a risk factor for SDB in older children (discussed later in the chapter), there are not enough data to reach a reliable conclusion about the role of prematurity (with or without BPD) in children prior to school age. Rates of symptoms of sleep-disordered breathing reported in cohorts of former premature infants in this age category range from approximately 8 % [29] to 20 % [30], and are not significantly different from rates in population-based studies of healthy toddlers [22]. In a study of preterm children at 9 months corrected age (mean gestational age of 31.6 weeks), birth weight and gestational age were not identified as risk factors for the presence of SDB symptoms [29]. In a study of slightly older toddlers (18–22 months) who had been born extremely prematurely (24–28 weeks gestation), no markers of severity of neonatal illness in the neonatal period were associated with SDB risk [30]. Surprisingly, several markers of neonatal illness severity were associated with a lower risk of reported SDB symptoms, including duration of caffeine treatment, duration of ventilator treatment, and hospital length of stay. The presence of BPD, necrotizing enterocolitis, and exposure to both hypoxia and hyperoxia were not associated with SDB symptoms in either direction. Female sex was the only risk factor identified, with females 2.7 times (95 % CI 1.13–6.5) more likely to have SDB symptoms [30]. These studies, however, are limited by the lack of accuracy of symptoms to identify SDB and potential parental reporting biases.

There have been two large population-based studies that have examined the relationship between prematurity and symptoms of SDB, with disparate findings. The first is a longitudinal study that enrolled over 14,000 children in Southwest England (Avon Longitudinal Study of Parents and Children) [31]. SDB was assessed using questionnaires administered at three time points, 1.5, 4.75, and 6 years of age. In this study, prematurity was not a risk factor for SDB symptoms (snoring, mouth-breathing, witnessed apneas) at ages 1.5 or 4.75 years. There was a modest relationship between gestational age and witnessed apneas only at age 6 (OR 1.23, 95 % CI 1.02, 1.47).

In a cross-sectional study using data from the medical records of nearly 400,000 Australian children ages 2.5–6, sleep apnea, as defined by the use of billing codes, was present in 4145 or 1 % of children [32]. Children born prematurely (gestational age <32 weeks) were more likely to have a diagnosis of sleep apnea (hazard ratio 2.74 (95 % CI 2.16, 3.49) in multivariate models. Children born small for gestational age did not have increased risk for sleep apnea.

The above studies, although quite large, used very different methodologies to classify children as having SDB, both of which may result in misclassification. The Avon Longitudinal Study of Parents and Children study [31] identified children with SDB symptoms via questionnaire, and based on other studies, less than half of these children would likely have PSG-documented OSAS. Conversely, the Australian study [32] identified sleep apnea using diagnostic codes, which requires a health care provider to elicit symptoms and often conduct follow-up testing, and then enter the code, likely underestimating the prevalence. This supposition is supported by the difference in the prevalence reported (1 %) and that reported in a meta-analysis of the prevalence of SDB symptoms such as snoring of around 8 % [22].

The studies discussed above used questionnaires or administrative data to assess for SDB symptoms. In-lab polysomnography (PSG) is expensive and may be burdensome to families, likely explaining the lack of published reports of cohorts of premature infants studied prospectively with PSG. We identified two retrospective studies that examined PSG findings in early childhood in former preterm infants. In a retrospective study of 62 children with BPD < 3 years of age (mean 10 months, range 2.5–31.4 months, mean gestational age of 25.8 ± 1.9 weeks) undergoing PSG for clinical indications including oxygen titration, McGrath-Morrow [33] reported that the mean respiratory disturbance index (RDI, sum of obstructive apneas, mixed apneas, central apneas, and hypopneas/hour of total sleep time) was 8.2 ± 10.1. Obstructive apneas were rare (average index of 0.7 ± 1.6). Similar to patterns seen in healthy children, central apneas made up the largest proportion of reported events (mean 3.6 + 4.6), followed by hypopneas (2.8 ± 6.1). Children who were 18 months or older when studied had a lower RDI (3.4 ± 2.9) than the entire cohort. A subset underwent a second PSG at a mean age of 13.4 + 5.2 months; RDI improved from 14.5 ± 13.3 to 5.2 ± 6.3. The authors did not report the number of children followed at the center who did not undergo PSG; so, prevalence estimates are not possible. There was no control population reported, but values are above published normal values, at least in the younger age groups. These findings suggest that former preterm infants with BPD may be more likely to have abnormal PSG findings, but the study design does not allow prevalence estimates nor does it distinguish between findings related strictly to lower respiratory tract disease versus upper airway obstruction.

Sharma and colleagues used a retrospective study design to study children with BPD followed at a single pulmonary center who had been diagnosed with OSAS [34]. Of 387 children with BPD, 12 (3 %) had PSG findings suggesting OSAS. Children with OSAS were characterized by a mean gestational age of 27 weeks (range 24–33); 10 out of 12 had been intubated in the neonatal period, and 9 out of 12 met criteria for BPD. The mean age at the time of the study was 19 months (range 9–28), and most presented with snoring. The mean apnea hypopnea index (AHI) was 29 (range 1–120). The degree of prematurity did not correlate with OSAS severity. All were treated with adenotonsillectomy. Three required additional treatment (positive pressure ventilation or supplemental oxygen), although most did not have follow-up PSGs. The PSGs were ordered based on clinical symptoms, and the authors do not report the number of children who were studied with PSG overall or the number with negative studies; so, it is not possible to estimate the prevalence of SDB in this sample of children.

Prematurity has been identified as a risk factor for PSG-defined OSAS in two retrospective studies of young children. In a single center retrospective study of 139 children ages 0–17 months with PSG-confirmed OSAS, prematurity was identified in 29 % of children [35]. More than half of the premature infants in this study had severe OSAS (AHI >10). Gestational age, the presence of BPD, or other comorbidities were not reported. In another single site retrospective study of children under 2 years of age who underwent adenotonsillectomy at a single institution over a 7-year period, the authors identified prematurity as a risk factor for PSG-defined OSAS as well as SDB as defined by symptoms prompting surgical treatment [36]. Prematurity (gestational age < 37 weeks) was present in 27 % of children with PSG-defined OSAS compared with 9 % of the statewide population of children under 2 years of age ($p < 0.0001$). In this study, prematurity was not associated with severe OSAS (AHI >10) in multivariate analyses, but this may have been limited by little statistical power.

In summary, in very young children, a number of studies have reported that prematurity is associated with SDB symptoms and/or PSG-identified OSAS. However, existing data are not fully consistent, with gaps in understanding whether SDB severity is associated with prematurity. There is also uncertainty over whether this relationship is explained by BPD.

Middle Childhood and Obstructive Sleep Apnea Syndrome

The published data suggesting prematurity is associated with an increased risk for sleep disordered breathing is more consistent in school-aged children than it is in younger children. The Cleveland Children's Sleep and Health Study (CCSHS) is a population-based study of 907 children aged 8–11 years of age that used stratified sampling to achieve over-representation of former preterm children (gestational age < 36 weeks) [24]. Children were studied in their homes with multichannel recordings of airflow, respiratory effort, electrocardiography, and oximetry. The primary definition used to define OSAS was an obstructive AHI ≥5. Snoring was more common in children born preterm (21 % vs. 14 %, $p = .0049$), as was OSAS (4.3 vs. 0.9 %, $p = .0013$). OSAS was five times (95 % CI 1.6–20.1) more likely in children born prematurely than those born at term in analyses adjusted for race, obesity, and sex. OSAS was also independently associated with African American race.

In a follow-up analysis that focused on the 383 children born preterm in the Cleveland Children's Sleep and Health Study cohort, researchers aimed to identify demographic and perinatal risk factors for SDB (defined as obstructive apnea index (AI) ≥1 or obstructive AHI ≥5) at school age [23] within this subgroup. Univariate analysis identified race, having a single mother, mild preeclampsia, cardiopulmonary resuscitation or intubation in the delivery room, and use of methylxanthines as risk factors. After adjusting for race, having a single mother was associated with a 2.45 (95 % CI 1.01–6.39) increase in odds of SDB, and maternal mild preeclampsia was associated with a 7.56 (1.66–34.48) increase. Severe preeclampsia was not associated in either unadjusted or adjusted analyses. The investigators speculated that differences in the putative pathophysiology of mild and severe preeclampsia could explain these findings, with mild preeclampsia reflecting influences of placental hypoxemia occurring independently of vascular and other changes characteristic of severe preeclampsia. Maternal smoking may have been a particularly important confounder, as maternal smoking may reduce the risk of severe preeclampsia, and smoking rates were much higher in those with mild preeclampsia. While the point estimates of the association between maternal smoking and SDB were elevated (2.1), this was a nonsignificant finding. There was no univariate or multivariate association between multiple markers of neonatal illness severity in this study, including gestational age, birth weight, BPD, duration of ventilatory support, and intraventricular hemorrhage.

The Cleveland Children's Sleep and Health Study investigators also quantified the association of SDB with impaired neurocognitive function and academic achievement [37]. In unadjusted analyses, SDB was associated with significant reductions in performance in six out of seven neurocognitive and achievement tests; these differences were attenuated after multivariate adjustments (age, sex, birth weight category, socioeconomic status), with most of the attenuation attributable to socioeconomic status (caregiver education, marital status, and income). Hypothesizing prematurity might confer increased vulnerability to adverse neurocognitive effects of SDB, investigators performed stratified analyses in children born preterm. There were similar findings to the full cohort in unadjusted analysis. The attenuation following multivariable adjustment, including that for socioeconomic status, was present but not as strong as it had been in the full cohort. Children born preterm with SDB had significantly lower performance on five out of seven neurocognitive and achievement tests compared to those without SDB after multivariate adjustments. Taken together, these findings suggest that preterm birth increases the risk for SDB at school age independently of severe neonatal illnesses such as BPD, and that prematurity may result in increased susceptibility to adverse neurocognitive and academic achievement effects.

Perinatal morbidity including premature birth is strongly associated with race and socioeconomic status. Race, socioeconomic status, and neighborhood level factors are also strong risk factors for SDB [24, 25]. As suggested by the attenuation of the association between SDB and neurocognitive consequences found by Emancipator and colleagues [37], the relationship between SDB and social determinants of health is complex. Calhoun and colleagues investigated the association between SDB and a wide range of prenatal and perinatal risk factors, and further attempted to understand the association between these complications and SES/race [38]. The authors compared a population of 105 children who were referred to a specialty sleep clinic and who were subsequently diagnosed with SDB based on a clinical PSG with an AHI ≥ 5. The control population included 508 children enrolled in a population-based cohort study of healthy children who had a negative research PSG. Therefore, while the control group was population based, the children with SDB were brought to medical attention by their caregivers, and were not drawn from a population-based cohort. Children with SDB were older, had a higher mean BMI, and were much more likely to be minority, of low SES, exposed to smoke during pregnancy, and have had perinatal complications including premature birth, preeclampsia, gestational diabetes, and neonatal respiratory distress. After controlling for race, SES, and BMI percentile, there remained a significant association between SDB and prematurity. SDB was also associated with maternal smoking during pregnancy, need for supplemental oxygen at birth, and delayed walking milestones in multivariate analyses [38]. In another study of 197 children ages 5–12 years who were born preterm and had participated in a neonatal study of caffeine use, chorio-amniotis and multiple gestation were associated with OSAS, while maternal white race and maternal age were protective [39]. Other risk factors, including birth weight, sex, and use of antenatal corticosteroids, were not related to OSAS. These studies [23, 24, 37–39] support using a low threshold to identify and test former preterm school-aged children for SDB, even without a history of significant lung disease, and particularly in those who are minorities or of lower SES status.

Adolescents and Young Adults and Sleep-Disordered Breathing

At least two studies have shown that SDB in middle childhood often regresses during the transition to adolescence [40, 41]. In the Cleveland Children's Sleep and Health Study, participants were studied using objective sleep apnea testing at ages 8–11 years and 16–19 years [26]. While OSAS prevalence was similar at each time point (4–5 %), OSAS largely did not persist from middle childhood into adolescence, that is, most of the children with OSAS at a young age did not have OSAS as adolescents, while adolescents with OSAS largely did not display OSAS during middle childhood. Preterm birth, which was a risk factor for OSAS in middle childhood, was not associated with OSAS in unadjusted or adjusted models at 16–19 years of age. Risk factors for SDB in postpubertal adolescents appear to be similar to risk factors for SDB in adults, including male sex, age, BMI, and metabolic derangements.

There are very little data available to determine the association between preterm birth and SDB in adults. Epidemiological studies that describe risk factors for the presence or development of OSAS in adults do not typically include perinatal events as putative risk factors [26, 42]. Even if they were included, these data would be subject to significant recall biases, and treatment practices for children born prematurely have changed significantly over the last several decades. There is one longitudinal cohort study of adults who have been followed prospectively from birth into their early 20s that provides some insight into the relationship between prematurity and SDB in young adults. The Helsinki Study of Very Low Birth Weight Adults is comprised of 335 consecutively born infants with a birth weight below 1500 g and treated in a tertiary neonatal center in Finland [43]. A control population of single-ton term infants born at the same centers was also recruited. Symptoms of SDB were assessed using a brief questionnaire, and the primary SDB outcome was snoring reported at least one or two times per week. While there was no difference in crude estimates of SDB, in analyses adjusted for age, sex, smoking, parental education, BMI, and depression, chronic snoring was 2.2 times more likely (85 % CI 1.1–4.5) in young adults born prematurely compared to those born at term. Maternal smoking during pregnancy was significantly associated with chronic snoring in those who had been born prematurely. Other perinatal risk factors including preeclampsia and mechanical ventilation were not associated with snoring. No objective measures of SDB were performed in this study.

In summary, disorders of respiratory control during sleep are very common in infants who were born prematurely. The risk of OSAS in middle childhood is increased in children who were born prematurely, but this risk appears to attenuate during adolescence. There are limited data exploring the relationship between prematurity and SDB in adulthood. The evidence of associations between premature birth and disordered breathing during sleep across the life span is summarized in Fig. 1.

Impact of Preterm Birth on Sleep Architecture and Circadian Rhythm (Fig. 2)

Overview of Circadian Entrainment in the Neonatal Period

A full discussion of the development of circadian rhythms in the immediate neonatal period is outside the scope of this chapter; interested readers are referred to a comprehensive review [8]. Circadian rhythm development begins in the fetal period and is responsive to maternal signals [44]. Studies in preterm primates demonstrate circadian clock responsiveness to light develops as early as 24 weeks gestation [45], and longitudinal studies of preterm infants show development of circadian oscillations in body temperature by 3 months corrected age [8]. There is evidence that nonphysiological exposure to light in the neonatal (NICU) period may disturb sleep wake patterns in infants. While there are conflicting reports about the effectiveness of cycled light-dark exposures in the neonatal intensive care unit on circadian entrainment, there are data that support this practice [46, 47].

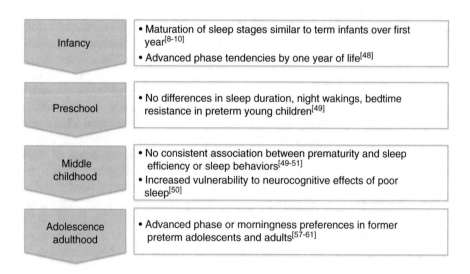

Fig. 2 Summary of associations between premature birth and sleep behaviors/circadian rhythms throughout the life span

Sleep Architecture in the First Year of Life

Infants born prematurely undergo maturation of sleep architecture from Active Sleep/REM-dominated to Quiet Sleep/NREM-dominated during the first year of life, similar to term infants. "Asymptomatic" preterm infants have sleep architecture that is nearly indistinguishable from full-term peers once they reach term postmenstrual age (PMA) [10]. Extreme prematurity and treatment with mechanical ventilation are associated with small reductions in the proportion of time in quiet sleep at term PMA. Maternal steroids and steroids given to the infant were not associated with delays or advances in sleep architecture [10]. In the early 1980s, Anders and Keener conducted a longitudinal study of term and preterm infants during their first year of life in which sleep architecture was assessed at seven time points in the home using video somnography [9]. They found similar sleep-wake state development in both groups, with consolidated sleep at night and quiet sleep dominating the primary sleep period by 1 year (corrected) of age. While the authors recruited preterm infants who had experienced "serious complications secondary to prematurity," the majority of the infants were 30 weeks gestation or greater, and half were over 1500 g at birth. To address how more extreme prematurity and modern treatments of prematurity may affect sleep architecture as infants approach 1 year of age, Guyer and colleagues used actigraphy to assess 24-h sleep-wake rhythms in 34 preterm infants (<32 weeks gestation) compared with 14 term infants at 5, 11, and 25 weeks corrected age [48]. Actigraphs are worn on the limb and measure movement in order to estimate sleep duration and other measures of sleep quality. Nighttime sleep and consolidated sleep between midnight and 6 am were longer at all ages studied in the preterm infants. In another study using actigraphy, Asaka and Takada assessed sleep-wake architecture in 14 children born at very low birth weight (VLBW, <1500 g) compared to a control population of children born at term [49] at approximately 1 year (corrected) age. Preterm infants fell asleep, woke earlier, and had a slightly shorter duration of nighttime sleep (approximately 20 min on average) compared with former full-term infants. Total sleep duration was similar, as were sleep efficiency and night awakenings.

Sleep Patterns and Behaviors in Preschool and School-Aged Children

Iglowstein and colleagues collected prospective data over a 10-year period on sleep patterns in children born preterm and compared them to a control population of children born at term [50]. The preterm cohort consisted of 130 children born in the mid-1970s, with a mean gestational age of 34 weeks (range 27–36), including 30 children considered extremely premature (<32 weeks). The term control group was comprised of 75 children born during the same period with a gestational age ≥ 37 weeks. The groups were matched by socioeconomic status. Sleep patterns and behaviors were elicited using structured face-to-face interviews that included questions about bedtime, wake time, night wakings, difficult behaviors around bedtime, and bed sharing. Sleep patterns and behaviors were remarkably similar between the two groups, with no differences found using linear and generalized mixed models. The authors also reported no difference between the children born very preterm (<32 week gestation) compared with those born at term. These findings should be interpreted cautiously given the small sample and the difference between neonatal practices to treat extreme prematurity in the mid-1970s and today. In a more contemporary study, sleep behaviors and cognitive function in 58 children aged 6–10 years who had been born at <32 weeks gestation were compared with 55 full-term children [51]. Children born preterm had increased night awakenings based on in-home PSG compared with term children, but otherwise showed similar sleep patterns. Cognitive test scores were lower in preterm compared to term children on average, and sleep efficiency was negatively associated with performance on cognitive tests in the children born preterm but not those born at term. While sleep measures were assessed using more objective measures, they were based on only a single night recording. In the context of this limitation, similar to the findings with respect to SDB [37], these findings raise concern that children born preterm may be more susceptible to adverse effects of impaired sleep quality due to nonrespiratory causes than their term peers.

In addition to concerns about the impact of treatment with corticosteroids on the maturation of sleep-wake patterns and the long-term risk of respiratory and nonrespiratory sleep disorders, Marcus and colleagues addressed the hypothesis that neonatal use of caffeine results in long-term abnormalities in sleep architecture and breathing during sleep [52]. Caffeine, a methylxanthine, is the most commonly used medication in infants born before 32 weeks gestation [53], and has clear short-term and medium-term benefits on a variety of neonatal outcomes including respiratory control, the development of BPD, and neurocognitive development [54, 55]. The short-term effects of caffeine on sleep are also well known, but citing animal data showing neonatal administration of caffeine affects ventilatory control in adult animals, these investigators hypothesized that there may be long-term effects of blocking adenosine receptors in the brain on sleep architecture and ventilatory control in children [52]. They addressed this hypothesis by obtaining subjective (questionnaire) and objective (2 weeks of actigraphy and one night in-home PSG) measures of sleep in a subset of children ages 5–12 years who had been randomized to caffeine or placebo as neonates in the Caffeine for Apnea of Prematurity (CAP) trial [54]. While the prevalence of OSAS (defined as an AHI ≥2) was high (24 % in the caffeine group and 29 % in the placebo group), there were no differences in the coprimary outcomes of AHI and sleep duration by actigraphy between the caffeine and placebo groups [52]. No group differences were apparent in other measures of sleep quality, including wake after sleep onset, bedtime, sleep onset latency, and sleep efficiency. Periodic limb movements during sleep were also common, but there were no group differences. This study confirms other studies demonstrating a high prevalence of SDB in former preterm children at school age, but suggests that high rates of SDB cannot be attributed to neonatal caffeine use. Caffeine also did not result in long-term differences in sleep architecture. While the objective of this study was not to compare sleep quality or behaviors to a control group of term children, actigraphy findings were similar to those reported in healthy school-aged children.

Preterm Birth and Circadian Rhythms in Adolescents and Adults

Adolescents typically develop a progressive phase delay in their circadian clocks during puberty [56], manifested by going to sleep and waking later than younger children or older adults. Animal models suggesting that circadian clock development can be impacted by perinatal stress and exposures [57] are supported by a small literature showing lasting impact of premature birth on sleep-wake rhythms [58, 59]. Using two questionnaires that assessed morningness versus eveningness preferences in two separate cohorts of 13-year-old children born preterm and term controls, Natale et al. found a shift in adolescents born preterm toward morningness preferences [58]. This study was limited by lack of assessment of objective measures of sleep-wake schedules. Hibbs et al. used actigraphy to objectively capture sleep and wake times in a cohort of 501 adolescents aged 16–19 years who were part of the longitudinal Cleveland Children's Sleep and Health Study [59]. While pubertal status was assessed in only 70 % of subjects, over 99 % of those assessed had completed puberty at the time of this study. Weekday bedtime in the 217 adolescents born preterm was approximately 30 min earlier than the 284 adolescents born at term as assessed by actigraphy and self-report. Wake times were also earlier by approximately 20 min. Sleep efficiency was similar, and adolescents born prematurely were more likely to report functioning best in the morning compared with term peers. After adjusting for age, race, maternal education, and household income, midsleep time remained earlier in preterm adolescents compared with term peers by 22 min. These findings support a relative phase advance in children born prematurely.

Researchers found similar patterns in young adults who had been born at very low birth weight in the Helsinki Study of Very Low Birth Weight Adults cohort [60]. These findings were reported in a prospective study that was designed to follow up on earlier reports from this cohort, suggesting an increased propensity toward morningness using questionnaires [61] and advanced phase tendencies found in a post hoc analysis [62]. Actigraphy was used to measure sleep in 75 subjects aged 21–29 years (40 VLBW and 35 controls) for at least 5 days. Young adults born prematurely woke 40 min earlier on average, with no differences in sleep duration or measures of sleep quality. Findings were not affected by adjustment for age, sex, parental education, employment status, use of antidepressants, and current smoking.

Disturbed sleep or insufficient sleep in childhood may negatively affect a range of behaviors, cognition, and health. Although children born preterm may be vulnerable to the adverse effects of insufficient sleep because of underlying health or cognitive, there is no current evidence indicating that former preterm infants have an increased prevalence of short or fragmented sleep, other than related to SDB. Interestingly, this group appears to display a tendency toward morningness or advanced phase circadian rhythm, which may be advantageous in relationship to adjusting to early school start times. Evidence for associations between premature birth and sleep behaviors across the life span is summarized in Fig. 2.

Summary

The maturation of sleep and breathing is vulnerable to significant impacts during critical periods of brain and respiratory system development. The trajectories of these critical developmental milestones may be adversely affected by the direct impact of premature birth, by comorbid conditions, by neonatal treatments, and by environmental exposures in the neonatal intensive care unit and during treatment. Disorders of respiratory control, including sudden infant death syndrome and obstructive sleep apnea syndrome are more common in children born prematurely. The effects of prematurity on disordered breathing during sleep appear to wane with age. However, given developmental plasticity, a high index of suspicion for SDB in the former preterm infant is needed. In contrast, effects on circadian rhythm persist into adulthood, and possibly may have beneficial effects. Further work is needed to understand the impact of systematic sleep assessments in preterm children, and how shared risk factors for prematurity and sleep disorders, particularly race and socioeconomic status, interact.

References

1. Di Fiore JM, Poets CF, Gauda E, Martin RJ, MacFarlane P. Cardiorespiratory events in preterm infants: etiology and monitoring technologies. J Perinatol. 2016;36(3):165–71.
2. Di Fiore JM, Poets CF, Gauda E, Martin RJ, MacFarlane P. Cardiorespiratory events in preterm infants: interventions and consequences. J Perinatol. 2016;36(4):251–8.
3. Darnall RA, Ariagno RL, Kinney HC. The late preterm infant and the control of breathing, sleep, and brainstem development: a review. Clinics in perinatology. 2006;33(4):883–914. ; abstract x.
4. Darnall RA. The role of CO(2) and central chemoreception in the control of breathing in the fetus and the neonate. Respir Physiol Neurobiol. 2010;173(3):201–12.
5. Ross KR, Rosen CL. Sleep and respiratory physiology in children. Clin Chest Med. 2014;35(3):457–67.
6. Visser GH, Poelmann-Weesjes G, Cohen TM, Bekedam DJ. Fetal behavior at 30 to 32 weeks of gestation. Pediatr Res. 1987;22(6):655–8.

7. Lehtonen L, Martin RJ. Ontogeny of sleep and awake states in relation to breathing in preterm infants. Semin Neonatol. 2004;9(3):229–38.

8. Mirmiran M, Maas YG, Ariagno RL. Development of fetal and neonatal sleep and circadian rhythms. Sleep Med Rev. 2003;7(4):321–34.

9. Anders TF, Keener M. Developmental course of nighttime sleep-wake patterns in full-term and premature infants during the first year of life. I. Sleep. 1985;8(3):173–92.

10. Hoppenbrouwers T, Hodgman JE, Rybine D, Fabrikant G, Corwin M, Crowell D, et al. Sleep architecture in term and preterm infants beyond the neonatal period: the influence of gestational age, steroids, and ventilatory support. Sleep. 2005;28(11):1428–36.

11. Curzi-Dascalova L, Christova-Gueorguieva L, Lebrun F, Firtion G. Respiratory pauses in very low risk prematurely born infants reaching normal term. A comparison to full-term newborns. Neuropediatrics. 1984;15(1):13–7.

12. Booth CL, Morin VN, Waite SP, Thoman EB. Periodic and non-periodic sleep apnea in premature and fullterm infants. Dev Med Child Neurol. 1983;25(3):283–96.

13. Albani M, Bentele KH, Budde C, Schulte FJ. Infant sleep apnea profile: preterm vs. term infants. Eur J Pediatr. 1985;143(4):261–8.

14. Calder NA, Williams BA, Smyth J, Boon AW, Kumar P, Hanson MA. Absence of ventilatory responses to alternating breaths of mild hypoxia and air in infants who have had bronchopulmonary dysplasia: implications for the risk of sudden infant death. Pediatr Res. 1994;35(6):677–81.

15. Katz-Salamon M, Jonsson B, Lagercrantz H. Blunted peripheral chemoreceptor response to hyperoxia in a group of infants with bronchopulmonary dysplasia. Pediatr Pulmonol. 1995;20(2):101–6.

16. Malloy MH, Hoffman HJ. Prematurity, sudden infant death syndrome, and age of death. Pediatrics. 1995;96:464–71.

17. Leach CE, Blair PS, Fleming PJ, Smith IJ, Platt MW, Berry PJ, et al. Epidemiology of SIDS and explained sudden infant deaths. CESDI SUDI Research Group. Pediatrics. 1999;104(4):e43.

18. Halloran DR, Alexander GR. Preterm delivery and age of SIDS death. Ann Epidemiol. 2006;16(8):600–6.

19. Garcia 3rd AJ, Koschnitzky JE, Ramirez JM. The physiological determinants of sudden infant death syndrome. Respir Physiol Neurobiol. 2013;189(2):288–300.

20. Beebe DW. Neurobehavioral morbidity associated with disordered breathing during sleep in children: a comprehensive review. Sleep. 2006;29(9):1115–34.

21. Bhattacharjee R, Kheirandish-Gozal L, Pillar G, Gozal D. Cardiovascular complications of obstructive sleep apnea syndrome: evidence from children. Prog Cardiovasc Dis. 2009; 51(5):416–33.

22. Lumeng JC, Chervin RD. Epidemiology of pediatric obstructive sleep apnea. Proc Am Thorac Soc. 2008;5(2):242–52.

23. Hibbs AM, Johnson NL, Rosen CL, Kirchner HL, Martin R, Storfer-Isser A, et al. Prenatal and neonatal risk factors for sleep disordered breathing in school-aged children born preterm. J Pediatr. 2008;153(2):176–82.

24. Rosen CL, Larkin EK, Kirchner HL, Emancipator JL, Bivins SF, Surovec SA, et al. Prevalence and risk factors for sleep-disordered breathing in 8- to 11-year-old children: association with race and prematurity. J Pediatr. 2003;142(4):383–9.

25. Spilsbury JC, Storfer-Isser A, Kirchner HL, Nelson L, Rosen CL, Drotar D, et al. Neighborhood disadvantage as a risk factor for pediatric obstructive sleep apnea. J Pediatr. 2006;149(3): 342–7.

26. Spilsbury JC, Storfer-Isser A, Rosen CL, Redline S. Remission and incidence of obstructive sleep apnea from middle childhood to late adolescence. Sleep. 2015;38(1):23–9.

27. Katz ES, D'Ambrosio CM. Pathophysiology of pediatric obstructive sleep apnea. Proc Am Thorac Soc. 2008;5(2):253–62.

28. Owens RL, Edwards BA, Eckert DJ, Jordan AS, Sands SA, Malhotra A, et al. An integrative model of physiological traits can be used to predict obstructive sleep apnea and response to non positive airway pressure therapy. Sleep. 2015;38(6):961–70.
29. Montgomery-Downs HE, Young ME, Ross MA, Polak MJ, Ritchie SK, Lynch SK. Sleep-disordered breathing symptoms frequency and growth among prematurely born infants. Sleep Med. 2010;11(3):263–7.
30. Wang K, Difiore JM, Martin RJ, Rosen CL, Hibbs AM. Markers for severity of illness associated with decreased snoring in toddlers born ELGA. Acta Paediatr. 2013;102(1):e39–43.
31. Bonuck KA, Chervin RD, Cole TJ, Emond A, Henderson J, Xu L, et al. Prevalence and persistence of sleep disordered breathing symptoms in young children: a 6-year population-based cohort study. Sleep. 2011;34(7):875–84.
32. Raynes-Greenow CH, Hadfield RM, Cistulli PA, Bowen J, Allen H, Roberts CL. Sleep apnea in early childhood associated with preterm birth but not small for gestational age: a population-based record linkage study. Sleep. 2012;35(11):1475–80.
33. McGrath-Morrow SA, Ryan T, McGinley BM, Okelo SO, Sterni LM, Collaco JM. Polysomnography in preterm infants and children with chronic lung disease. Pediatr Pulmonol. 2012;47(2):172–9.
34. Sharma PB, Baroody F, Gozal D, Lester LA. Obstructive sleep apnea in the formerly preterm infant: an overlooked diagnosis. Front Neurol. 2011;2:73.
35. Qubty WF, Mrelashvili A, Kotagal S, Lloyd RM. Comorbidities in infants with obstructive sleep apnea. J Clin Sleep Med. 2014;10(11):1213–6.
36. Cote V, Ruiz AG, Perkins J, Sillau S, Friedman NR. Characteristics of children under 2 years of age undergoing tonsillectomy for upper airway obstruction. Int J Pediatr Otorhinolaryngol. 2015;79(6):903–8.
37. Emancipator JL, Storfer-Isser A, Taylor HG, Rosen CL, Kirchner HL, Johnson NL, et al. Variation of cognition and achievement with sleep-disordered breathing in full-term and preterm children. Arch Pediatr Adolesc Med. 2006;160(2):203–10.
38. Calhoun SL, Vgontzas AN, Mayes SD, Tsaoussoglou M, Sauder K, Mahr F, et al. Prenatal and perinatal complications: is it the link between race and SES and childhood sleep disordered breathing? J Clin Sleep Med. 2010;6(3):264–9.
39. Tapia IE, Shults J, Doyle LW, Nixon GM, Cielo CM, Traylor J, et al. Perinatal risk factors associated with the obstructive sleep apnea syndrome in school-aged children born preterm. Sleep. 2016;39(4):737–42.
40. Tishler PV, Larkin EK, Schluchter MD, Redline S. Incidence of sleep-disordered breathing in an urban adult population: the relative importance of risk factors in the development of sleep-disordered breathing. JAMA. 2003;289(17):2230–7.
41. Young T, Shahar E, Nieto FJ, Redline S, Newman AB, Gottlieb DJ, et al. Predictors of sleep-disordered breathing in community-dwelling adults: the Sleep Heart Health Study. Arch Intern Med. 2002;162(8):893–900.
42. Bixler EO, Fernandez-Mendoza J, Liao D, Calhoun S, Rodriguez-Colon SM, Gaines J, et al. Natural history of sleep disordered breathing in prepubertal children transitioning to adolescence. Eur Respir J. 2016;47(5):1402–9.
43. Paavonen EJ, Strang-Karlsson S, Raikkonen K, Heinonen K, Pesonen AK, Hovi P, et al. Very low birth weight increases risk for sleep-disordered breathing in young adulthood: the Helsinki Study of Very Low Birth Weight Adults. Pediatrics. 2007;120(4):778–84.
44. Reppert SM, Schwartz WJ. Functional activity of the suprachiasmatic nuclei in the fetal primate. Neurosci Lett. 1984;46(2):145–9.
45. Hao H, Rivkees SA. The biological clock of very premature primate infants is responsive to light. Proc Natl Acad Sci U S A. 1999;96(5):2426–9.
46. Mirmiran M, Ariagno RL. Influence of light in the NICU on the development of circadian rhythms in preterm infants. Semin Perinatol. 2000;24(4):247–57.
47. Mann NP, Haddow R, Stokes L, Goodley S, Rutter N. Effect of night and day on preterm infants in a newborn nursery: randomised trial. Br Med J. 1986;293(6557):1265–7.

48. Guyer C, Huber R, Fontijn J, Bucher HU, Nicolai H, Werner H, et al. Very preterm infants show earlier emergence of 24-hour sleep-wake rhythms compared to term infants. Early Hum Dev. 2015;91(1):37–42.

49. Asaka Y, Takada S. Activity-based assessment of the sleep behaviors of VLBW preterm infants and full-term infants at around 12 months of age. Brain Dev. 2010;32(2):150–5.

50. Iglowstein I, Latal Hajnal B, Molinari L, Largo RH, Jenni OG. Sleep behaviour in preterm children from birth to age 10 years: a longitudinal study. Acta Paediatr. 2006;95(12):1691–3.

51. Hagmann-von Arx P, Perkinson-Gloor N, Brand S, Albert D, Holsboer-Trachsler E, Grob A, et al. In school-age children who were born very preterm sleep efficiency is associated with cognitive function. Neuropsychobiology. 2014;70(4):244–52.

52. Marcus CL, Meltzer LJ, Roberts RS, Traylor J, Dix J, D'Ilario J, et al. Long-term effects of caffeine therapy for apnea of prematurity on sleep at school age. Am J Respir Crit Care Med. 2014;190(7):791–9.

53. Clark RH, Bloom BT, Spitzer AR, Gerstmann DR. Reported medication use in the neonatal intensive care unit: data from a large national data set. Pediatrics. 2006;117(6):1979–87.

54. Schmidt B, Roberts RS, Davis P, Doyle LW, Barrington KJ, Ohlsson A, et al. Caffeine therapy for apnea of prematurity. N Engl J Med. 2006;354(20):2112–21.

55. Schmidt B, Roberts RS, Davis P, Doyle LW, Barrington KJ, Ohlsson A, et al. Long-term effects of caffeine therapy for apnea of prematurity. N Engl J Med. 2007;357(19):1893–902.

56. Carskadon MA, Vieira C, Acebo C. Association between puberty and delayed phase preference. Sleep. 1993;16(3):258–62.

57. Koehl M, Barbazanges A, Le Moal M, Maccari S. Prenatal stress induces a phase advance of circadian corticosterone rhythm in adult rats which is prevented by postnatal stress. Brain Res. 1997;759(2):317–20.

58. Natale V, Sansavini A, Trombini E, Esposito MJ, Alessandroni R, Faldella G. Relationship between preterm birth and circadian typology in adolescence. Neurosci Lett. 2005;382(1–2): 139–42.

59. Hibbs AM, Storfer-Isser A, Rosen C, Ievers-Landis CE, Taveras EM, Redline S. Advanced sleep phase in adolescents born preterm. Behav Sleep Med. 2014;12(5):412–24.

60. Bjorkqvist J, Paavonen J, Andersson S, Pesonen AK, Lahti J, Heinonen K, et al. Advanced sleep-wake rhythm in adults born prematurely: confirmation by actigraphy-based assessment in the Helsinki Study of Very Low Birth Weight Adults. Sleep Med. 2014;15(9):1101–6.

61. Strang-Karlsson S, Kajantie E, Pesonen AK, Raikkonen K, Hovi P, Lahti J, et al. Morningness propensity in young adults born prematurely: the Helsinki study of very low birth weight adults. Chronobiol Int. 2010;27(9–10):1829–42.

62. Strang-Karlsson S, Raikkonen K, Kajantie E, Andersson S, Hovi P, Heinonen K, et al. Sleep quality in young adults with very low birth weight – the Helsinki study of very low birth weight adults. J Pediatr Psychol. 2008;33(4):387–95.

Airway Outcomes

Wade G. McClain, Gita M. Fleischman, and Amelia F. Drake

Introduction

Airway obstruction in the premature infant is a common cause of respiratory distress and can result from a wide array of structural and physiological problems. Although congenital problems can cause obstruction, many cases are directly related to supportive treatment of pulmonary immaturity, such as prolonged endotracheal intubation. In some patients, the residual effects are minimal; in other cases, the ongoing care that they need is substantial and long term. Most of the positive outcomes relate to success in achieving normal breathing and airway patency. Treatment cannot be undertaken without identification of the anatomical site(s) of obstruction, and this chapter will discuss pathophysiology, treatment, and outcomes based on anatomical subsite.

The heterogeneity of pathophysiology of upper airway obstruction makes systematic study of outcomes for specific disease processes difficult, and the literature specifically relating to outcomes among premature infants is relatively sparse. Where available, data for outcomes among premature infants have been included and identified as such. In other cases, many studies include term infants with similar pathology, which are discussed to provide an overview of current knowledge.

From a historical perspective, the literature in the 1980s and 1990s in pediatric surgery and otolaryngology journals contained articles from a number of leaders in this area around the world, reporting the occurrence of laryngeal stenosis in infants who had been ventilated and included recommendations for its prevention, which was key. In 1981, a landmark article first mentioned the anterior cricoid split

W.G. McClain, DO • G.M. Fleischman, MD • A.F. Drake, MD (✉)
Department of Otolaryngology/Head and Neck Surgery, University of North Carolina School of Medicine, Chapel Hill, NC, 27599-7070, USA
e-mail: Amelia_Drake@unc.edu; Gitanjali.Fleischman@unchealth.unc.edu; Wade_McClain@med.unc.edu

© Springer International Publishing AG 2017
A.M. Hibbs, M. S. Muhlebach (eds.), *Respiratory Outcomes in Preterm Infants*, Respiratory Medicine, DOI 10.1007/978-3-319-48835-6_11

procedure as an alternative to tracheostomy in infants with subglottic stenosis [1]. This article demonstrated that a simple procedure, though it did require ongoing support of the infant, could lyse the area of stenosis and achieve reasonable success (~90 %). The subglottic area was now accessible to surgeons to enlarge. As the numbers and complexity of laryngeal stenosis increased, so did the procedures, with anterior and posterior grafting described. Authors in many countries reported their outcomes in large numbers during this era of rapid reporting and surgical treatment, and innovation elapsed. Centers of excellence were recognized as those who had increasing success in the surgical and medical management of these difficult problems. This chapter hopes to delineate some of the more common airway outcomes of prematurity that are known, and to explore options for their successful management.

Base of Tongue

The base of tongue extends from the circumvallate papillae to the vallecula. When displaced posteriorly, either because of enlargement due to macroglossia or mass such as lingual thyroid or by retrognathia, airway obstruction can occur. Syndromes such as trisomy 21 and Beckwith-Wiedemann syndrome exhibit macroglossia and resultant glossoptosis. Such syndromes when occurring in premature infants may be diagnosed later, secondary to other problems, but do complicate further management. Even in term infants, the Pierre Robin sequence (PRS) can present with severe and even life-threatening upper airway obstruction in the perinatal period due to retrognathia. Approximately 50 % of cases of PRS are associated with an identifiable syndrome or chromosomal abnormality. Early identification of syndromic cases is important as these are associated with worse airway and feeding outcomes [2]. Management of the airway in PRS ranges from positioning changes to nasopharyngeal airway placement to surgical intervention such as tongue-lip adhesion, mandibular distraction osteogenesis, or tracheostomy. As with many of the airway lesions discussed in this text, tracheostomy definitively establishes a patent airway in PRS, but morbidity associated with tracheostomy means that its avoidance is the goal of the other interventions discussed here.

Airway obstruction in PRS can be managed nonsurgically in 40–84 % of cases [3]. Failures of nonsurgical management, as defined by continuing respiratory distress or abnormal polysomnogram, were traditionally treated with tracheostomy or tongue-lip adhesion. Recent literature suggests that mandibular distraction osteogenesis is well tolerated and has superior outcomes to tongue-lip adhesion [4]. The idea of "catch-up growth" of the mandible postnatally may be erroneous, as studies do not show an improvement in polysomnographic findings with advancing age [5]. Distraction osteogenesis outcomes in premature infants with PRS do not appear worse than those in term infants in limited studies [6].

Supraglottis

The supraglottis is the most common subsite of the upper airway for lesions that present with stridor in the newborn and is usually associated with inspiratory stridor. Congenital laryngomalacia is the single most common cause of stridor in newborns and infants. It is diagnosed in 50–75 % of all infants with stridor [7, 8]. This stridor is distinctly high-pitched, inspiratory, and worsens with supine position and sleep. The noise is attributed to prolapse of supraglottic structures into the airway and subsequent turbulent airflow.

Laryngomalacia is a disease spectrum, ranging from intermittent positional stridor to life-threatening airway compromise, with the development of cor pulmonale. Historically, the etiology of laryngomalacia was postulated to be secondary to cartilaginous immaturity and anatomical abnormality; however, it is now understood that laryngeal hypotonicity resulting from neuromuscular immaturity is the most accepted hypothesis (Figs. 1 and 2).

Laryngomalacia is most easily diagnosed endoscopically, with a simple bedside flexible fiberoptic laryngoscopic exam, which allows for direct visualization of the airway during dynamic respiration, from the oropharynx to the hypopharynx and larynx. Large-scale studies have shown that endoscopy is more sensitive at diagnosing laryngomalacia than radiographic evaluation [9]. Additionally, flexible bronchoscopy performed under sedation by pediatric pulmonology should be considered, because laryngomalacia may be associated with additional lower airway lesions, with reports ranging from 10–41 % of secondary lesions [10, 11]. Diagnosis of laryngomalacia in

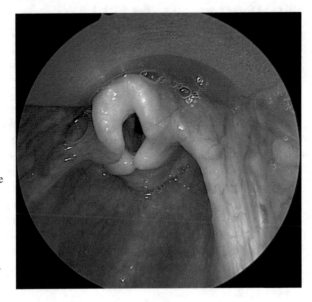

Fig. 1 Direct laryngoscopic view of laryngomalacia. Note the curled appearance of the epiglottis and the medial prolapse of the arytenoids. The laryngoscope blade's position in the vallecula has elevated the epiglottis and moderated the appearance of supraglottic collapse

Fig. 2 Immediate postoperative appearance of the patient from Fig. 1 after aryepiglottic fold division. Note the expanded supraglottic airway. Removal of redundant arytenoid soft tissue could be subsequently performed to further open the airway

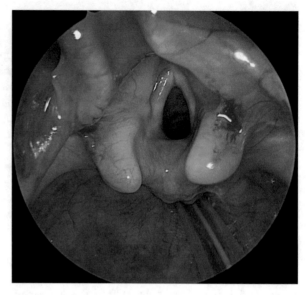

premature infants is important, as it may be a large contributor to failure to extubate, or alternatively these children may require prolonged CPAP.

Gastroesophageal reflux (GER) and laryngomalacia have been shown to be strongly correlated. In one study, GERD was found in 64 % of patients with laryngomalacia, and was significantly associated with severe symptoms and complicated clinical course including increased rates of hospitalization, poor weight gain, and the need for surgical intervention [12].

Glottis

Obstruction at the level of the glottis can be caused by a failure of recannulation of the airway during fetal development, as seen in laryngeal webs or atresia (Fig. 3), as well as by vocal cord immobility. Vocal cord paralysis can be either unilateral or bilateral. Unilateral paralysis is most commonly iatrogenic and is associated with birth trauma or repair of cardiac abnormalities. The extended course of the left recurrent laryngeal nerve exposes it to iatrogenic damage during cardiovascular surgery and esophageal surgery. Because of this, unilateral paralysis is predominantly left-sided. The right vagus nerve can be injured during placement and decannulation of ECMO cannulas [13]. Unilateral paralysis can present with a hoarse, breathy cry, and can be associated with aspiration and dysphagia. Therefore, diagnosis should be sought early, and further management should ideally involve speech therapy in joint consultation with ENT or pulmonology.

Fig. 3 A congenital laryngeal web in an infant with 22q11.2 microdeletion syndrome

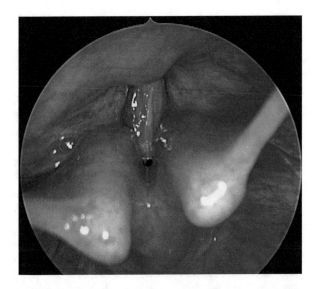

A 2014 meta-analysis estimated the rate of unilateral vocal fold paralysis after congenital cardiac surgery to be approximately 9 %, but a subset of the analyzed studies in which all patients were prospectively evaluated by laryngoscopy reported a rate of 30 % [14]. Risk of unilateral paralysis after patent ductus arteriosus ligation was reported in 5–17 % of preterm and low birth weight infants [15, 16]. Risk of unilateral vocal fold *dysfunction* is even higher, approximately 58 %, in infants that undergo more complex repairs such as Norwood or aortic arch reconstruction [17]. Younger age, underlying airway or genetic abnormalities are further risks, and may warrant formal airway evaluation, for instance, at the time of extubation [18]. Interestingly, left vocal cord dysfunction during exercise was demonstrated in 26 % of such former premature infants with history of PDA ligation when they were adults [19].

A majority of congenital vocal fold paralysis is bilateral. Bilateral paralysis can be congenital acquired in the early neonatal period due to hydrocephalus or Arnold-Chiari malformation, but is often idiopathic. Premature infants who required intubation at delivery may only be diagnosed with vocal fold paralysis at the time of extubation. Bilateral vocal fold paralysis causing airway compromise normally presents with high-pitched inspiratory or biphasic stridor. The cry often sounds relatively normal, and this can delay diagnosis.

Diagnosis of unilateral or bilateral vocal cord dysfunction is best accomplished either by laryngoscopy or bronchoscopy. Further evaluation of their swallowing and feeding will determine treatment options ranging from watchful waiting in patients who can maintain adequate oxygenation and avoid significant aspiration to tracheostomy in those that cannot.

Subglottis

Description/Classification

Subglottic stenosis (SGS) is defined as narrowing of the subglottic airway to <3.5 mm in premature infants and 4.0 mm in term neonates. It can be caused by neoplasms such as hemangioma (Fig. 4), but in the premature infant, it is most often iatrogenic or congenital.

The vast majority (~95 %) of cases are acquired due to airway trauma, most commonly endotracheal intubation. SGS without a history of airway manipulation is considered congenital. The proportion of SGS that is congenital is likely underestimated because of the frequency of intubation before formal endoscopy in the setting of respiratory distress.

Congenital SGS can be due to cartilaginous or membranous stenosis. Congenital cartilaginous SGS can be due to a flattened (short anterior/posterior diameter), elliptical (shortened lateral diameter) (Fig. 5), or a "trapped" first tracheal ring that telescopes into the subglottis, narrowing the airway. Membranous stenosis results from hypertrophy of the submucosal tissues or mucous glands and appears soft on rigid endoscopy (Fig. 6). Congenital SGS is more likely to be amenable to observation and avoidance of surgical intervention. Because it does not result from an inflammatory process, it is also more likely to be successfully treated if surgical intervention becomes necessary.

Fig. 4 Classic appearance of a subglottic hemangioma. Red irregular mass in the lateral posterior portion of the subglottis

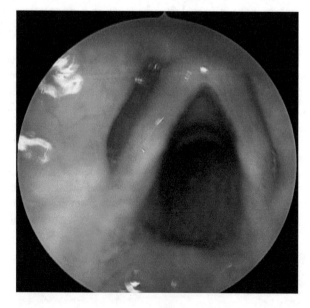

Fig. 5 Elliptical cricoid showing narrowed horizontal diameter of the subglottis

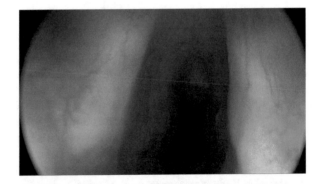

Fig. 6 Subglottic cysts can arise after even transient endotracheal intubation

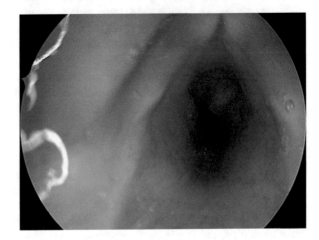

Epidemiology

The emergence and rapid advance of the specialty of neonatology since the 1960s has allowed the survival of premature infants with their associated pulmonary diseases of prematurity. Along with the increased survival of extreme premature infants, the incidence of prolonged endotracheal intubation may increase, causing ongoing prevalence despite the measures taken to minimize risks. As the understanding of the pathophysiology of subglottic/laryngotracheal stenosis has improved, techniques designed to minimize tissue damage have been developed, and the incidence of SGS associated with endotracheal intubation has decreased.

The true incidence of SGS specifically in premature infants is difficult to quantify. Available series include all intubated neonates and fail to specify whether they are premature or term. Reported incidence of SGS in intubated neonates has decreased from 4 % in the early 1980s to 0.63 % in more recent series [20].

Pathophysiology

Several factors combine to make to the level of the cricoid cartilage in the subglottis the site of the majority of instances of acquired LTS. The cricoid is the only complete cartilaginous ring in the normal airway, thus eliminating the ability of the airway to dilate to reduce pressure on the mucosa and submucosa. Additionally, the cricoid is the narrowest portion of the infant airway, creating the greatest levels of hydrostatic pressure along a fixed-diameter endotracheal tube. Hydrostatic pressure exceeding capillary pressure creates relative ischemia and leads to mucosal and submucosal damage. Reduced thickness of submucosal tissue at the level of the cricoid also leads to early exposure of the perichondrium and subsequent increase in inflammation. In postmortem anatomical examinations of low birth weight infants, exposure of the perichondrium at the level of the cricoid is seen in as few as 8 days in many specimens. Depth and size of mucosal scarring increases with the duration of intubation [21].

The same pathophysiological process of scar formation that leads to SGS frustrates attempts to surgically treat the condition. The increased scar deposition after mucosal trauma from intubation can also occur after endoscopic and open surgical treatment.

Treatment

Tracheostomy is in most cases a successful treatment modality for subglottic stenosis, allowing normal feeding and providing a safe airway. It is associated with significant morbidity and is generally not undertaken in infants under 2000g, as complications increase in smaller patients. The overarching goal of other modalities is to either prevent tracheostomy in the first place or allow decannulation. The majority of studies investigating these techniques define success as allowing for extubation while avoiding tracheostomy or allowing for decannulation.

The technique of dividing the cricoid ring to allow for expansion of the subglottic airway dates to Réthi's description in 1956, but was popularized by the description of the anterior cricoid split by Cotton and Seid [1]. This technique involves a midline division of the anterior cricoid lamina and first tracheal ring without graft placement. A stent, either an endotracheal tube in the nontracheotomized patient or an Aboulker or Rutter stent or Montgomery T-tube in a patient with previously placed tracheostomy, is left in place temporarily to allow for healing. In well-selected patients without significant comorbidities, the success of this operation is quite good, with extubation/decannulation rates of approximately 70% [22]. Patients with a longer total period of preoperative intubation and with multiple medical or neurological comorbidities fare worse with success rates around 40–50 % [23].

The development by Cotton and colleagues of laryngotracheal reconstruction (LTR) in the 1970s led to improvement in outcomes by combining division of the cricoid with placement of cartilage grafts harvested from the thyroid ala or costal cartilage. When compared with anterior cricoid split, LTR is more successful and reduces complications [24]. Success rates of up to 83 % are reported [25]. Outcomes of this procedure are worse in the setting of stenosis that extends superiorly to the glottis or supraglottis and in patients under 4 kg [26, 27].

Some evidence that single stage procedure (i.e., leaving an endotracheal tube in place postoperatively rather than a tracheostomy with a second procedure to decannulate) is more likely to result in decannulation when controlling for severity of disease and previous surgery [28].

Before the development of open airway reconstruction techniques in the 1970s by Cotton and colleagues, the mainstay of treatment for SGS was serial anterograde rigid dilation (bougienage). This proved unsatisfactory and was rapidly supplanted in many cases by the newer open techniques. Shearing trauma to the mucosa inherent to the technique of bougienage could induce inflammation and fibrosis and worsen stenosis. The adoption of balloon dilation coupled with newer endoscopic techniques has brought endoscopic treatment as a primary modality back to the forefront of treatment for SGS. Balloon dilation offers the benefit of circumferential compression that limits shearing forces and theoretically reduces mucosal damage and resulting in inflammatory response. As with previous dilation techniques, balloon dilation typically requires multiple procedures to establish a durable improvement in airway diameter as discussed below. This can be contrasted with open repair techniques which aim to establish an adequate airway with one procedure. Both techniques require close follow-up and serial bronchoscopy to ensure continued patency.

Early descriptions of the technique employed angioplasty balloon catheters under fluoroscopy [29]. Most surgeons currently performing the procedure currently employ bronchoscopic visualization for placement. More recently, noncompliant balloons able to deliver pressure directly to a stenotic segment without deformation have been developed and widely adopted. Reported success rates, as defined as avoidance of tracheostomy or decannulation, vary between 39 and 100 %. Studies with longer term follow-up report success of approximately 50–60 % [30–32].

There are currently no studies directly examining outcomes of rigid dilation versus balloon dilation. Published studies show similar success rates between the two techniques despite the theoretical advantages of balloon dilation detailed earlier [33]. As with other airway reconstruction techniques, overall patient numbers analyzed in these studies are limited enough to make meaningful statistical analysis difficult.

Outcomes of all endoscopic techniques are improved in the setting of acute, or evolving, stenosis. After the development of submucosal fibrosis, dilation is less successful in both the initial improvement in airway cross-sectional area and the durability of the improvement. Avelino et al. reported a 100 % success rate in acute stenosis, defined as stenosis treated 30 days after extubation or tracheostomy for failed extubation, versus 39 % for those treated more than 30 days after extubation or tracheotomy (Fig. 7).

Fig. 7 An "early" or
evolving stenosis. Note the
translucence of the thin
subglottic web. This was
successfully treated with a
single endoscopic procedure

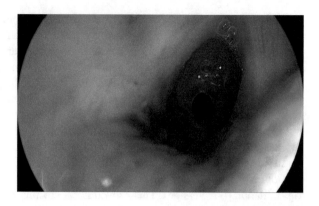

Recently, techniques combining endoscopic cricoid (anterior, posterior, and anterior/posterior) splits with balloon dilation have been reported with good success rates [34]. It is possible that these combined techniques may lead to improved outcomes over simple balloon dilation in chronic or congenital stenosis.

Trachea

The most common cause of stridor arising from the trachea in infants is tracheomalacia (TM) [35]. Tracheomalacia refers to a weakness of the structure of the trachea and can present variably depending on the location of the lesion. Most often, it is intrathoracic and causes expiratory wheeze and stridor that are particularly exacerbated by cough or Valsalva. The cough has a brassy quality; yet, collapse of the trachea during cough impedes effective airway clearance. If the malacic segment is extrathoracic, it can present as inspiratory or biphasic stridor. The terms "tracheomalacia" and "tracheobronchomalacia" are often used interchangeably in the literature, but the former can refer more precisely to disease that is isolated to the trachea and the latter to more widely distributed disease [36].

Tracheomalacia can be divided into primary and secondary types. Primary TM results from an inherent weakness of the tracheal framework and is commonly seen in otherwise normal premature infants [37]. It can also be associated with a number of conditions, including congenital abnormalities of the cartilage such as chondrodysplasia, polychondritis, and Ehlers-Danlos syndrome, the mucopolysaccharidoses, trisomy 21, and tracheoesophageal fistulas as discussed below. Primary TM without other associated abnormalities is often a self-limited disease that often improves or resolves by 2 years of age and can be managed expectantly. In some children, it is severe enough, however, to require ongoing noninvasive positive pressure ventilation. Prematurity *per se* does not worsen outcomes in TM [37]; however, the course of the premature infant may be complicated by tracheomalacia. Primary TM associated with connective tissue disease is more likely to be problematic and require surgical intervention.

Currently available and used surgical interventions include tracheostomy, aorto-pexy, and in some cases stenting. Tracheostomy allows for long-term positive pressure ventilation that can address diffuse weakness and airway collapse. Aortopexy can provide relief in severe localized tracheomalacia without significant involvement of the bronchi [38]. Although traditionally performed via thoracotomy, recent descriptions of successful thoracoscopic aortopexy may allow the procedure to be performed with less morbidity [39]. Other interventions such as airway stenting are used in some centers, but can lead to troublesome and sometimes dangerous granulation tissue formation and bleeding along with the possibility of erosion of the airway by the stent.

Tracheomalacia is also nearly universally present to some degree in cases of tracheoesophageal fistula (TEF). Whether this should be considered a primary or secondary form is open to debate [40]. TM associated with TEF can persist with mild symptoms and increased frequency of cough and respiratory infection often occurring to the age of 5 years [41]. Prolonged cough and bacterial infections following usual childhood viruses are likely to be secondary to impaired cough clearance, as the malacic segment cannot propel secretions upward.

Secondary tracheobronchomalaica (TBM), that is, malacia involving trachea and extending to the bronchi, can be caused by extrinsic compression, most commonly by vascular abnormalities, and also due to cardiac and skeletal abnormalities as well as solid masses such as tumors, cysts, and goiters. Secondary TBM can also be caused by damage to the tracheobronchial framework (Fig. 8). Premature infants that undergo prolonged intubation are particularly vulnerable to development of TBM. Ninety-six percent of infants diagnosed with secondary TBM in one series were former premature infants that had undergone prolonged endotracheal intubation. This same series also reported that premature infants were more likely (75 % vs. 39 %) to require tracheostomy for treatment compared to their term peers [42] (Fig. 9).

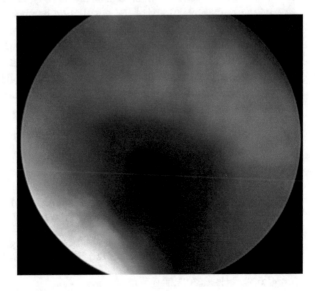

Fig. 8 Tracheomalacia secondary to extrinsic compression from a double aortic arch

Fig. 9 Endoscopic appearance of complete tracheal rings. Critical airway narrowing can be exacerbated in the premature infant if the tracheal segment with complete rings is manipulated and must be avoided

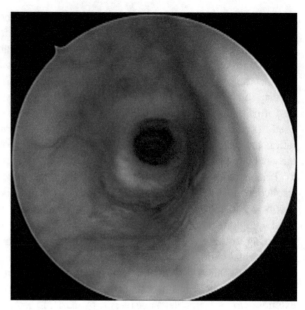

Summary

A wide array of anatomical and physiological abnormalities can lead to symptomatic upper airway of obstruction in the premature infant. Modern techniques have led to improved outcomes in this population, but management continues to be a challenge. Successful outcomes are contingent upon early identification of the site(s) and pathophysiology of obstruction, and this relies on close collaboration between neonatologists, pulmonologists, and airway surgeons.

Once the pathophysiology of the obstruction has been identified, treatment can be tailored to the patient. Milder cases are often self-limited with continued growth of the infant and can be treated with supportive care. More severe and even life-threatening cases can require multiple complex surgical interventions over many years. Outcomes continue to improve as medical and surgical techniques are refined, but there remain significant challenges in maximizing survival and quality of life in the premature infant with airway obstruction.

References

1. Cotton RT, Seid AB. Management of the extubation problem in the premature child. Anterior cricoid split as an alternative to tracheotomy. Ann Otol Rhinol Laryngol. 1980;89(6 I):508–11.
2. Izumi K, Konczal LL, Mitchell AL, Jones MC. Underlying genetic diagnosis of pierre robin sequence: retrospective chart review at two children's hospitals and a systematic literature review. J Pediatr [Internet]. 2012;160(4):645–50.e2. Available from: http://dx.doi.org/10.1016/j.jpeds.2011.09.021. Mosby, Inc.

3. Reddy VS. Evaluation of upper airway obstruction in infants with Pierre Robin sequence and the role of polysomnography – review of current evidence. Paediatr Respir Rev [Internet]. Elsevier Ltd; 2016;17:80–7. Available from: http://www.ncbi.nlm.nih.gov/pubmed/26563513.

4. Papoff P, Guelfi G, Cicchetti R, Caresta E, Cozzi DA, Moretti C, et al. Outcomes after tongue-lip adhesion or mandibular distraction osteogenesis in infants with Pierre Robin sequence and severe airway obstruction. Int J Oral Maxillofac Surg [Internet]. International Association of Oral and Maxillofacial Surgery. 2013;42(11):1418–23. Available from: http://dx.doi.org/10.1016/j.ijom.2013.07.747.

5. Lee JJ, Thottam PJ, Ford MD, Jabbour N. Characteristics of sleep apnea in infants with Pierre-Robin sequence: is there improvement with advancing age?. Int J Pediatr Otorhinolaryngol [Internet]. 2015;79(12):2059–2067. Elsevier Ireland Ltd. Available from: http://dx.doi.org/10.1016/j.ijporl.2015.09.014.

6. Murage KP, Tholpady SS, Friel M, Havlik RJ, Flores RL. Outcomes analysis of mandibular distraction osteogenesis for the treatment of Pierre Robin sequence. Plast Reconstr Surg [Internet]. 2013;132(2):419–21. Available from: http://www.ncbi.nlm.nih.gov/pubmed/23897339.

7. Olney DR, Greinwald JH, Smith RJ, Bauman NM. Laryngomalacia and its treatment. Laryngoscope. 1999;109(11):1770–5.

8. Richter GT, Thompson DM. The surgical management of laryngomalacia. Otolaryngol Clin North Am. 2008 Oct;41(5):837–64.

9. Yuen HW, Tan HKK, Balakrishnan A. Synchronous airway lesions and associated anomalies in children with laryngomalacia evaluated with rigid endoscopy. Int J Pediatr Otorhinolaryngol. 2006;70(10):1779–84.

10. Rifai HA, Benoit M, El-Hakim H. Secondary airway lesions in laryngomalacia: a different perspective. Otolaryngol Head Neck Surg [Internet]. 2011;144(2):268–73. Available from: http://www.ncbi.nlm.nih.gov/pubmed/21493429.

11. Adil E, Rager T, Carr M. Location of airway obstruction in term and preterm infants with laryngomalacia. Am J Otolaryngo Head Neck Med Surg. Am J Otolaryngol. 2012 Jul–Aug;33(4):437–40.

12. Giannoni C, Sulek M, Friedman EM, Duncan III NO. Gastroesophageal reflux association with laryngomalacia: a prospective study. Int J Pediatr Otorhinolaryngol [Internet]. 1998;43(1):11–20. Available from: http://dx.doi.org/10.1016/S0165-5876(97)00151-1.

13. Schumacher RE, Weinfeld IJ, Bartlett RH. Neonatal vocal cord paralysis following extracorporeal membrane oxygenation. Pediatrics [Internet]. 1989;84(5):793–6. Available from: http://www.ncbi.nlm.nih.gov/pubmed/2797975.

14. Strychowsky JE, Rukholm G, Gupta MK, Reid D. Unilateral vocal fold paralysis after congenital cardiothoracic surgery: a meta-analysis. Pediatrics [Internet]. 2014;133(6):e1708–23. Available from: http://pediatrics.aappublications.org/cgi/doi/10.1542/peds.2013-3939.

15. Rukholm G, Farrokhyar F, Reid D. Vocal cord paralysis post patent ductus arteriosus ligation surgery: risks and co-morbidities. Int J Pediatr Otorhinolaryngol [Internet]. 2012;76(11):1637–41. Elsevier Ireland Ltd. Available from: http://dx.doi.org/10.1016/j.ijporl.2012.07.036.

16. Zbar RIS, Chen AH, Behrendt DM, Bell EF, Smith RJH. Incidence of vocal fold paralysis in infants undergoing ligation of patent ductus arteriosus. Ann Thorac Surg. 1996;61(3):814–6.

17. Pham V, Connelly D, Wei JL, Sykes KJ, O'Brien J. Vocal cord paralysis and Dysphagia after aortic arch reconstruction and Norwood procedure. Otolaryngol Head Neck Surg [Internet]. 2014;150(5):827–33. Available from: http://www.ncbi.nlm.nih.gov/pubmed/24515967. http://www.pubmedcentral.nih.gov/articlerender.fcgi?artid=PMC4262533.

18. Wilson MN, Bergeron LM, Kakade A, Simon LM, Caspi J, Pettitt T, et al. Airway management following pediatric cardiothoracic surgery. Otolaryngol Head Neck Surg. 2013;149(4):621–7.

19. Røksund OD, Clemm H, Heimdal JH, Aukland SM, Sandvik L, Markestad T, et al. Left vocal cord paralysis after extreme preterm birth, a new clinical scenario in adults. Pediatrics [Internet]. 2010;126(6):e1569–77. Available from: http://www.ncbi.nlm.nih.gov/pubmed/21098147.

20. Walner DL, Loewen MS, Kimura RE. Neonatal subglottic stenosis – incidence and trends. Laryngoscope. 2001;111(1):48–51.
21. Sato K, Nakashima T. Histopathologic changes in laryngeal mucosa of extremely low-birth .... Ann Otol Rhinol Laryngol. 2006;115(11):816.
22. Cotton RT, Myer CM, Bratcher GO, Fitton CM. Anterior cricoid split, 1977-1987: evolution of a technique. Arch Otolaryngol Head Neck Surg [Internet]. 1988;114(11):1300–2. Available from: http://archotol.jamanetwork.com/article.aspx?articleid=616678.
23. Rotenberg BW, Berkowitz RG. Changing trends in the success rate of anterior cricoid split. Ann Otol Rhinol Laryngol [Internet]. 2006 [cited 2016 Feb 2];115(11):833–6. Available from: http://www.ncbi.nlm.nih.gov/pubmed/17165666.
24. Richardson MA, Inglis AF. A comparison of anterior cricoid split with and without costal cartilage graft for acquired subglottic stenosis. Int J Pediatr Otorhinolaryngol. 1991;22(2):187–93.
25. Younis RT, Lazar RH, Astor F. Posterior cartilage graft in single-stage laryngotracheal reconstruction. Otolaryngol Head Neck Surg. 2003;129(03):168–75.
26. Morita K, Yokoi A, Bitoh Y, Fukuzawa H, Okata Y, Iwade T, et al. Severe acquired subglottic stenosis in children: analysis of clinical features and surgical outcomes based on the range of stenosis. Pediatr Surg Int [Internet]. Springer Berlin Heidelberg; 2015;31(10):943–7. Available from: http://link.springer.com/10.1007/s00383-015-3773-1.
27. McQueen CT, Shapiro NL, Leighton S, Guo XG, Albert DM.. Single-stage laryngotracheal reconstruction: the great ormond street experience and guidelines for patient selection. Arch Otolaryngol Neck Surg [Internet]. 1999;125(3):320–2. Available from: http://dx.doi.org/10.1001/archotol.125.3.320.
28. Saunders MW, Thirlwall A, Jacob A, Albert DM. Single-or-two-stage laryngotracheal reconstruction; comparison of outcomes. Int J Pediatr Otorhinolaryngol [Internet]. 1999;50(1):51–4. Available from: http://www.ncbi.nlm.nih.gov/pubmed/10596887.
29. Cohen Mervyn D, Weber TR, Rao CC. Balloon dilatational of tracheal and bronchial stenosis. AJR Am J Roentgenol. 1984;142(3):477–8.
30. Hebra A, Powell DD, Smith CD, Biemann OH. Balloon tracheoplasty in children: Results of a 15-year experience. J Pediatr Surg [Internet]. 1991;26(8):957–61. Available from: http://linkinghub.elsevier.com/retrieve/pii/002234689190843I.
31. Avelino M, Maunsell R, Jubé WI. Predicting outcomes of balloon laryngoplasty in children with subglottic stenosis. Int J Pediatr Otorhinolaryngol [Internet]. 2015;79(4):532–6. Available from: http://linkinghub.elsevier.com/retrieve/pii/S0165587615000385.
32. Whigham AS, Howell R, Choi S, Peña M, Zalzal G, Preciado D. Outcomes of balloon dilation in pediatric subglottic stenosis. Ann Otol Rhinol Laryngol [Internet]. 2012;121(7):442–8. Available from: http://www.ncbi.nlm.nih.gov/pubmed/24711947.
33. Chueng K, Chadha NK. Primary dilatation as a treatment for pediatric laryngotracheal stenosis: a systematic review. Int J Pediatr Otorhinolaryngol [Internet]. Elsevier Ireland Ltd; 2013;77(5):623–8. Available from: http://dx.doi.org/10.1016/j.ijporl.2013.02.003.
34. Mirabile L, Serio PP, Baggi RR, Couloigner VV. Endoscopic anterior cricoid split and balloon dilation in pediatric subglottic stenosis. Int J Pediatr Otorhinolaryngol [Internet]. Elsevier Ireland Ltd; 2010;74(12):1409–14. Available from: http://dx.doi.org/10.1016/j.ijporl.2010.09.020.
35. Zoumalan R, Maddalozzo J, Holinger LD. Etiology of stridor in infants. Ann Otol Rhinol Laryngol. 2007;116(5):329–34.
36. Carden KA, Boiselle PM, Waltz DA, Ernst A. Tracheomalacia and tracheobronchomalacia in children and adults. Chest. 2005;127(3):984–1005. PMID: 15764786.
37. Doull IJ, Mok Q, Tasker RC. Tracheobronchomalacia in preterm infants with chronic lung disease. Arch Dis Child Fetal Neonatal Ed [Internet]. 1997;76(3):F203–5. Available from: http://www.pubmedcentral.nih.gov/articlerender.fcgi?artid=1720642&tool=pmcentrez&rendertype=abstract.

38. Dave S, Currie BG. The role of aortopexy in severe tracheomalacia. J Pediatr Surg. 2006 Mar;41(3):533–7.
39. Van Der Zee DC, Straver M. Thoracoscopic aortopexy for tracheomalacia. World J Surg. 2015;39(1):158–64.
40. Greenholz SK, Karrer FM, Lilly JR. Contemporary surgery of tracheomalacia. J Pediatr Surg. 1986;21(6):511–4.
41. Chetcuti P, Phelan PD. Respiratory morbidity after repair of oesophageal atresia and tracheo-oesophageal fistula. Arch Dis Child. 1993;68(2):167–70.
42. Jacobs IN, Wetmore RF, Tom LWC, Handler SD, Potsic WP. Tracheobronchomalacia in children. Arch Otolaryngol Head Neck Surg [Internet]. 1994;120(2):154–8. Available from: http://archotol.jamanetwork.com/article.aspx?articleid=622075.

Pulmonary Hypertension
in Bronchopulmonary Dysplasia

Steven H. Abman

Introduction

As first characterized nearly five decades ago, bronchopulmonary dysplasia (BPD) was described as severe chronic respiratory disease with high mortality in relatively late-gestation preterm infants, as infants below 28 weeks gestation rarely survived in that era [1]. With surfactant therapy, improved ventilator care, more aggressive nutrition, and other interventions, the increases in survival of even the most immature newborns at gestational ages between 23 and 28 weeks have been remarkable [2–6]. However, these successes have not led to a reduction in the incidence of BPD, which remains a major problem, occurring in an estimated 10,000–15,000 infants per year in the USA alone [7]. Thus, developing novel approaches that target disease prevention or attenuating disease severity is of critical importance, as infants with established BPD require prolonged NICU courses, have frequent readmissions during the first 2 years after hospital discharge for respiratory infections, asthma, and related problems, and have persistent lung function abnormalities and exercise intolerance as adolescents and young adults [8].

Funding Source This work was supported in part by grants from the NHLBI HL085703 (S.H.A.), HL068702 (S.H.A.), and U01 HL102235 (S.H.A.). The author has no conflicts of interest with this work, but has received grant funding from Shire Pharmaceuticals for laboratory research

S.H. Abman, MD
Pediatric Heart Lung Center, Sections of Pediatric Pulmonary Medicine, University of Colorado School of Medicine and Children's Hospital Colorado, Aurora, CO 80045, USA

Critical Care Medicine, University of Colorado School of Medicine and Children's Hospital Colorado, Aurora, CO 80045, USA

Department of Pediatrics, University of Colorado School of Medicine and Children's Hospital Colorado, Mail Stop B395, 13123 East 16th Avenue, Aurora, CO 80045, USA
e-mail: steven.abman@ucdenver.edu

© Springer International Publishing AG 2017
A.M. Hibbs, M. S. Muhlebach (eds.), *Respiratory Outcomes in Preterm Infants*,
Respiratory Medicine, DOI 10.1007/978-3-319-48835-6_12

197

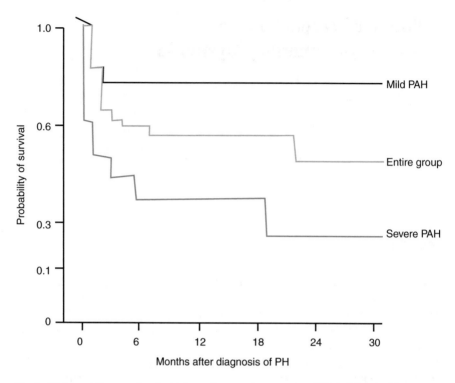

Fig. 1 High mortality associated with late pulmonary hypertension (PH) in BPD. As illustrated in this schematic, mortality is higher in the severe PH group than BPD infants with lower levels of PH (Adapted from reference [15])

Although outcomes have improved since the late 1960s, pulmonary hypertension (PH) and related pulmonary vascular disease (PVD) continue to cause significant morbidity and mortality in prematurely born children [1, 9–12]. Despite striking changes in the nature and epidemiology of BPD over time, PH continues to contribute significantly to high morbidity and mortality in BPD, and is present early in the course of disease [12–15]. Even the original descriptions of BPD noted striking pulmonary hypertensive vascular remodeling in severe cases, and that the presence of PH beyond 3 months of age was associated with high mortality (40 %; 11). Now, in the "postsurfactant era" or the "new BPD," late PH continues to be strongly linked with poor survival [15] (Fig. 1). This chapter briefly discusses our current understanding and approach for PH management in preterm infants with BPD, including discussion of recent guidelines from the joint American Heart Association and American Thoracic Society report on the care of children with PH [16].

The Abnormal Pulmonary Circulation in BPD

The lung circulation in infants with BPD is characterized by abnormalities of vascular tone and reactivity, structure, and growth, which include a reduction of small pulmonary arteries and a "dysmorphic" pattern of vessel branching within the lung interstitium [5, 9] (Fig. 2). Impaired vascular growth, or angiogenesis, is associated with disruption of alveolarization and reduces the alveolar–capillary surface area, which impairs gas exchange, increases the need for prolonged oxygen and ventilator therapy, causes poor exercise tolerance, and increases the risk for developing PH [17–22].

Mechanisms that coordinate normal vascular growth and alveolarization during development or cause abnormal lung growth in BPD are poorly understood. Disruption of key signals between airway epithelium and endothelial cells can alter vascular and alveolar growth, resulting in decreased arterial and airspace development. Experimental studies have shown that early antenatal or postnatal injury to the developing lung can impair angiogenesis, which further contributes to decreased alveolarization and simplification of distal lung airspace (the "vascular hypothesis" [23–25]). Angiogenic signaling pathways, including those involving vascular

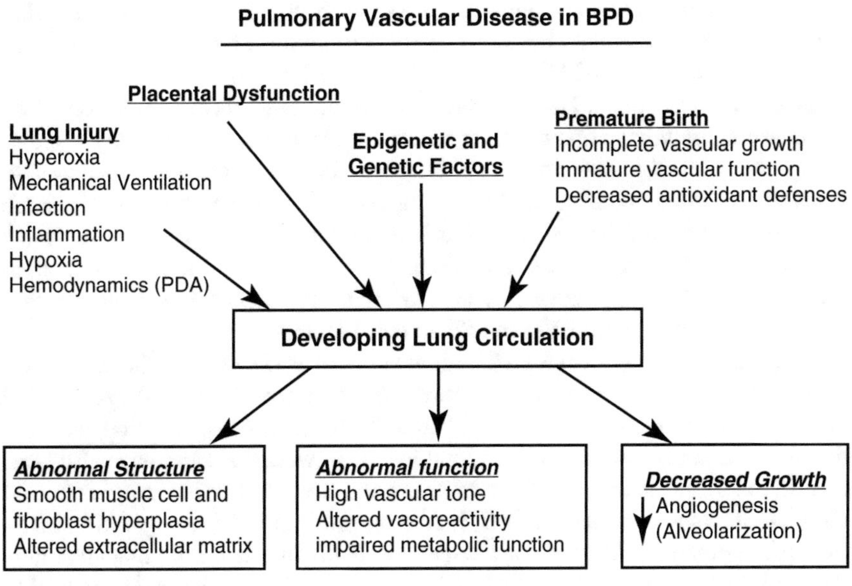

Fig. 2 Schematic illustration of the pathogenesis and pathobiology of pulmonary vascular disease in BPD (From reference [22])

endothelial growth factor (VEGF) and nitric oxide are important mediators of normal pulmonary vascular development [25]. Disruption of vascular growth and signaling markedly reduces alveolar–capillary surface area, which contributes to impaired lung diffusion capacity in BPD [26]. Placental overproduction of soluble VEGF receptor-1, which inhibits VEGF signaling, mainly causes maternal endothelial dysfunction and plays a central role in the pathogenesis of pre-eclampsia and can impair pulmonary vascular growth in utero and throughout infancy, even without hyperoxia, mechanical ventilation, or other postnatal insults [27–30]. Intrauterine growth restriction is another condition that has been associated with the disruption of VEGF signaling [25, 31] and an increased risk for BPD and PH in preterm infants [32]. Thus, abnormalities of the lung circulation in BPD are not only related to the presence or absence of PH, but more broadly, PVD, after premature birth as manifested by decreased vascular growth and structure, also contributes to the pathogenesis and abnormal cardiopulmonary physiology of BPD.

These laboratory concepts have recently been demonstrated in a prospective clinical study in which early echocardiogram findings of PVD at day 7 of life was strongly associated with the subsequent diagnosis of BPD and poor respiratory outcomes [13]. Past clinical studies have suggested that sustained elevations of pulmonary artery pressure as assessed by serial echocardiograms may be associated with increased risk for BPD [13, 14, 33–36], supporting the hypothesis that PVD or PH in premature newborns may be an early clinical marker for predicting BPD. Early echocardiographic signs of PVD in preterm infants have now been associated with increased risk for both BPD and late PH as well as with prolonged oxygen treatment [13, 14]. Sustained evidence of elevated right ventricular pressure through the first week after birth may reflect early pulmonary vascular injury that increases risk for BPD. Whether these changes are secondary to delayed transition to extrauterine life, injury due to excessive hemodynamic stress from PDA or other shunts as has been previously reported, or other forms of vascular injury remains to be determined. Understanding the drivers behind these early vascular changes will be crucial to developing novel intervention strategies to prevent both BPD and PH in these infants.

In addition to early hemodynamic indicators of PVD, clinical factors associated with late PH in most studies include lower gestational age, birth weight, and longer periods of respiratory support. Patent ductus arteriosus, infection, oligohydramnios, small for gestational age, and low birth weight z-score have also been identified as risk factors for PH in infants born preterm. Further examination of clinical factors associated with PH, including prenatal risks, along with translational investigations and rigorous screening of infants, will help elucidate how these clinical factors impair normal pulmonary vascular development and lead to BPD and PH.

Early injury to the lung circulation leads to the rapid development of PH after premature birth. Abnormalities of the pulmonary circulation in BPD include increased vascular tone and vasoreactivity, hypertensive remodeling, and decreased growth. Physiological abnormalities of the pulmonary circulation in BPD include elevated PVR and abnormal vasoreactivity, as evidenced by the marked vasoconstrictor response to acute hypoxia [37]. Cardiac catheterization studies have shown that even mild hypoxia can cause marked elevations in pulmonary artery pressure in some infants with BPD, including infants with only modest basal elevations of PH [37]. Increased pulmonary vascular tone contributes to high PVR even in older children with BPD without hypoxia, suggesting that abnormal vascular function persists even late in the course [38].

Abnormal pulmonary vascular structure also contributes to high PVR due to increased smooth muscle cell hyperplasia and altered vascular compliance caused by increased production of an abnormal extracellular matrix. Growth of the distal lung circulation is impaired in infants with severe BPD, and decreased arterial growth reduces vascular surface area that further impairs gas exchange and increases the risk for the development of PH and impaired exercise capacity in older children. Prominent bronchial or other systemic-to-pulmonary collateral vessels were noted in early morphometric studies of infants with BPD, and can be readily identified in many infants during cardiac catheterization. Although these collateral vessels are generally small, large collaterals may contribute to significant shunting of blood flow to the lung, causing edema and need for higher FiO_2.

In addition, recent autopsy studies suggest the presence of striking intrapulmonary anastomotic, or "shunt," vessels that link the distal pulmonary and bronchial vessels, and may contribute to poor oxygenation [39]. Past clinical studies have further shown that metabolic function of the pulmonary vasculature is impaired in BPD, as reflected by the lack of pulmonary clearance of circulating norepinephrine during passage through the lung, which may contribute to left ventricular dysfunction and systemic hypertension [40]. Reduced vascular surface area implies that even relatively minor increases in left-to-right shunting of blood flow through a patent foramen ovale, atrial septal defect (ASD), or patent ductus arteriosus may induce a far greater hemodynamic injury in infants with BPD than in infants with normal lung vascular growth.

Persistent abnormalities of pulmonary vascular growth and/or failure of the lung vasculature to "catch-up" to infants born at term may contribute to PVD that becomes increasingly symptomatic later in life. BPD infants have reduced pulmonary diffusing capacity compared to age-matched term controls, suggesting that BPD infants have decreased alveolar surface area available for gas exchange [26]. These differences were also found in children at 11 years of age who had been born extremely preterm and in adult survivors of BPD. Thus, reduced arterial number, structural abnormalities of the vessel wall, and abnormal vascular function, together with impairments in respiratory mechanics and cardiac function, can contribute to increased PVR and PVD in BPD, leading to significant morbidity and mortality.

Diagnostic Approach to PH in BPD

PH is not only a marker of more severe BPD, but high PVR can also cause right ventricular dysfunction, impaired cardiac output, limited oxygen delivery, increased pulmonary edema, and possibly a higher risk for sudden death. Recent

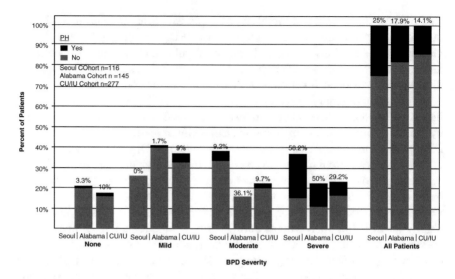

Fig. 3 Relationship of pulmonary hypertension to severity of BPD. As shown, three distinct studies show that the incidence of PH by echocardiogram is highest in infants with severe BPD (From reference [22])

Table 1 Diagnostic approach to infants with pulmonary hypertension in BPD

Evaluation of underlying lung disease
Prolonged monitoring of O_2 (awake, asleep, feeds)
$PaCO_2$ contribution to PH or marker of disease severity, need for chronic (effective) ventilation?
Chronic aspiration (barium swallow, swallowing study, pH probe, impedance study)
Sleep study
Structural airway disease: flexible bronchoscopy
Reactive airway disease
Chest CT scan
Cardiac catheterization

studies suggest that between 15 and 25 % of preterm infants may develop echocardiogram signs of PH or PVD, which strongly relates to disease severity [8, 41, 42] (Fig. 3). Prospective data regarding the precise incidence and natural history of PH in BPD are relatively limited, and most information on diagnostic and therapeutic strategies are based on clinical observations, rather than rigorous, randomized clinical trials.

In general, it is recommended that early echocardiograms be obtained for the diagnosis of PH in preterm infants with severe RDS who require high levels of ventilator support and supplemental oxygen, especially in the setting of oligohydramnios and intrauterine growth restriction (IUGR) ([16]; Table 1; Fig. 4). Infants with more severe prematurity (<26 weeks) are at highest risk for late PH, and infants with

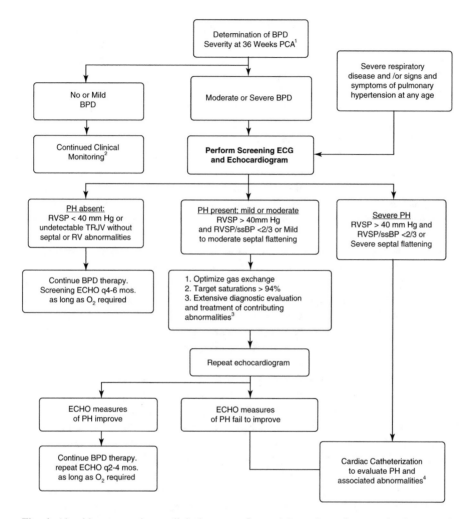

Fig. 4 Algorithm suggesting a clinical strategy for applying echocardiograms in the care of infants with BPD (From reference [22])

a particularly slow rate of clinical improvement, as manifested by persistent or progressively increased need for high levels of respiratory support, should be assessed for PH. In the setting of established BPD, preterm infants, who, at 36 weeks postconceptual age, still require positive pressure ventilation support, are not weaning consistently from oxygen, have oxygen needs at levels disproportionate to their degree of lung disease, or have recurrent cyanotic episodes warrant screening for PH or related cardiovascular sequelae. Other clinical markers often associated with more severe disease include feeding dysfunction and poor growth, recurrent hospitalizations, and elevated $PaCO_2$. High $PaCO_2$, is a marker of disease severity and reflects significant airways obstruction, abnormal lung compliance with heterogeneous parenchymal disease, or reduced surface area, and is an indication for PH screening. Another strategy would be to use echocardiograms to screen every patient at 36 weeks of age who is diagnosed with moderate or severe BPD, but how often clinically significant PH would be missed in patients with milder BPD is uncertain.

Serial electrocardiograms have inadequate sensitivity and positive predictive value for identification of right ventricular hypertrophy (RVH) as a marker of PH. As a result, obtaining serial echocardiograms for screening for PH in patients with BPD is generally recommended. Estimated systolic pulmonary artery pressure (sPAP) derived from the tricuspid regurgitant jet (TRJV) measured by echocardiogram has become one of the most utilized findings for evaluating PH. Past studies have shown excellent correlation coefficients (r values between 0.93 and 0.97) when compared with cardiac catheterization measurements in children < 2 years old with congenital heart disease [43]. However, these studies evaluated echocardiogram and cardiac catheterization performed simultaneously under the same hemodynamic conditions, and the utility of echocardiograms in predicting disease severity as applied in the clinical setting is less clear.

The utility of echocardiogram assessments of PH in infants with BPD has been compared with subsequent cardiac catheterization measurements of pulmonary artery pressure [44]. Systolic PAP could be estimated in only 61 % of studies, and there was poor correlation between echocardiogram and cardiac catheterization measures of sPAP in these infants. Echocardiogram estimates of sPAP correctly identified the presence or absence of PH in 79 % of these studies, but the severity of PH was correctly assessed in only 47 % of those studies. Seven of 12 children (58 %) without PH by echocardiogram had PH during subsequent cardiac catheterization. In the absence of a measurable TRJV, qualitative echocardiogram findings of PH, including right atrial enlargement, right ventricular hypertrophy, right ventricular dilation, pulmonary artery dilation, and septal flattening, either alone or in combination have relatively poor predictive value. Factors associated with chronic lung disease, specifically marked pulmonary hyperinflation, expansion of the thoracic cage, and alteration of the position of the heart, adversely effect the ability to detect and measure TRJV. As used in clinical practice, echocardiography often identifies PH in infants with BPD, but estimates of sPAP were not obtained consistently and were often not reliable for determining disease severity. Other measures of right ventricular strain and PH, including AT/ET ratio and the Tei index, could be helpful in the absence of a measurable TRJV, but have not been fully evaluated in infants with BPD. Despite its limitations, echocardiography remains the best available screening tool for PH in BPD patients.

In patients with PH by echocardiogram, we generally recommend cardiac catheterization for patients with BPD who: (1) have persistent signs of severe cardiorespiratory disease or clinical deterioration not directly related to airways disease; (2) are suspected of having significant PH despite optimal management of their lung disease and associated morbidities; (3) are candidates for chronic PH

Table 2 Guidelines for PH management in BPD[a]

Screening for PH by echocardiogram is recommended in infants with *established BPD* (Class I, Level B)
Evaluation and treatment of lung disease, including assessments for hypoxemia, aspiration, structural airways disease, and the need for changes in respiratory support, is recommended in infants with BPD and PH *before initiation* of PAH-targeted therapy (Class I, Level B)
Evaluation for chronic therapy for PH in infants with BPD should follow recommendations for all children with PH and include *cardiac catheterization* to diagnose disease severity and potential contributing factors such as LV diastolic dysfunction, anatomical shunts, pulmonary vein stenosis, and systemic collaterals (Class I, Level B)
Supplemental oxygen therapy is reasonable to avoid episodic or sustained hypoxemia and with the goal of maintaining O_2 saturations between *92 and 95 %* in patients with established BPD and PH (Class IIa, Level C)
PAH-targeted therapy can be useful for infants with BPD and PH on optimal treatment of underlying respiratory and cardiac disease (Class IIa, Level C)

[a]From reference [16]

drug therapy; (4) have unexplained, recurrent pulmonary edema; or (4) respond poorly to PAH-targeted therapies (Table 2).

The goals of cardiac catheterization are to: assess the severity of PH; exclude or document the severity of associated anatomical cardiac lesions; define the presence of systemic–pulmonary collateral vessels; pulmonary venous obstruction; or left heart dysfunction; and to assess pulmonary vascular reactivity in patients who fail to respond to oxygen therapy alone (Table 2). Other critical information can be acquired during cardiac catheterization that may significantly aid in the management of infants with BPD. In particular, assessment of shunt lesions, especially atrial septal defects; the presence, size, and significance of bronchial or systemic collateral arteries; determining the presence of pulmonary artery stenosis; and structural assessments of the pulmonary arterial and venous circulation by angiography, including pulmonary vein stenosis, are among several key factors that may affect cardiopulmonary function [45].

Most importantly, elevated pulmonary capillary wedge or left atrial pressure may signify left-sided systolic or diastolic dysfunction. LV diastolic dysfunction can contribute to PH, recurrent pulmonary edema, or poor iNO responsiveness in infants with BPD, and measuring changes in PCWP and LAP during acute vaso-reactivity testing may help with this assessment. In addition to high pulmonary vascular tone, abnormal vasoreactivity, hypertensive vascular remodeling, decreased surface area, and left ventricular diastolic dysfunction (LVDD) can also contribute to high pulmonary artery pressure in infants with BPD [46]. Up to 25 % of BPD infants with PH who were evaluated by cardiac catheterization had hemodynamic signs of LVDD in one retrospective study [47]. Some infants with LVDD present with persistent requirements for frequent diuretic therapy to treat recurrent pulmonary edema, even in the presence of only mild PH.

Treatment of PH in BPD

The initial clinical strategy for the management of PH in infants with BPD begins with treating the underlying lung disease. This includes an extensive evaluation for chronic reflux and aspiration, structural airway abnormalities (such as tonsillar and adenoidal hypertrophy, vocal cord paralysis, subglottic stenosis, tracheomalacia, and other lesions), assessments of bronchoreactivity, improving lung edema and airway function, and others. Periods of acute hypoxia, whether intermittent or prolonged, are common causes of late PH in BPD (Tables 1 and 2). Brief assessments of oxygenation ("spot checks") are not sufficient for decisions on the level of supplemental oxygen needed. Targeting oxygen saturations to 92–95 % should be sufficient to prevent the adverse effects of hypoxia in most infants, without increasing the risk of additional lung inflammation and injury. A sleep study may be necessary to determine the presence of noteworthy episodes of hypoxia and whether hypoxemia has predominantly obstructive, central, or mixed causes.

Additional studies that may be required include flexible bronchoscopy for the diagnosis of anatomical and dynamic airway lesions (such as tracheomalacia) that may contribute to hypoxemia and poor clinical responses to oxygen therapy. Upper gastrointestinal series, pH or impedance probe, and swallow studies may be indicated to evaluate for gastroesophageal reflux and aspiration that can contribute to ongoing lung injury. For patients with BPD and severe PH who fail to maintain near-normal ventilation or require high levels of FiO_2 despite conservative treatment, consideration should be given to chronic mechanical ventilatory support. Despite the growing use of pulmonary vasodilator therapy for the treatment of PH in BPD, data demonstrating efficacy are extremely limited, and the use of these agents should only follow thorough diagnostic evaluations and aggressive management of the underlying lung disease. Current therapies used for PH therapy in infants with BPD generally include inhaled NO, sildenafil, endothelin-receptor antagonists (ERA), prostacyclin analogs, and calcium channel blockers.

Inhaled nitric oxide (iNO) causes selective pulmonary vasodilation and improves oxygenation in infants with established BPD [38, 48] (Table 3). Although long-term iNO therapy has been used in BPD infants, especially for those who require continued mechanical ventilator support, efficacy data are not available. Although iNO for PH therapy is often initiated at doses of 10–20 ppm, most patients subsequently tolerate weaning of the iNO dose below 10 ppm. The lower dose may further enhance ventilation–perfusion matching, allowing for better oxygenation at lower FiO_2, whereas higher doses (20 ppm) may further enhance pulmonary hemodynamics.

Sildenafil, a highly selective type 5 phosphodiesterase (PDE-5) inhibitor, augments cyclic GMP content in vascular smooth muscle, and has been approved for adults with PH alone and in combination with standard treatment regimens. Studies of sildenafil therapy in children with PH have been limited, but include a demonstration of its efficacy in the treatment of persistent PH of the newborn [49]

Table 3 PAH-targeted drug therapies for children

Drug class	Drug and dosing	Adverse effects	Comments
Anticoagulation	*Warfarin* (dosage to generally target INR between 1.5 and 2.0)	Bleeding complications, difficulty maintaining INR at target range	Use in children before walking well or with developmental or neurological problems increases risk for serious bleeding
Calcium channel blockers	*Nifedipine* (starting dose: 0.1–0.2 mg/kg PO daily) *Diltiazem* (starting dose: 0.3–0.5 mg/kg PO daily) *Amlodipine* (starting dose: 0.1–0.3 mg/kg PO daily)	Bradycardia, hypotension Decreased cardiac function Peripheral edema Rash, gum hyperplasia, constipation	Urge cautious use with close monitoring, especially with drug initiation, in infants and young children with suspected cardiac (especially RV) dysfunction; most strongly supported if children shown to have positive testing for acute vasoreactivity during cardiac catheterization.
NO-cGMP pathway	*Inhaled NO:* 5–20 ppm	Rebound with drug withdrawal	Higher doses (>5–10 ppm) may worsen V–Q matching in setting of lung disease
	Sildenafil: starting dose for infants <1 year: 0.5–1 mg/kg three times daily PO; Dosage by body weight: <20 kg: 10 mg three times daily >20 kg: 20 mg three times daily; *Tadalafil* (starting dose: 0.5–1 mg/day)	Headache, nasal congestion, flushing, agitation, hypotension, hypoxemia, priapism, potential for visual changes or hearing loss.	Avoid higher doses in children due to report of increased mortality in STARTS-2 study in young children with IPAH (ref. [11]); FDA urges caution and close monitoring of its use. EMA supports use in children, but with lower dose range. Limited experience with tadalafil in younger children, often switch from sildenafil after stable period of time.

(continued)

Table 3 (continued)

Drug class	Drug and dosing	Adverse effects	Comments
Endothelin blockade	*Bosentan* (dual ETA and ETB receptor inhibitor): starting dose is half of maintenance dose, which is based on body weight: 　<10 kg: 2 mg/kg PO BID 　10–20 kg: 31.25 mg PO BID 　>20–40 kg: 62.5 PO BID 　> 40 kg: 125 PO BID *Ambrisentan* (ETA inhibitor): 5–10 mg PO daily	Hepatotoxicity HCG and pregnancy test required per age Fluid retention Teratogenicity	Requires liver function testing monthly Growing experience in children for bosentan, but extremely limited published experience for ambrisentan in young children
Prostacyclin analogs	*Epoprostenol* (Flolan; Veletri- (thermostable): continuous iv infusion, starting dose: 1–2 ng/kg/min iv, with incremental increases as tolerated and ongoing changes due to tachyphylaxis; typical dose is 50–80 ng/kg/min *Treprostinil* (Remodulin): iv or subcutaneous: starting dose is 2 ng/kg/min, with incremental increases over time to achieve or sustain benefit; *Inhaled and oral forms* available and under investigation as well *Iloprost* (intermittent inhalation) – initially 2.5 ug dose, increase to 5 ug, as tolerated; usually requires 6–9 inhalations daily	Hypotension Flushing Diarrhea Jaw pain Central line complications (sepsis) Rebound PH if stopped suddenly Can cause high cardiac output syndrome Half-lives: epoprostenol, short (2–5 min), and Flolan requires cooling; *treprostinil*, longer (4–5 h) and stable in room temperature Flushing, headache common Can cause cough, wheeze	Ventilation–perfusion mismatch may complicate use in setting of lung disease; Nonselective vasodilator, can cause systemic hypotension Subcutaneous route causes site pain, but usually manageable Pretreatment with inhaled bronchodilators or steroid can attenuate respiratory side effects

and its safety and possible efficacy during long-term therapy in older children with PH [50]. By prolonging cGMP levels during iNO-induced vasodilation, PDE-5 inhibitors may be useful to augment the response to iNO therapy or to prevent rebound PH after abrupt withdrawal of iNO. In a study of 25 infants with chronic lung disease and PH (18 with BPD), prolonged sildenafil therapy, as part of an aggressive program to treat PH, was associated with improvement in PH by echocardiogram in most (88 %) patients without significant rates of adverse events [51]. Although the time to improvement was variable, many patients were able to wean off mechanical ventilator support and other PH therapies, especially iNO, during the course of sildenafil treatment without worsening of PH. The recommended starting dose for sildenafil is 0.5 mg/kg/dose every 8 hours, and systemic blood pressure should be closely monitored. If there is no evidence of systemic hypotension, this dose can be gradually increased over 2 weeks to achieve desired pulmonary hemodynamic effect or a maximum of 2 mg/kg/dose every 8 hours.

Bosentan, a nonselective ET receptor antagonist, is commonly used in older patients with PH. A retrospective study suggested that bosentan may be safe and effective for the treatment of PH in children as young as 9 months [52], but data are limited to case reports regarding its use in BPD infants. Monthly liver function testing is required to monitor for hepatotoxicity.

Calcium channel blockers (CCB) benefit some patients with PH, and short-term effects of CCB in infants with BPD have been reported [53, 54]. Nifedipine can acutely lower pulmonary artery pressure and PVR in children with BPD; however, some patients were acutely hypoxemic during in this study, and the effects of nifedipine on pulmonary artery pressure were not different from the effects of supplemental oxygen alone. In comparison with an acute study of iNO reactivity in infants with BPD, the acute response to CCB was poor, and some infants developed systemic hypotension [38]. Concerns persist that young infants with PH, especially with evidence of impaired myocardial contractility, may worsen with CCB therapy, and caution is urged, especially with the initiation of CCB therapy [15]. The use of sildenafil or bosentan for chronic therapy of PH in infants with BPD is generally favored over CCB therapy [15].

Intravenous prostacyclin analogs (PGI_2; epoprostenol, treprostinil) therapy has been used extensively in older patients with severe PH, and has been shown to improve survival of patients with advanced disease. PGI_2 has been used in some infants with BPD and late PH, but concerns regarding its potential to worsen gas exchange due to increased ventilation–perfusion mismatching in the setting of chronic lung disease and systemic hypotension have limited its use in this setting. Subcutaneous infusions of treprostinil may be safe and effective in infants with severe BPD, but concerns persist regarding the potential for worsening oxygenation [55]. Although iloprost, another stable PGI_2 analog, is available for inhalational use, the need for frequent treatments (6–8 times daily) and occasional bronchospasm may be significant factors restricting its use in the setting of BPD.

Currently, there is limited evidence on how long these therapies need to be continued [41, 51]. If PH gradually resolves with lung growth as expected, the medications may be either gradually tapered off, or the infant allowed to "outgrow the dose" before discontinuation of PH-targeted drugs. In addition to close monitoring of pulmonary status, infants with BPD and PH should be followed by serial echocardiograms, which should be obtained at least every 2–4 weeks with the acute initiation of therapy and at 4–6 month intervals with stable disease. Abrupt worsening of PH may reflect several factors, including the lack of compliance with oxygen therapy or medication use, but can be related to the progressive development of pulmonary vein stenosis or veno-occlusive disease). Some infants with resolved PH have signs and echocardiogram findings of worsening during acute viral infection. With these infants, PAH-targeted drug therapy is generally initiated and continued until serial echocardiograms show resolution of disease. Concurrent use of brain natriuretic peptide (BNP) or NT-pro-BNP may further aid clinical decision-making, but do not specifically diagnose PH, or should be used to direct therapy in isolation from clinical and echocardiogram findings.

Repeat cardiac catheterization may be indicated for patients being treated for PH with vasodilator therapy who experience clinical deterioration, worsening PH by echocardiogram, or when echocardiogram measurements fail to provide adequate hemodynamic assessment of sicker patients. We recommend weaning medications with serial normal or near-normal echocardiogram findings, and that the addition of biomarkers, such as pro-NT brain natriuretic peptide levels, may be useful for long-term follow-up.

Conclusions

In summary, PVD and PH contribute to the pathophysiology and cardiorespiratory outcomes of infants with BPD. Data are extremely limited regarding many aspects of the care of PH in BPD, including the need to learn more about its natural history and prevalence, mechanisms that cause PH or contribute to progressive disease, and the relative risks and benefits of current therapeutic strategies. Although new therapies are now available for the treatment of PH, their role in the clinical care of severe BPD and improving long-term outcomes requires more thorough investigation. Finally, strategies that specifically target the preservation of endothelial survival and function may also lead to novel approaches for the prevention of BPD and late PH.

References

1. Northway WH, Rosan RC, Porter DY. Pulmonary disease following respirator therapy of hyaline membrane disease. Bronchopulonary dysplasia. N Engl J Med. 1967;276:357–68.
2. Jobe AH, Bancalari E. Bronchopulmonary dysplasia. Am J Respir Crit Care Med. 2001;163:1723–9.

3. Jobe AH. The new BPD: an arrest of lung development. Pediatr Res. 1999;46:641–3.
4. Baraldi E, Filippone M. Chronic lung disease after premature birth. N Engl J Med. 2007;357(19):1946–55.
5. Hussain AN, Siddiqui NH, Stocker JT. Pathology of arrested acinar development in postsurfactant BPD. Hum Pathol. 1998;29:710–7.
6. McEvoy C, Jain L, Schmidt B, Abman SH, Bancalari E, Aschner J. Bronchopulmonary dysplasia: NHLBI Workshop on the Primary Prevention of Chronic Lung Diseases. Ann Am Thorac Soc. 2014;Suppl 3:S146–53.
7. Stoll BJ, Hansen NI, Bell EF, et al. Trends in care practices, morbidity and mortality of extremely preterm neonates. JAMA. 2015;314:1039–51.
8. Wong PM, Lees AN, Louw J, et al. Emphysema in young adult survivors of moderate-to-severe bronchopulmonary dysplasia. Eur Respir J. 2008;32(2):321–8.
9. Hislop AA, Haworth SG. Pulmonary vascular damage and the development of cor pulmonale following hyaline membrane disease. Pediatr Pulmonol. 1990;9:152–161.
10. Bush A, Busst CM, Knight WB, Hislop AA, Haworth SG, Shinebourne EA. Changes in the pulmonary circulation in BPD. Arch Dis Child. 1990;65:739–45.
11. Fouron JC, Le Guennec JC, Villemant D, et al. Value of echocardiography in assessing the outcome of bronchopulmonary dysplasia of the newborn. Pediatrics. 1980;65(3):529–35.
12. Abman SH. Pulmonary hypertension in chronic lung disease of infancy. Pathogenesis, pathophysiology and treatment. In: Bland RD, Coalson JJ, editors. Chronic lung disease of infancy. New York: Marcel Dekker; 2000. p. 619–68.
13. Mourani PM, Sontag MK, Younoszai A, Miller JI, Kinsella JP, Baker CD, Poindexter BB, Ingram DA, Abman SH. Early pulmonary vascular disease in preterm infants at risk for BPD. Am J Respir Crit Care Med. 2015;191:87–95.
14. Mirza H, Ziegler J, Ford S, Padbury J, Tucker R, Laptook A. Pulmonary hypertension in preterm infants: prevalence and association with bronchopulmonary dysplasia. J Pediatr. 2014;165(5):909–14.e1.
15. Khemani E, McElhinney DB, Rhein L, et al. Pulmonary artery hypertension in formerly premature infants with bronchopulmonary dysplasia: clinical features and outcomes in the surfactant era. Pediatrics. 2007;120(6):1260–9.
16. Abman SH, Hansmann G, Archer S, et al. American Heart Association and American Thoracic Society Joint Guidelines for Pediatric Pulmonary Hypertension. Circulation. 2015;132:2037–99.
17. Stenmark KR, Abman SH. Lung vascular development: implications for the pathogenesis of bronchopulmonary dysplasia. Annu Rev Physiol. 2005;67:623–61.
18. Thebaud B, Abman SH. Bronchopulmonary dysplasia: where have all the vessels gone? Roles of angiogenic growth factors in chronic lung disease. Am J Respir Crit Care Med. 2007;175(10):978–85.
19. Bhatt AJ, Pryhuber GS, Huyck H, et al. Disrupted pulmonary vasculature and decreased VEGF, flt-1, and Tie 2 in human infants dying with BPD. Am J Respir Crit Care Med. 2000;164:1971–80.
20. Lassus P, Turanlahti M, Heikkila P, et al. Pulmonary vascular endothelial growth factor and Flt-1 in fetuses, in acute and chronic lung disease, and in persistent pulmonary hypertension of the newborn. Am J Respir Crit Care Med. 2001;164(10 Pt 1):1981–7.
21. De Paepe ME, Mao Q, Powell J, et al. Growth of pulmonary microvasculature in ventilated preterm infants. Am J Respir Crit Care Med. 2006;173(2):204–11.
22. Mourani PM, Abman SH. Pulmonary vascular disease in BPD: physiology, diagnosis and treatment. In: Abman SH, editor. Bronchopulmonary dysplasia. New York: Informa; 2010. p. 347–63.
23. Jakkula M, Le Cras TD, Gebb S, et al. Inhibition of angiogenesis decreases alveolarization in the developing rat lung. Am J Physiol Lung Cell Mol Physiol. 2000;279:L600–7.
24. Abman SH. BPD: a vascular hypothesis. Am J Respir Crit Care Med. 2001;164:1755–6.

25. Abman SH. Impaired vascular endothelial growth factor signaling in the pathogenesis of neonatal pulmonary vascular disease. Adv Exp Med Biol. 2010;661:323–35.
26. Balinotti JE, Chakr VC, Tiller C, et al. Growth of lung parenchyma in infants and toddlers with chronic lung disease of infancy. Am J Respir Crit Care Med. 2010;181(10):1093–7.
27. Hansen AR, Barnes CM, Folkman J, McElrath TF. Maternal preeclampsia predicts the development of bronchopulmonary dysplasia. J Pediatr. 2010;156(4):532–6.
28. Foidart JM, Schaaps JP, Chantraine F, Munaut C, Lorquet S. Dysregulation of anti-angiogenic agents (sFlt-1, PLGF, and sEndoglin) in preeclampsia – a step forward but not the definitive answer. J Reprod Immunol. 2009;82(2):106–11.
29. Tang JR, Karumanchi SA, Seedorf G, Markham N, Abman SH. Excess soluble vascular endothelial growth factor receptor-1 in amniotic fluid impairs lung growth in rats: linking preeclampsia with bronchopulmonary dysplasia. Am J Physiol Lung Cell Mol Physiol. 2012;302(1):L36–46.
30. Li F, Hagaman JR, Kim HS, et al. eNOS deficiency acts through endothelin to aggravate sFlt-1-induced pre-eclampsia-like phenotype. J Am Soc Nephrol. 2012;23(4):652–60.
31. Rozance PJ, Seedorf GJ, Brown A, et al. Intrauterine growth restriction decreases pulmonary alveolar and vessel growth and causes pulmonary artery endothelial cell dysfunction in vitro in fetal sheep. Am J Physiol Lung Cell Mol Physiol. 2011;301(6):L860–71.
32. Check J, Gotteiner N, Liu X, et al. Fetal growth restriction and pulmonary hypertension in premature infants with bronchopulmonary dysplasia. J Perinatol. 2013;33:553–7.
33. Evans NJ, Archer LNJ. Doppler assessment of pulmonary artery pressure during recovery from hyaline membrane disease. Arch Dis Child. 1991;66:802–4.
34. Subhedar NV, Shaw NJ. Changes in pulmonary arterial pressure in preterm infants with chronic lung disease. Arch Dis Child. 2000;82:F243–7.
35. Czernik C, Rhode S, Metze B, Schmalisch G, Buhrer C. Persistently elevated right ventricular index of myocardial performance in preterm infants with incipient bronchopulmonary dysplasia. PLoS One. 2012;7(6):e38352.
36. Skinner JR, Boys RJ, Hunter S, Hey EN. Pulmonary and systemic arterial pressure in hyaline membrane disease. Arch Dis Child. 1992;67(4 Spec No):366–73.
37. Abman SH, Wolfe RR, Accurso FJ, Koops BL, Wiggins JW. Pulmonary vascular response to to oxygen in infants with severe BPD. Pediatrics. 1985;75:80–4.
38. Mourani P, Ivy DD, Gao D, Abman SH. Pulmonary vascular effects of inhaled NO and oxygen tension in older children and adolescents with bronchopulmonary dysplasia. Am J Respir Crit Care Med. 2004;170:1006–13.
39. Galambos C, Sims-Lucas S, Abman SH. Histologic evidence of intrapulmonary arteriovenous shunt vessels in premature infants with severe bpd. Ann Am Thorac Soc. 2013;10:474–81.
40. Abman SH, Schaffer MS, Wiggins JW, et al. Pulmonary vascular extraction of circulating norepinephrine in infants with BPD. Pediatr Pulmonol. 1987;3:386–91.
41. An HS, Bae EJ, Kim GB, et al. Pulmonary hypertension in preterm infants with BPD. Korean Circ J. 2010;40:131–6.
42. Slaughter JR, Pakradhi T, Lones DE et al. Echocardiographic detection of pulmonary hypertension in extremely low birth weight infants with BPD requiring prolonged positive pressure ventilation. J Perinatol. 2011;31:1–6.
43. Currie PJ, Seward JB, Chan KL, et al. Continuous wave Doppler determination of right ventricular pressure: a simultaneous Doppler-catheterization study in 127 patients. J Am Coll Cardiol. 1985;6(4):750–6.
44. Mourani PM, Sontag MK, Younoszai A, et al. Clinical utility of echocardiography for the diagnosis and management of pulmonary vascular disease in young children with chronic lung disease. Pediatrics. 2008;121(2):317.
45. Drossner DM, Kim DW, Maher KO, et al. Pulmonary vein stenosis: prematurity and associated conditions. Pediatrics. 2008;122:e656–61.

46. Mourani PM, Fagan T, Ivy DD, Rosenberg A, Abman SH. Left ventricular diastolic dysfunction in bronchopulmonary dysplasia. J Pediatr. 2008;152:291–3.
47. Del Cerro MJ, Sabate-Rotes A, Carton A, et al. Pulmonary hypertension in BPD: clinical findings, cardiovascular abnormalities and outcomes. Pediatr Pulmonol. 2014;49:49–59.
48. Banks BA, Seri I, Ischiropoulos H, et al. Changes in oxygenation with inhaled nitric oxide in severe bronchopulmonary dysplasia. Pediatrics. 1999;103(3):610–8.
49. Baquero H, Soliz A, Neira F, et al. Oral sildenafil in infants with persistent pulmonary hypertension of the newborn: a pilot randomized blinded study. Pediatrics. 2006;117(4):1077–83.
50. Humpl T, Reyes JT, Holtby H, et al. Beneficial effect of oral sildenafil therapy on childhood pulmonary arterial hypertension: twelve-month clinical trial of a single-drug, open-label, pilot study. Circulation. 2005;111(24):3274–80.
51. Mourani PM, Sontag MK, Lui G, et al. Effects of long-term sildenafil treatment for pulmonary hypertension in infants with chronic lung disease. J Pediatr. 2008;121:317–25.
52. Rosenzweig EB, Ivy DD, Widlitz A, et al. Effects of long-term bosentan in children with pulmonary arterial hypertension. J Am Coll Cardiol. 2005;46(4):697–704.
53. Brownlee JR, Beekman RH, Rosenthal A. Acute hemodynamic effects of nifedipine in infants with bronchopulmonary dysplasia and pulmonary hypertension. Pediatr Res. 1988;24(2):186–90.
54. Johnson CE, Beekman RH, Kostyshak DA, et al. Pharmacokinetics and pharmacodynamics of nifedipine in children with bronchopulmonary dysplasia and pulmonary hypertension. Pediatr Res. 1991;29(5):500–3.
55. Ferdman DJ, Rosenzweig EB, Zuckerman WA, Krishnan U. Subcutaneous treprostinil for pulmonary hypertension in chronic lung disease of infancy. Pediatrics. 2014;134:e274–8.

Infection and Inflammation: Catalysts of Pulmonary Morbidity in Bronchopulmonary Dysplasia

Phillip S. Wozniak, Mohannad Moallem, and Pablo J. Sánchez

Introduction

Despite improvements in the care of preterm infants with gentler ventilation techniques, antenatal glucocorticoid therapy, and surfactant treatment, bronchopulmonary dysplasia (BPD) remains a major public health problem worldwide. BPD, as defined by the need for supplemental oxygen at 36 weeks' postmenstrual age [1–3], is the most frequent pulmonary morbidity among survivors of prematurity—a chronic lung condition that affects more than 10,000 premature infants in the United States alone each year [4, 5]. Before the surfactant era, BPD was primarily a structural injury of the preterm lung characterized by decreased alveolarization and surface area, alternating atelectasis with hyperinflation, pulmonary lesions, and fibrosis

P.S. Wozniak, BA
Department of Pediatrics, Division of Neonatology, Nationwide Children's Hospital – The Ohio State University, Columbus, OH, USA

Nationwide Children's Hospital – The Ohio State University, Center for Perinatal Research, The Research Institute at Nationwide Children's Hospital, 700 Children's Drive, RB3, WB5245, Columbus, OH 43205-2664, USA

M. Moallem, MD
Department of Pediatrics, Division of Neonatology, Nationwide Children's Hospital – The Ohio State University, Columbus, OH, USA

P.J. Sánchez, MD (✉)
Department of Pediatrics, Division of Neonatology, Nationwide Children's Hospital – The Ohio State University, Columbus, OH, USA

Pediatric Infectious Diseases, Nationwide Children's Hospital – The Ohio State University, Columbus, OH, USA

Nationwide Children's Hospital – The Ohio State University, Center for Perinatal Research, The Research Institute at Nationwide Children's Hospital, 700 Children's Drive, RB3, WB5245, Columbus, OH 43205-2664, USA
e-mail: Pablo.Sanchez@nationwidechildrens.org

© Springer International Publishing AG 2017
A.M. Hibbs, M. S. Muhlebach (eds.), *Respiratory Outcomes in Preterm Infants*,
Respiratory Medicine, DOI 10.1007/978-3-319-48835-6_13

[6]. Today, BPD represents a developmental arrest of the preterm lung with interruption of the pulmonary septation, alveolarization, and vascularization during the saccular and alveolar stages of lung development [7].The result is a lung with fewer, larger alveoli and a corresponding decrease in surface area available for gas exchange.

The 2014 National Institutes of Health Heart, Lung, and Blood Institute workshop on prevention of BPD identified six possible causative factors associated with BPD: structurally and biochemically immature lungs, hyperoxia and oxidant injury, mechanical injury associated with positive pressure respiratory support, poor respiratory drive and apnea, poor nutrition, and importantly, infection and inflammation [5]. Any or all of these factors, possibly in concert with genetic predisposition or epigenetic factors, could contribute to its occurrence, even though recent genome-wide association studies (GWAS) failed to identify any specific loci associated with moderate to severe BPD [8, 9]. Clearly, the pathophysiology of BPD is complex and likely multifactorial, but a central role for *pulmonary inflammation* seems critical to its development.

Antenatal Infection and Inflammation

There is a substantial body of literature associating "chorioamnionitis" with the development of BPD, with recent meta-analyses demonstrating odds ratios of 3.0 and 2.2 for the occurrence of BPD at 28 days of age and 36 weeks postmenstrual age, respectively [10]. How chorioamnionitis contributes to the development of BPD, however, remains a topic of ongoing debate.

Chorioamnionitis is diagnosed often as symptomatic maternal disease with intrapartum fever in association with clinical and laboratory signs of infection or inflammation, but more appropriately, by histopathology [11]. The so-called histological chorioamnionitis can be acute or chronic based on neutrophilic or lymphocytic infiltration of the fetal membranes, respectively. Both neutrophils and lymphocytes may be of either maternal or fetal origins [12]. Unlike acute cases, chronic chorioamnionitis has both cellular (innate) and humoral (adaptive) immune responses, which could indicate maternal antibody-mediated antifetal rejection that has been associated with preterm birth [13]. The suggestion by Goldenberg et al. [14] that intrauterine infection and/or inflammation accounts for up to 90 % of preterm births before 28 weeks' gestation lends credence to the theory that predisposition of preterm infants to BPD may occur in utero.

Ureaplasma parvum and *Ureaplasma urealyticum*, both genital mycoplasmas, are the most common bacteria isolated from placentas with histological chorioamnionitis as well as from amniotic fluid [15, 16, 17]. These organisms are typically of low virulence, and thus capable of producing a chronic infection of the uterine cavity and fetal compartment [14, 18]. In fact, neonatal colonization with *Ureaplasma spp.* has been associated with chorioamnionitis [19].

Prospective cohort studies have associated *Ureaplasma* colonization with the development of BPD [20, 21]. Respiratory tract colonization with *Ureaplasma spp.* occurs in 28–33 % of infants with birth weight <1500 g, and among those < 26 weeks' gestation, as many as 65 % of infants are culture-positive or polymerase chain reaction (PCR)-positive for *Ureaplasma spp.* at least once in the first month of age [22]. *Ureaplasma* colonization increases with decreasing gestational age, a finding that correlates with the risk of developing BPD [23].

Several mechanisms for the association of *Ureaplasma* colonization of preterm infants and BPD have been proposed. The ability of *Ureaplasma spp.* to hydrolyze urea as their sole source of energy results in the generation of ammonium ions that interact with lung water to form ammonium hydroxide and potentially result in mucosal/epithelial injury and inflammation [24]. However, the major virulence factor that has been identified experimentally is the *Ureaplasma* multiple banded antigen (MBA), a surface-exposed lipoprotein [22]. *Ureaplasma spp.* have been shown to evade the host immune response by varying the size of MBA and *mba* gene [22, 24]. Both MBA and *mba* gene size variants have been detected in infected sheep amniotic fluid and fetal lung, and the size variation also has correlated with the severity of chorioamnion inflammation.

Clearance of *Ureaplasma* species from the lung also appears to be dependent on local host immune response mediators, such as surfactant protein-A (SPA) [15]. Okugbule-Wonodi et al. [25] demonstrated that SPA increased phagocytosis and killing of *Ureaplasma spp.* by macrophages. In a mouse model, SPA-deficient mice showed delayed clearance of *Ureaplasma* from the lungs, increased inflammatory cells, and increased proinflammatory cytokine expression [26]. These findings are particularly relevant for preterm infants who lack robust immune responses and endogenous SPA production in the first 48 h of age.

Does Chorioamnionitis Cause BPD?

Intra-amniotic inflammation (IAI) secondary to histological chorioamnionitis can result in premature maturation of the fetal lung that is mediated by such proinflammatory cytokines as interleukin (IL)-1α, IL-1β, IL-6, IL-8, and tumor necrosis factor (TNF)-α. These can act directly on fetal lung cells, including the Type II alveolar cells that produce surfactant [27, 28]. In rabbits, Bry et al. [29] demonstrated that IL-1α enhanced messenger RNA transcription of both surfactant proteins and lipids resulted in improved lung compliance [12, 29]. Although the proinflammatory cytokines protected against the development of respiratory distress syndrome (RDS), the fetal inflammation has been associated subsequently with increased incidence of BPD [12, 27, 30, 31].

While the signaling pathways responsible for lung development have been well characterized, the effects of chorioamnionitis and/or antenatal inflammation on those pathways have not [32, 33]. Bacterial antigens such as lipopolysaccharide can cause altered distribution of elastin, the mesenchymal structural protein responsible for proper septation of the lung [12, 34, 35]. Intra-amniotic inflammation also can cause dysregulation of critical growth factors necessary for lung development. Fibroblast growth factor (FGF)-10 expression is inhibited by nuclear factor kappa-light-chain-enhancer of activated B cells (NF-κB), the major proinflammatory signaling pathway stimulated by IL-1 and TNF-α [36, 37]. FGF-10 plays a key role in lung branching morphogenesis, remodeling, repair, and regeneration [12, 38]. Inhibition or dysregulation of these key functions as a consequence of histological chorioamnionitis or inflammation has resulted in a lung condition in animals that is similar to BPD in humans [35].

The effects of antenatal inflammation are not limited to the developing airway. The developing pulmonary vasculature also is susceptible to adverse remodeling due to antenatal inflammation, limiting the capacity for gas exchange in the preterm lung. Antenatal inflammation can inhibit vascular endothelial growth factor (VEGF), angiopoietin-1, transforming growth factor-β (TGF-β), endoglin, connective tissue growth factor (CTGF), endothelial nitric oxide synthase (eNOS), platelet endothelial cell adhesion molecule-1 (PECAM-1), and VEGF-receptor 2 (VEGF-R2) [12, 39, 40]. In addition, antenatal inflammation can cause smooth muscle hypertrophy in the pulmonary vasculature, predisposing to pulmonary hypertension that is a major complication of BPD [12, 39]. VEGF is responsible for the regulation of eNOS, which plays a crucial role in the regulation of pulmonary vascular tone and modulation of pulmonary vascular development. PECAM-1 and VEGF-R2 are essential for proper development of pulmonary endothelial cells [39].

It seems clear that antenatal inflammation alone has the potential to cause both impaired alveolarization and reduced development of the pulmonary vasculature leading to the development of BPD in some at-risk preterm infants, even in the absence of mechanical ventilation [39, 41]. However, other indirect mechanisms linking chorioamnionitis and/or inflammation to BPD may be involved.

Does Chorioamnionitis Make the Lung Susceptible to BPD?

Exposure of the preterm fetus to chorioamnionitis may result in a systemic fetal inflammatory response syndrome (FIRS) with activation of the innate immune system [42, 43] and manifested by histological chorioamnionitis with funisitis and increased umbilical cord blood concentrations of proinflammatory cytokines [42]. Such infants have a decreased clinical response to exogenous surfactant, more frequent use of exogenous surfactant, increased need for mechanical ventilation, longer time to extubation, longer supplemental oxygen use, and more frequently develop BPD [43, 44, 45].

Mechanical factors also contribute to the development of BPD. Hillman et al. [46] showed that as few as six breaths at high tidal volumes were sufficient to eliminate the surfactant response in fetal sheep. Furthermore, 15 min of ventilation at escalating tidal volumes has been associated with a substantial inflammatory response in the preterm lung that is characterized by production of multiple classes of cytokines and other proinflammatory markers, increased mRNA for IL-1β and IL-6, increased inflammatory cell infiltrates, increased alveolar wall thickening, and decreased alveolar expansion, with a concomitant delayed or deficient release of the anti-inflammatory cytokine, IL-10 [47, 48]. Of note, stretch injury overlapped consistently with the maturational effects induced by chorioamnionitis and prolonged LPS exposure in utero [46].

Supplemental oxygen supplied to the preterm infant, whether by mechanical ventilation or other support measures, such as continuous positive airway pressure (CPAP) or nasal cannula, also has injurious effects on the preterm lung by inducing an inflammatory response [45]. This inflammation stimulates the activity of VEGF and causes breakdown of the alveolar–capillary barrier, vascular leakage, introduction of proinflammatory mediators, pulmonary edema, and, ultimately, endothelial apoptosis [45, 49]. An animal study of hyperoxia-induced BPD in preterm rabbits identified 2217 dysregulated pathophysiological pathways affecting inflammation, vascular development, and reactive oxygen species (ROS) metabolism [50]. Because antioxidant defense do not develop until much later in gestation, preterm infants receiving high concentrations of oxygen are particularly susceptible to ROS-mediated injury [51, 52].

Antenatal inflammation due to chorioamnionitis also has been linked to the development of BPD through immune tolerance due to the preterm lung's structural immaturity and the preterm infant's immature immune system [12, 53]. Several in vitro and animal studies have indicated that intrauterine endotoxin/LPS exposure can downregulate immune responses akin to tolerance [54–57]. LPS-induced immune paralysis may be caused by reduced expression of major histocompatibility complex II (MHC) antigen on fetal blood monocytes and increased expression of the immunosuppressive cytokines, IL-10 and TGF-β [12, 57].

Repeated exposure to LPS in *Ureaplasma*-infected fetal sheep induces both endotoxin tolerance and tolerance of other toll-like receptor (TLR) agonists [55]. Since TLRs are major activators of the immune system, cross-tolerance of toll-like agonists may enhance immune suppression in the preterm infant and increase the vulnerability to a "second hit"—sepsis, ventilator-mediated injury, or hyperoxia [12, 55]. On the other hand, Kramer and Jobe [56] hypothesized that this immunosuppressive fetal response may be an advantageous adaptation to chronic exposure to chorioamnionitis that prevents more serious inflammation-mediated lung injury. Indeed, Kallapur et al. [58] lent weight to this theory when they showed that chronic exposure to intra-amniotic endotoxin did not lead to progressive lung injury and extensive structural abnormalities in fetal sheep, but only to mild, persistent inflammation. However, chorioamnionitis leading to prolonged immune dysfunction may subsequently increase susceptibility to postnatal infections.

Bacterial Sepsis and BPD

Early-onset sepsis (≤72 h after birth) has been shown to initiate an inflammatory cascade in preterm infants similar to that seen with exposure to histological chorioamnionitis. Similarly, late-onset sepsis (LOS; >72 h of age) causes both proinflammatory and profibrotic responses in the preterm lung, increasing its susceptibility to BPD [45, 59, 60].

In a retrospective study of 7509 infants born at <32 weeks' gestation in 29 neonatal intensive care units (NICUs) of the Canadian Neonatal Network from 2010 to 2011, Shah et al. [59] identified 1104 (15 %) infants with LOS, defined as a positive blood and/or cerebrospinal fluid bacterial culture. Of these 1104 infected infants, 909 (82 %) had Gram-positive and 195 (18 %) had Gram-negative infections. As compared with no infection, the odds ratio (OR) of mortality/BPD was higher in infants who had Gram-negative (OR, 2.79; 95 % confidence interval [CI], 1.96–3.97) and Gram-positive (OR, 1.44; 95 % CI, 1.21–1.71) sepsis. Infants with Gram-negative sepsis were significantly more likely to have been born to mothers with chorioamnionitis than uninfected infants ($p = 0.004$) or those with Gram-positive infections ($p = 0.04$). This study supports the contention that the proinflammatory cascade that occurs with LOS can exacerbate preexisting inflammatory conditions associated with chorioamnionitis exposure or initiate an inflammatory and fibrotic response that results in BPD [45, 59, 61, 62]. Prevention of postnatal sepsis must remain a high priority for prevention of BPD.

Cytomegalovirus Infection and BPD

Congenital cytomegalovirus (CMV) infection is the most common congenital viral infection in developed nations, occurring in approximately 0.1–2.0 % of all live births [63, 64]. CMV is a *Betaherpesvirinae* virus that infects human leukocytes, and transmission to the infant occurs transplacentally following primary maternal infection, reactivation of latent maternal infection, or maternal reinfection with a different viral strain [64]. In addition, infants can acquire the virus during birth from exposure to infected vaginal and cervical secretions, or postnatally by either blood transfusion or, more commonly, ingestion of human milk from a CMV-seropositive mother [65, 66]. Intrapartum and postnatal acquisition of CMV, defined as detection of CMV in body fluids at ≥21 days of age, and to a lesser extent congenital infection, can result in pneumonitis and increased likelihood for development of BPD in preterm infants [64, 67].

In 1976, Whitley et al. [68] first noted the association of perinatally acquired CMV infection with protracted pneumonitis in two infants with lower respiratory tract obstruction at 1 month of age [68]. Virological, serological, immunological, and electron microscopic studies indicated that CMV was a major causative factor. Subsequently, case reports associated multicystic lung disease, fibrosis, and pulmonary hypertension with postnatal CMV infection [1, 69–71].

Two recent studies provide new evidence for an association between postnatal acquisition of CMV and BPD. Mukhopadhyay et al. [72] conducted a retrospective review of 145 very low birth weight (VLBW, ≤1500 g) infants who were tested for CMV infection while in the NICU at Brigham and Women's Hospital, Boston from 1999 to 2013. Of the 145 infants, 27 (19 %) had postnatal detection of CMV defined as diagnosis at ≥21 days of age; all had birth weight <1250 g and were born at <32 weeks' gestation. Sixteen (59 %) infants presented with acute respiratory decompensation, and importantly, CMV-infected infants had significantly more exposure to mechanical ventilation ($p = 0.03$) and a higher incidence of BPD (OR 4.0; 95 % CI, 1.3–12.4; $p = 0.02$). The authors suggested that postnatal symptomatic

CMV infection, like late-onset bacterial sepsis, may predispose to development of BPD by a combination of direct pathogen effects on the lung, inflammation, and/or increased exposure to mechanical ventilation and supplemental oxygen.

Similarly, in a propensity-matched retrospective cohort study of 101,111 VLBW infants at 348 NICUs managed by the Pediatrix Medical Group from 1997 to 2012, 328 (0.3 %) infants had a diagnosis or detection of CMV at ≥21 days of age [73]. Postnatal CMV infection was associated with an increased risk for death or BPD at 36 weeks' postmenstrual age (risk ratio, 1.21; 95 % CI, 1.10–1.32) and BPD (risk ratio, 1.33; 95 % CI, 1.19–1.50). Changes in cardiorespiratory status associated with postnatal CMV infection included a new requirement for vasopressor medications (9 %; $n = 29$), intubation for mechanical ventilation (15 %; $n = 49$), a new oxygen requirement (28 %; $n = 91$), and death (1.2 %; $n = 4$).

Given the association of postnatal acquisition of CMV with BPD, the key challenge remains development of preventative measures against CMV acquisition in extremely low gestational age infants. Transmission of CMV by blood transfusion to preterm infants has been virtually eliminated by the use of CMV antibody-negative donors, freezing red blood cells in glycerol before administration, or leukoreduction. Ingestion of human milk now is the primary means by which preterm infants acquire CMV postnatally [74]. While pasteurization of human milk inactivates CMV, it also may reduce its known cognitive, immunological, and nutritional benefits. Freezing milk at −20 °C decreases CMV viral titers, but does prevent transmission [75, 76].

Respiratory Viral Infection and BPD

The occurrence of respiratory viral infections in preterm infants in the NICU has been documented in a prospective surveillance study performed in two NICUs in Syracuse, NY during a 1-year period [77]. Fifty preterm infants <33 weeks' gestation who were in the NICU since birth underwent nasopharyngeal swab testing for detection of respiratory viruses (influenza A/B; respiratory syncytial virus [RSV] A/B; parainfluenza [PIV] 1–4; coronavirus, human rhinovirus/enterovirus [hRV]; adenovirus; human metapneumovirus [HMPV]) by multiplex PCR testing twice weekly within 3 days of birth and up to the time of discharge. Fifty two percent (26/50) of infants tested positive for a respiratory virus at least once during the NICU stay. Of 708 specimens obtained, the following viruses were detected: PIV-3, 13; hMPV, 9; RSV-B, 8; RSV-A, 7; PIV-2, 7; hRV, 7; and influenza B, 4. Of note, 18 samples (28 % of the positive swabs) included more than one virus, similar to studies performed in older infants with bronchiolitis where viral codetection is relatively common. Fourteen infants had sequentially positive specimens for the same virus over 3 to 13 days, suggesting that these were true positive results. Compared to infants who did not have a respiratory viral pathogen detected, virus-positive infants had significantly longer length of stay (70 d vs. 35 d, $p = 0.002$), need for intubation (65 % vs. 29 %, $p = 0.01$), duration of intubation (19 vs. 5 d, $p = 0.03$), duration of oxygen requirement (51 vs. 13 d, $p = 0.002$), more episodes of desaturation ($p < 0.0001$), and clinical deterioration episodes ($p = 0.0001$), and importantly, BPD (46 % vs. 21 %, $p = 0.05$).

In a single-site prospective study performed in a German NICU from 8/2010–3/2014, Kidszun et al. [78] performed respiratory viral multiplex PCR testing on 88 infants (median gestational age, 27 weeks; median birth weight, 852 g) who underwent 137 evaluations for late-onset sepsis. A respiratory virus was detected in the nasopharynx of six (7 %) infants (2, RSV; 4, picornavirus). Similarly, Ronchi et al. [79] conducted a 1-year study (1/15/12–1/31/13) for the detection of respiratory viruses by multiplex PCR testing in infants evaluated for possible sepsis and in whom intravenous antibiotic therapy was initiated. During the 13-month study, 100 infants (mean gestational age, 31 weeks; mean birth weight, 1698 g) had 135 sepsis evaluations, and 8 infants (8 %), or 6 % ($n = 8$) of sepsis evaluations, had a respiratory virus detected from nasopharyngeal swabs. These included hRV($n = 4$), coronaviruses (1, HKU-1; 1, OC43), and PIV-3 ($n = 2$). These studies suggest that respiratory viral infections are under-recognized in premature infants in the NICU; yet, they are associated with acute morbidity. Their contribution to long-term respiratory and neurodevelopmental outcomes, however, remains unknown.

It is likely that respiratory viral infections can exacerbate the underlying lung abnormalities of infants with BPD and result in impairment of lung function through early childhood and possibly adolescence. Longitudinal studies of mice who received supplemental oxygen have found a lifelong increased susceptibility to infection with respiratory viruses, and in particular, influenza A virus, compared to preterm controls exposed only to room air [80–82]. Higher oxygen concentrations led to a dose-dependent inflammatory response to influenza A exposure [45, 52, 83], with enhanced recruitment of macrophages, neutrophils, and lymphocytes, as well as increased alveolar fibrosis, increased monocyte chemoattractant protein (MCP-1), and greater mortality [80]. O'Reilly et al. [80] demonstrated that alveolar type II cells that are responsible for surfactant production can express viral receptors on their surface, with surfactant protein-deficient mice having decreased viral clearance. Pulmonary outcomes of preterm infants infected with a respiratory virus early in life—and especially with RSV, hRV, PIV, and hMPV—bear striking resemblance to outcomes of very premature infants with BPD [84, 85]. Both BPD and early respiratory infection with RSV have been associated with recurrent wheeze and lung function abnormalities that persist to school age [64, 86]. In addition, viral lower respiratory tract infections (LRTIs) may be a marker for preexisting abnormal lung function in neonates [64, 87]. Infants with BPD have substantially more rehospitalizations due to RSV and hRV infection than age-matched controls without BPD [88, 89].

Similar to BPD, RSV also has been shown to cause persistently diminished lung function among preterm infants and increased wheezing throughout childhood [90, 91–94]. Preterm infants hospitalized with RSV infection are significantly more likely to require supplemental oxygen and mechanical ventilation, exposing them to additional pulmonary injury [88]. In 2015, the SPRING study demonstrated that among children born at 32–35 weeks' gestation, RSV hospitalization was associated with increased wheezing through 6 years of age, as well as increased utilization of health care resources and decreased self-reported quality of life [95].

The humanized monoclonal antibody, palivizumab, has been shown to significantly reduce RSV hospitalizations in infants and children at high risk for severe RSV infection [96]. Simoes et al. [97] conducted a cohort study of 421 preterm infants who had received palivizumab and were not hospitalized for RSV ($n = 191$) or who never received palivizumab ($n = 230$; 76 hospitalized for RSV). Infants who received palivizumab had significantly less parent-documented and physician-diagnosed recurrent wheezing. Similarly, the Dutch RSV Neonatal Network conducted a multicenter, double-blind, placebo-controlled trial of palivizumab prophylaxis in 429 otherwise healthy preterm infants of 33 to 35 weeks' gestation and demonstrated that palivizumab prophylaxis significantly reduced wheezing days during the first year of age [98]. These studies continue to implicate RSV infection as an important mechanism of recurrent wheeze during the first year of life in preterm infants.

Future Directions

As the direction of causality between infection, inflammation, and BPD remains unanswered, research is needed to better elucidate their interaction and contribution to long-term pulmonary morbidity in preterm infants, with the ultimate goal of developing and implementing novel therapies and interventions. Nonetheless, a central role for pulmonary inflammation seems key, and the factors that contribute to its evolution need to be explored.

Early and prolonged antibiotic therapy in preterm infants has been associated with BPD [99], suggesting an important role of the airway microbiome as a mediator of the inflammatory process [100]. Recently, Lal et al. [101] reported temporal dysbiotic changes in the airway microbiome from birth to the development of BPD in preterm infants. They noted decreased *Lactobacillus spp.* in endotracheal aspirates of preterm infants who developed BPD and infants born to mothers with chorioamnionitis. How the airway microbiome is established, and the possible factors such as chorioamnionitis, antibiotic use, and postnatal infection that potentially contribute to its dysregulation need further exploration [102].

The human virome, or the viral component of the human microbiome, represents the collection of all viruses that are found in or on humans, including viruses that cause acute, persistent, or latent infection, and viruses that integrate into the human genome, such as endogenous retroviruses [103]. The human virome includes both eukaryotic and prokaryotic viruses (bacteriophages), the latter of which can infect the broad array of bacteria that inhabit the body and influence bacterial population structure or virulence. Its impact on human health has received less attention than that of the bacterial microbiome, even though it is likely to be equally important in homeostasis and disease. The potential importance of the human virome in the development of BPD is not known, and our current lack of understanding of its ontogeny in preterm infants constitutes a major knowledge gap in our continuing efforts to decrease the incidence of BPD and its consequences.

Finally, genome-wide transcriptional profiles of the infant's inflammatory response to conditions associated with prematurity could provide new key evidence about the pathogenesis of BPD [104]. Analysis of the infant's transcriptome also could be used to support the clinical significance of detecting bacterial or viral sequences in clinical specimens by detecting expression of immune/inflammatory genes that may contribute to the development of BPD [105]. Importantly, such technology could aid in the identification and subsequent validation of candidate biosignatures and biomarkers for BPD in preterm infants with bacterial and respiratory viral infections.

References

1. Nijman J, de Vries LS, Koopman-Esseboom C, Uiterwaal CS, van Loon AM, Verboon-Maciolek MA. Postnatally acquired cytomegalovirus infection in preterm infants: a prospective study on risk factors and cranial ultrasound findings. Arch Dis Child Fetal Neonatal Ed. 2012;97(4):F259–63. Epub 2012/01/17.
2. Shennan AT, Dunn MS, Ohlsson A, Lennox K, Hoskins EM. Abnormal pulmonary outcomes in premature infants: prediction from oxygen requirement in the neonatal period. Pediatrics. 1988;82(4):527–32. Epub 1988/10/01.
3. Poindexter BB, Feng R, Schmidt B, Aschner JL, Ballard RA, Hamvas A, et al. Comparisons and limitations of current definitions of bronchopulmonary dysplasia for the prematurity and respiratory outcomes program. Ann Am Thorac Soc. 2015;12(12):1822–30. Epub 2015/09/24.
4. Jobe AH, Bancalari E. Bronchopulmonary dysplasia. Am J Respir Crit Care Med. 2001;163(7):1723–9. Epub 2001/06/13.
5. McEvoy CT, Jain L, Schmidt B, Abman S, Bancalari E, Aschner JL. Bronchopulmonary dysplasia: NHLBI Workshop on the Primary Prevention of Chronic Lung Diseases. Ann Am Thorac Soc. 2014;11(Suppl 3):S146–53. Epub 2014/04/24.
6. Northway Jr WH, Rosan RC, Porter DY. Pulmonary disease following respirator therapy of hyaline-membrane disease. Bronchopulmonary dysplasia. N Engl J Med. 1967;276(7):357–68. Epub 1967/02/16.
7. Baraldi E, Filippone M. Chronic lung disease after premature birth. N Engl J Med. 2007;357(19):1946–55. Epub 2007/11/09.
8. Wang H, St Julien KR, Stevenson DK, Hoffmann TJ, Witte JS, Lazzeroni LC, et al. A genome-wide association study (GWAS) for bronchopulmonary dysplasia. Pediatrics. 2013;132(2):290–7. Epub 2013/07/31.
9. Lal CV, Ambalavanan N. Genetic predisposition to bronchopulmonary dysplasia. Semin Perinatol. 2015;39(8):584–91. Epub 2015/10/17.
10. Lowe J, Watkins WJ, Edwards MO, Spiller OB, Jacqz-Aigrain E, Kotecha SJ, et al. Association between pulmonary ureaplasma colonization and bronchopulmonary dysplasia in preterm infants: updated systematic review and meta-analysis. Pediatr Infect Dis J. 2014;33(7):697–702. Epub 2014/01/22.
11. Higgins RD, Saade G, Polin RA, Grobman WA, Buhimschi IA, Watterberg K, et al. Evaluation and management of women and newborns with a maternal diagnosis of chorioamnionitis: summary of a workshop. Obstet Gynecol. 2016;127(3):426–36. Epub 2016/02/09.
12. Kunzmann S, Collins JJ, Kuypers E, Kramer BW. Thrown off balance: the effect of antenatal inflammation on the developing lung and immune system. Am J Obstet Gynecol. 2013;208(6):429–37. Epub 2013/01/15.

13. Lee J, Romero R, Xu Y, Kim JS, Topping V, Yoo W, et al. A signature of maternal anti-fetal rejection in spontaneous preterm birth: chronic chorioamnionitis, anti-human leukocyte antigen antibodies, and C4d. PLoS One. 2011;6(2):e16806.Epub 2011/02/18.
14. Goldenberg RL, Culhane JF, Iams JD, Romero R. Epidemiology and causes of preterm birth. Lancet. 2008;371(9606):75–84. Epub 2008/01/08.
15. Viscardi RM, Kallapur SG. Role of ureaplasma respiratory tract colonization in bronchopulmonary dysplasia pathogenesis: current concepts and update. Clin Perinatol. 2015;42(4):719–38. Epub 2015/11/26.
16. Murtha AP, Edwards JM. The role of Mycoplasma and Ureaplasma in adverse pregnancy outcomes. Obstet Gynecol Clin North Am. 2014;41(4):615–27. Epub 2014/12/03.
17. Waites KB, Xiao L, Paralanov V, Viscardi RM, Glass JI. Molecular methods for the detection of Mycoplasma and ureaplasma infections in humans: a paper from the 2011 William Beaumont Hospital Symposium on molecular pathology. J Mol Diagn. 2012;14(5):437–50. Epub 2012/07/24.
18. Goldenberg RL, Hauth JC, Andrews WW. Intrauterine infection and preterm delivery. N Engl J Med. 2000;342(20):1500–7. Epub 2000/05/18.
19. Sanchez PJ. Perinatal transmission of Ureaplasma urealyticum: current concepts based on review of the literature. Clin Infect Dis. 1993;17(Suppl 1):S107–11. Epub 1993/08/01.
20. Schelonka RL, Katz B, Waites KB, Benjamin Jr DK. Critical appraisal of the role of Ureaplasma in the development of bronchopulmonary dysplasia with metaanalytic techniques. Pediatr Infect Dis J. 2005;24(12):1033–9. Epub 2005/12/24.
21. Sanchez PJ, Regan JA. Ureaplasma urealyticum colonization and chronic lung disease in low birth weight infants. Pediatr Infect Dis J. 1988;7(8):542–6. Epub 1988/08/01.
22. Zheng X, Teng LJ, Watson HL, Glass JI, Blanchard A, Cassell GH. Small repeating units within the Ureaplasma urealyticum MB antigen gene encode serovar specificity and are associated with antigen size variation. Infect Immun. 1995;63(3):891–8. Epub 1995/03/01.
23. Sung TJ, Xiao L, Duffy L, Waites KB, Chesko KL, Viscardi RM. Frequency of ureaplasma serovars in respiratory secretions of preterm infants at risk for bronchopulmonary dysplasia. Pediatr Infect Dis J. 2011;30(5):379–83. Epub 2010/11/26.
24. Robinson JW, Dando SJ, Nitsos I, Newnham J, Polglase GR, Kallapur SG, et al. Ureaplasma parvum serovar 3 multiple banded antigen size variation after chronic intra-amniotic infection/colonization. PLoS One. 2013;8(4):e62746.Epub 2013/05/03.
25. Okogbule-Wonodi AC, Chesko KL, Famuyide ME, Viscardi RM. Surfactant protein-A enhances ureaplasmacidal activity in vitro. Innate Immun. 2011;17(2):145–51. Epub 2010/03/04.
26. Famuyide ME, Hasday JD, Carter HC, Chesko KL, He JR, Viscardi RM. Surfactant protein-A limits Ureaplasma-mediated lung inflammation in a murine pneumonia model. Pediatr Res. 2009;66(2):162–7. Epub 2009/04/25.
27. Arntzen KJ, Kjollesdal AM, Halgunset J, Vatten L, Austgulen R. TNF, IL-1, IL-6, IL-8 and soluble TNF receptors in relation to chorioamnionitis and premature labor. J Perinat Med. 1998;26(1):17–26. Epub 1998/05/22.
28. D'Angio CT, Ambalavanan N, Carlo WA, McDonald SA, Skogstrand K, Hougaard DM, et al. Blood cytokine profiles associated with distinct patterns of bronchopulmonary dysplasia among extremely low birth weight infants. J Pediatr. 2016;174:45–51.e5. Epub 2016/04/28.
29. Bry K, Lappalainen U, Hallman M. Intraamniotic interleukin-1 accelerates surfactant protein synthesis in fetal rabbits and improves lung stability after premature birth. J Clin Invest. 1997;99(12):2992–9. Epub 1997/06/15.
30. Watterberg KL, Demers LM, Scott SM, Murphy S. Chorioamnionitis and early lung inflammation in infants in whom bronchopulmonary dysplasia develops. Pediatrics. 1996;97(2):210–5. Epub 1996/02/01.
31. Been JV, Zimmermann LJ. Histological chorioamnionitis and respiratory outcome in preterm infants. Arch Dis Child Fetal Neonatal Ed. 2009;94(3):F218–25. Epub 2009/01/10.
32. Morrisey EE, Hogan BL. Preparing for the first breath: genetic and cellular mechanisms in lung development. Dev Cell. 2010;18(1):8–23. Epub 2010/02/16.

33. Kramer BW, Kallapur S, Newnham J, Jobe AH. Prenatal inflammation and lung development. Semin Fetal Neonatal Med. 2009;14(1):2–7. Epub 2008/10/11.
34. Charafeddine L, D'Angio CT, Phelps DL. Atypical chronic lung disease patterns in neonates. Pediatrics. 1999;103(4 Pt 1):759–65. Epub 1999/04/02.
35. Kramer BW, Ladenburger A, Kunzmann S, Speer CP, Been JV, van Iwaarden JF, et al. Intravenous lipopolysaccharide-induced pulmonary maturation and structural changes in fetal sheep. Am J Obstet Gynecol. 2009;200(2):195.e1–10. Epub 2008/12/27.
36. Benjamin JT, Carver BJ, Plosa EJ, Yamamoto Y, Miller JD, Liu JH, et al. NF-kappaB activation limits airway branching through inhibition of Sp1-mediated fibroblast growth factor-10 expression. J Immunol. 2010;185(8):4896–903. Epub 2010/09/24.
37. Lawrence T. The nuclear factor NF-kappaB pathway in inflammation. Cold Spring Harb Perspect Biol. 2009;1(6):a001651. Epub 2010/05/12.
38. Beers MF, Morrisey EE. The three R's of lung health and disease: repair, remodeling, and regeneration. J Clin Invest. 2011;121(6):2065–73. Epub 2011/06/03.
39. Kallapur SG, Bachurski CJ, Le Cras TD, Joshi SN, Ikegami M, Jobe AH. Vascular changes after intra-amniotic endotoxin in preterm lamb lungs. Am J Physiol Lung Cell Mol Physiol. 2004;287(6):L1178–85. Epub 2004/08/24.
40. Thomas W, Seidenspinner S, Kramer BW, Kawczynska-Leda N, Chmielnicka-Kopaczyk M, Marx A, et al. Airway concentrations of angiopoietin-1 and endostatin in ventilated extremely premature infants are decreased after funisitis and unbalanced with bronchopulmonary dysplasia/death. Pediatr Res. 2009;65(4):468–73. Epub 2009/01/08.
41. Choi CW, Lee J, Oh JY, Lee SH, Lee HJ, Kim BI. Protective effect of chorioamnionitis on the development of bronchopulmonary dysplasia triggered by postnatal systemic inflammation in neonatal rats. Pediatr Res. 2016;79(2):287–94. Epub 2015/11/10.
42. Thomas W, Speer CP. Chorioamnionitis is essential in the evolution of bronchopulmonary dysplasia – the case in favour. Paediatr Respir Rev. 2014;15(1):49–52. Epub 2013/10/17.
43. Dessardo NS, Mustac E, Dessardo S, Banac S, Peter B, Finderle A, et al. Chorioamnionitis and chronic lung disease of prematurity: a path analysis of causality. Am J Perinatol. 2012;29(2):133–40. Epub 2011/12/08.
44. Been JV, Rours IG, Kornelisse RF, Jonkers F, de Krijger RR, Zimmermann LJ. Chorioamnionitis alters the response to surfactant in preterm infants. J Pediatr. 2010;156(1):10–5.e1. Epub 2009/10/17.
45. Balany J, Bhandari V. Understanding the impact of infection, inflammation, and their persistence in the pathogenesis of bronchopulmonary dysplasia. Front Med (Lausanne). 2015;2:90. Epub 2016/01/07.
46. Hillman NH, Polglase GR, Pillow JJ, Saito M, Kallapur SG, Jobe AH. Inflammation and lung maturation from stretch injury in preterm fetal sheep. Am J Physiol Lung Cell Mol Physiol. 2011;300(2):L232–41. Epub 2010/12/07.
47. Carvalho CG, Silveira RC, Procianoy RS. Ventilator-induced lung injury in preterm infants. Rev Bras Ter Intensiva. 2013;25(4):319–26. Epub 2014/02/21.
48. Beresford MW, Shaw NJ. Detectable IL-8 and IL-10 in bronchoalveolar lavage fluid from preterm infants ventilated for respiratory distress syndrome. Pediatr Res. 2002;52(6):973–8. Epub 2002/11/20.
49. Thickett DR, Armstrong L, Christie SJ, Millar AB. Vascular endothelial growth factor may contribute to increased vascular permeability in acute respiratory distress syndrome. Am J Respir Crit Care Med. 2001;164(9):1601–5. Epub 2001/11/24.
50. Salaets T, Richter J, Brady P, Jimenez J, Nagatomo T, Deprest J, et al. Transcriptome analysis of the preterm rabbit lung after seven days of hyperoxic exposure. PLoS One. 2015;10(8):e0136569.Epub 2015/09/01.
51. Weinberger B, Laskin DL, Heck DE, Laskin JD. Oxygen toxicity in premature infants. Toxicol Appl Pharmacol. 2002;181(1):60–7. Epub 2002/05/29.
52. Yee M, Chess PR, McGrath-Morrow SA, Wang Z, Gelein R, Zhou R, et al. Neonatal oxygen adversely affects lung function in adult mice without altering surfactant composition or activity. Am J Physiol Lung Cell Mol Physiol. 2009;297(4):L641–9. Epub 2009/07/21.

53. Kramer BW. Chorioamnionitis - new ideas from experimental models. Neonatology. 2011;99(4):320–5. Epub 2011/06/28.
54. Kallapur SG, Jobe AH, Ball MK, Nitsos I, Moss TJ, Hillman NH, et al. Pulmonary and systemic endotoxin tolerance in preterm fetal sheep exposed to chorioamnionitis. J Immunol. 2007;179(12):8491–9. Epub 2007/12/07.
55. Kallapur SG, Kramer BW, Knox CL, Berry CA, Collins JJ, Kemp MW, et al. Chronic fetal exposure to Ureaplasma parvum suppresses innate immune responses in sheep. J Immunol. 2011;187(5):2688–95. Epub 2011/07/26.
56. Kramer BW, Jobe AH. The clever fetus: responding to inflammation to minimize lung injury. Biol Neonate. 2005;88(3):202–7. Epub 2005/10/08.
57. Azizia M, Lloyd J, Allen M, Klein N, Peebles D. Immune status in very preterm neonates. Pediatrics. 2012;129(4):e967–74. Epub 2012/03/28.
58. Kallapur SG, Nitsos I, Moss TJ, Kramer BW, Newnham JP, Ikegami M, et al. Chronic endotoxin exposure does not cause sustained structural abnormalities in the fetal sheep lungs. Am J Physiol Lung Cell Mol Physiol. 2005;288(5):L966–74. Epub 2005/01/11.
59. Shah J, Jefferies AL, Yoon EW, Lee SK, Shah PS. Risk factors and outcomes of late-onset bacterial sepsis in preterm neonates born at < 32 weeks' gestation. Am J Perinatol. 2015;32(7):675–82. Epub 2014/12/09.
60. Shane AL, Stoll BJ. Neonatal sepsis: progress towards improved outcomes. J Infect. 2014;68(Suppl 1):S24–32. Epub 2013/10/22.
61. Kramer BW, Kramer S, Ikegami M, Jobe AH. Injury, inflammation, and remodeling in fetal sheep lung after intra-amniotic endotoxin. Am J Physiol Lung Cell Mol Physiol. 2002;283(2):L452–9. Epub 2002/07/13.
62. Adams-Chapman I. Long-term impact of infection on the preterm neonate. Semin Perinatol. 2012;36(6):462–70.
63. Alford CA, Stagno S, Pass RF, Britt WJ. Congenital and perinatal cytomegalovirus infections. Rev Infect Dis. 1990;12(Suppl 7):S745–53. Epub 1990/09/01.
64. Pryhuber GS. Postnatal infections and immunology affecting chronic lung disease of prematurity. Clin Perinatol. 2015;42(4):697–718. Epub 2015/11/26.
65. de Cates CR, Gray J, Roberton NR, Walker J. Acquisition of cytomegalovirus infection by premature neonates. J Infect. 1994;28(1):25–30. Epub 1994/01/01.
66. Capretti MG, Lanari M, Lazzarotto T, Gabrielli L, Pignatelli S, Corvaglia L, et al. Very low birth weight infants born to cytomegalovirus-seropositive mothers fed with their mother's milk: a prospective study. J Pediatr. 2009;154(6):842–8. Epub 2009/02/24.
67. Maschmann J, Hamprecht K, Dietz K, Jahn G, Speer CP. Cytomegalovirus infection of extremely low-birth weight infants via breast milk. Clin Infect Dis. 2001;33(12):1998–2003. Epub 2001/11/17.
68. Whitley RJ, Brasfield D, Reynolds DW, Stagno S, Tiller RE, Alford CA. Protracted pneumonitis in young infants associated with perinatally acquired cytomegaloviral infection. J Pediatr. 1976;89(1):16–22. Epub 1976/07/01.
69. Neuberger P, Hamprecht K, Vochem M, Maschmann J, Speer CP, Jahn G, et al. Case-control study of symptoms and neonatal outcome of human milk-transmitted cytomegalovirus infection in premature infants. J Pediatr. 2006;148(3):326–31. Epub 2006/04/18.
70. Bradshaw JH, Moore PP. Perinatal cytomegalovirus infection associated with lung cysts. J Paediatr Child Health. 2003;39(7):563–6. Epub 2003/09/13.
71. Koklu E, Karadag A, Tunc T, Altun D, Sarici SU. Congenital cytomegalovirus infection associated with severe lung involvement in a preterm neonate: a causal relationship? Eur J Pediatr. 2009;168(11):1409–12. Epub 2009/02/19.
72. Mukhopadhyay S, Meyer SA, Permar SR, Puopolo KM. Symptomatic postnatal cytomegalovirus testing among very low-birth-weight infants: indications and outcomes. Am J Perinatol. 2016; Epub 2016/04/09.
73. Kelly MS, Benjamin DK, Puopolo KM, Laughon MM, Clark RH, Mukhopadhyay S, et al. Postnatal cytomegalovirus infection and the risk for bronchopulmonary dysplasia. JAMA Pediatr. 2015;169(12):e153785.Epub 2015/12/08.

74. Josephson CD, Caliendo AM, Easley KA, Knezevic A, Shenvi N, Hinkes MT, et al. Blood transfusion and breast milk transmission of cytomegalovirus in very low-birth-weight infants: a prospective cohort study. JAMA Pediatr. 2014;168(11):1054–62. Epub 2014/09/23.
75. Hayashi S, Kimura H, Oshiro M, Kato Y, Yasuda A, Suzuki C, et al. Transmission of cytomegalovirus via breast milk in extremely premature infants. J Perinatol. 2011;31(6):440–5. Epub 2010/12/18.
76. Lombardi G, Garofoli F, Manzoni P, Stronati M. Breast milk-acquired cytomegalovirus infection in very low birth weight infants. J Matern Fetal Neonatal Med. 2012;25(Suppl 3):57–62. Epub 2012/10/04.
77. Bennett NJ, Tabarani CM, Bartholoma NM, Wang D, Huang D, Riddell SW, et al. Unrecognized viral respiratory tract infections in premature infants during their birth hospitalization: a prospective surveillance study in two neonatal intensive care units. J Pediatr. 2012;161(5):814–8. Epub 2012/06/15.
78. Kidszun A, Klein L, Winter J, Schmeh I, Grondahl B, Gehring S, et al. Viral infections in neonates with suspected late-onset bacterial sepsis – a Prospective Cohort Study. Am J Perinatol. 2016; Epub 2016/05/18.
79. Ronchi A, Michelow IC, Chapin KC, Bliss JM, Pugni L, Mosca F, et al. Viral respiratory tract infections in the neonatal intensive care unit: the VIRIoN-I study. J Pediatr. 2014;165(4):690–6. Epub 2014/07/17.
80. O'Reilly MA, Marr SH, Yee M, McGrath-Morrow SA, Lawrence BP. Neonatal hyperoxia enhances the inflammatory response in adult mice infected with influenza A virus. Am J Respir Crit Care Med. 2008;177(10) Epub 2008/02/23.:1103–10.
81. Buczynski BW, Yee M, Martin KC, Lawrence BP, O'Reilly MA. Neonatal hyperoxia alters the host response to influenza A virus infection in adult mice through multiple pathways. Am J Physiol Lung Cell Mol Physiol. 2013;305(4):L282–90. Epub 2013/06/12.
82. Buczynski BW, Yee M, Paige Lawrence B, O'Reilly MA. Lung development and the host response to influenza A virus are altered by different doses of neonatal oxygen in mice. Am J Physiol Lung Cell Mol Physiol. 2012;302(10):L1078–87. Epub 2012/03/13.
83. Maduekwe ET, Buczynski BW, Yee M, Rangasamy T, Stevens TP, Lawrence BP, et al. Cumulative neonatal oxygen exposure predicts response of adult mice infected with influenza A virus. Pediatr Pulmonol. 2014; doi:10.1002/ppul.23063. Epub 2014/05/23.
84. Lee KK, Hegele RG, Manfreda J, Wooldrage K, Becker AB, Ferguson AC, et al. Relationship of early childhood viral exposures to respiratory symptoms, onset of possible asthma and atopy in high risk children: the Canadian Asthma Primary Prevention Study. Pediatr Pulmonol. 2007;42(3):290–7.
85. Jacob SV, Coates AL, Lands LC, MacNeish CF, Riley SP, Hornby L, et al. Long-term pulmonary sequelae of severe bronchopulmonary dysplasia. J Pediatr. 1998;133(2):193–200.
86. Greenough A. Long term respiratory outcomes of very premature birth (<32 weeks). Semin Fetal Neonatal Med. 2012;17(2):73–6. Epub 2012/02/04.
87. Stein RT, Martinez FD. Respiratory syncytial virus and asthma: still no final answer. Thorax. 2010;65(12):1033–4. Epub 2010/10/28.
88. Resch B, Kurath-Koller S, Eibisberger M, Zenz W. Prematurity and the burden of influenza and respiratory syncytial virus disease. World J Pediatr. 2016;12(1):8–18. Epub 2015/11/20.
89. Miller EK, Bugna J, Libster R, Shepherd BE, Scalzo PM, Acosta PL, et al. Human rhinoviruses in severe respiratory disease in very low birth weight infants. Pediatrics. 2012;129(1):e60–7. Epub 2011/12/28.
90. Broughton S, Bhat R, Roberts A, Zuckerman M, Rafferty G, Greenough A. Diminished lung function, RSV infection, and respiratory morbidity in prematurely born infants. Arch Dis Child. 2006;91(1):26–30. Epub 2005/09/29.
91. Stein RT, Sherrill D, Morgan WJ, Holberg CJ, Halonen M, Taussig LM, et al. Respiratory syncytial virus in early life and risk of wheeze and allergy by age 13 years. Lancet. 1999;354(9178):541–5. Epub 1999/09/02.
92. Martinez FD, Wright AL, Taussig LM, Holberg CJ, Halonen M, Morgan WJ. Asthma and wheezing in the first six years of life. The Group Health Medical Associates. N Engl J Med. 1995;332(3):133–8. Epub 1995/01/19.

93. Darveaux JI, Lemanske Jr RF. Infection-related asthma. J Allergy Clin Immunol Pract. 2014;2(6):658–63. Epub 2014/12/03.
94. de Winter JJ, Bont L, Wilbrink B, van der Ent CK, Smit HA, Houben ML. Rhinovirus wheezing illness in infancy is associated with medically attended third year wheezing in low risk infants: results of a healthy birth cohort study. Immun Inflamm Dis. 2015;3(4):398–405. Epub 2016/01/07.
95. Carbonell-Estrany X, Perez-Yarza EG, Garcia LS, Guzman Cabanas JM, Boria EV, Atienza BB. Long-term burden and respiratory effects of respiratory syncytial virus hospitalization in preterm infants-The SPRING Study. PLoS One. 2015;10(5):e0125422.Epub 2015/05/09.
96. Palivizumab, a humanized respiratory syncytial virus monoclonal antibody, reduces hospitalization from respiratory syncytial virus infection in high-risk infants. The IMpact-RSV Study Group. Pediatrics. 1998;102(3 Pt 1):531–7. Epub 1998/09/17.
97. Simoes EA, Groothuis JR, Carbonell-Estrany X, Rieger CH, Mitchell I, Fredrick LM, et al. Palivizumab prophylaxis, respiratory syncytial virus, and subsequent recurrent wheezing. J Pediatr. 2007;151(1):34–42.e1. Epub 2007/06/26.
98. Blanken MO, Rovers MM, Molenaar JM, Winkler-Seinstra PL, Meijer A, Kimpen JL, et al. Respiratory syncytial virus and recurrent wheeze in healthy preterm infants. N Engl J Med. 2013;368(19):1791–9. Epub 2013/05/10.
99. Novitsky A, Tuttle D, Locke RG, Saiman L, Mackley A, Paul DA. Prolonged early antibiotic use and bronchopulmonary dysplasia in very low birth weight infants. Am J Perinatol. 2015;32(1):43–8. Epub 2014/05/06.
100. Imamura T, Sato M, Go H, Ogasawara K, Kanai Y, Maeda H, et al. The microbiome of the lower respiratory tract in premature infants with and without severe bronchopulmonary dysplasia. Am J Perinatol. 2016; Epub 2016/05/31.
101. Lal CV, Travers C, Aghai ZH, Eipers P, Jilling T, Halloran B, et al. The airway microbiome at birth. Sci Rep. 2016;6:31023. Epub 2016/08/05.
102. Lohmann P, Luna RA, Hollister EB, Devaraj S, Mistretta TA, Welty SE, et al. The airway microbiome of intubated premature infants: characteristics and changes that predict the development of bronchopulmonary dysplasia. Pediatr Res. 2014;76(3):294–301. Epub 2014/06/19.
103. Cadwell K. The virome in host health and disease. Immunity. 2015;42(5):805–13. Epub 2015/05/21.
104. Ramilo O, Mejias A. Shifting the paradigm: host gene signatures for diagnosis of infectious diseases. Cell Host Microbe. 2009;6(3):199–200. Epub 2009/09/15.
105. Heinonen S, Jartti T, Garcia C, Oliva S, Smitherman C, Anguiano E, et al. Rhinovirus detection in symptomatic and asymptomatic children: value of host transcriptome analysis. Am J Respir Crit Care Med. 2016;193(7):772–82. Epub 2015/11/17.

Index

© Springer International Publishing AG 2017
A.M. Hibbs, M. S. Muhlebach (eds.), *Respiratory Outcomes in Preterm Infants*,
Respiratory Medicine, DOI 10.1007/978-3-319-48835-6

Printed in the United States
By Bookmasters